# When to Call the Surgeon:
# Decision Making for
# Primary Care Providers

# When to Call the Surgeon: Decision Making for Primary Care Providers

**Robert A. Kozol, MD**
Chief of Surgery
Detroit Veterans Administration Hospital
Detroit, Michigan

**David Fromm, MD**
Chairman, Department of Surgery
Wayne State University School of Medicine
Detroit, Michigan

**Joseph C. Konen, MD**
Chair, Department of Family Medicine
Carolinas Medical Center
Charlotte, North Carolina

F. A. DAVIS COMPANY • Philadelphia

F. A. Davis Company
1915 Arch Street
Philadelphia, PA 19103

Printed in the United States of America
Last digit indicates print number: 10 9 8 7 6 5 4 3 2 1

*Senior Medical Editor:* Robert W. Reinhardt
*Developmental Editor:* Bernice M. Wissler
*Cover Designer:* Louis J. Forgione

**Library of Congress Cataloging-in-Publication Data**

When to call the surgeon : decision making for primary care providers /
   [edited by] Robert A. Kozol, David Fromm, Joseph C. Konen.
      p.  cm.
   Includes bibliographical references and index.
   ISBN 0-8036-0336-3
    1. Primary care (Medicine)—Decision making.  2. Surgery,
Operative.  3. Medical referral.  I. Kozol, Robert A.  II. Fromm,
David, 1939–   .  III. Konen, Joseph C.
   [DNLM: 1. Primary Health Care.  2. Surgical Procedures, Operative.
3. Referral and Consultation.  4. Decision Making.  W 84.6 W567
1998]
  R727.8.W47  1998
  616—dc21
  DNLM/DLC
  for Library of Congress                98-21038
                                 CIP

To Jill, Barbara, and Joan, for their unending support.

# Acknowledgments

A project of this size and complexity requires the efforts of many talented people. Many of the illustrations are the work of Jay Knipstein. Jacqueline Weisman managed hundreds of phone calls, faxes, and letters. In addition, she typed most of the book. Thanks also to the content reviewers, especially Dr. Thomas Lakata and Dr. Wayne Hale. Finally, we appreciate the personal attention that this project received from Sandy Reinhardt and Bernice Wissler of the F. A. Davis Company.

# Contributors

Alan M. Adelman, MD
Pennsylvania State University/Hershey
  Medical Center
Department of Family & Community
  Medicine
Hershey, Pennsylvania

Chenicheri Balakrishnan, MD
Assistant Professor
Wayne State University School of
  Medicine
Division of Plastic Surgery
Detroit, Michigan

Lee Beatty, MD
East Gaston Family Physicians
Carolinas Healthcare System
Mount Holly, North Carolina

Richard Blondell, MD
University of Louisville
Louisville, Kentucky

David Bouwman, MD
Professor of Surgery
Wayne State University School of
  Medicine
Detroit, Michigan

Don Burgio, MD
Assistant Professor
Department of Otolaryngology—Head
  and Neck Surgery
Wayne State University School of
  Medicine
Detroit, Michigan

Frank Celestino, MD
Wake Forest University School of
  Medicine
Winston-Salem, North Carolina

Jason Chao, MD
Assistant Professor of Family Medicine
Case Western Reserve University
Department of Family Practice
Cleveland, Ohio

Medical Director
Qual Choice Health Plan
Cleveland, Ohio

Max M. Cohen, MD
Chief of Surgery
Grace Hospital
Detroit, Michigan

Professor of Surgery
Wayne State University School of
  Medicine
Detroit, Michigan

Michael Dahn, MD, PhD
Professor of Surgery
Wayne State University School of
  Medicine
Detroit, Michigan

Veterans Administration Medical Center
Detroit, Michigan

Charles Driscoll, MD
Private Practice
West Branch, Iowa

Clinical Professor
University of Iowa
College of Medicine
Iowa City, Iowa

Charles Eaton, MD, MS
Associate Professor of Family Medicine
Brown University/Memorial Hospital of
    Rhode Island
Department of Family Medicine
Pawtucket, Rhode Island


Mark S. Friedland, MD
Assistant Professor
Wayne State University School of
    Medicine
Division of Vascular Surgery
Detroit, Michigan


David Fromm, MD
Chairman, Department of Surgery
Wayne State University School of
    Medicine
Detroit, Michigan


Rebecca Gladhu, MD
Assistant Professor
Department of Family Practice and
    Community Medicine
University of Texas Medical School at
    Houston
Houston, Texas


Gerald Goodenough, MD
Emory University School of Medicine
Department of Family & Preventive
    Medicine
Atlanta, Georgia


Cheryl Grigorian, MD
Assistant Professor of Radiology
Wayne State University School of
    Medicine
Detroit, Michigan

Staff Radiologist
Harper Hospital
Detroit, Michigan


Marko R. Gudziak, MD
Assistant Professor
Wayne State University School of
    Medicine
Department of Urology
Detroit, Michigan

David Jackson, MD
Associate Professor and Interim Chair
Wake Forest University School of
    Medicine
Winston-Salem, North Carolina


Mark P. Knudson, MD, MSPH
Associate Professor in Family Practice
Wake Forest University School of
    Medicine
Winston-Salem, North Carolina

Director, Residency Training
Wake Forest University School of
    Medicine
Winston-Salem, North Carolina


Joseph C. Konen, MD
Carolinas Medical Center
Chair, Department of Family Medicine
Charlotte, North Carolina


Mary Ann Kosir, MD
Assistant Professor of Surgery
Wayne State University School of
    Medicine

John D. Dingell VA Medical Center
Detroit, Michigan


Robert A. Kozol, MD
Associate Professor
Wayne State University School of
    Medicine
Detroit, Michigan

Chief of Surgery
VA Medical Center
Detroit, Michigan


WJ Krompinger, MD
Assistant Clinical Professor
Department of Orthopedic Surgery
University of Connecticut
School of Medicine
Farmington, Connecticut

Orthopedic Associate of Hartford
Hartford, Connecticut


Howard B. McNeely, MD
Board Certified, Diplomat
American Academy of Family Physicians
Norris, Tennessee

S. Gene McNeely, Jr, MD
Professor
Department of Obstetrics & Gynecology
Wayne State University School of
    Medicine
Detroit, Michigan

Chief, Department of Gynecology
Detroit Receiving Hospital—University
    Health Center
Detroit, Michigan

Daniel B. Michael, MD, PhD
Assistant Professor
Wayne State University School of
    Medicine
Detroit, Michigan

Chief, Neurosurgery
Detroit Receiving Hospital and University
    Health Center
Detroit, Michigan

Venita Morell, MD
Director, Predoctoral Education
Family and Community Medicine
Wake Forest University Baptist Medical
    Center
Winston-Salem, North Carolina

Sam Nasser, MD, PhD
Associate Professor of Orthopedics
Wayne State University School of
    Medicine
Detroit, Michigan

Marcus Plescia, MD, MPH
Associate Professor
Carolinas Medical Center
Department of Family Practice
Charlotte, North Carolina

Gregory Pomeroy, MD
Director, Portland Orthopedic Foot
    & Ankle Center
Portland, Maine

Lawrence Raymond, MD, ScM
University of North Carolina
Chapel Hill, North Carolina

Carolina Medical Center
Director, Occupational and
    Environmental Medicine
Charlotte, North Carolina

Paul Lee Salisbury, III, DDS
Department of Dentistry
Wake Forest University School of
    Medicine
Winston-Salem, North Carolina

Walter Salwen, MD
Assistant Professor of Surgery
Wayne State University School of
    Medicine
Veterans Administration Medical Center
Detroit, Michigan

John G. Spangler, MD, MPH
Wake Forest University School of
    Medicine
Department of Family & Community
    Medicine
Winston-Salem, North Carolina

Christopher Steffes, MD
Assistant Professor of Surgery
Wayne State University School of
    Medicine
Detroit, Michigan

Steven Tennenberg, MD
Assistant Professor of Surgery
Wayne State University School of
    Medicine
Detroit Veterans Affairs Medical Center
Detroit, Michigan

Joseph A. Troncale, MD
Lancaster General Hospital
Medical Director, Susquehanna
    Addictions Unit
Lancaster, Pennsylvania

Milton Hershey Medical School
Department of Family Practice
Hershey, Pennsylvania

James Tyburski, MD
Assistant Professor of Surgery
Wayne State University School of
    Medicine
Detroit, Michigan

George Yoo, MD
Assistant Professor
Department of Otolaryngology—Head
    and Neck Surgery
Wayne State University School of
    Medicine
Detroit, Michigan

# Preface

The American health care system is evolving rapidly, driven by the public's growing expectations of improved health status and a successful outcome in every situation, and by the need to balance technological advances with economic restraints. A renewed interest in primary care as the foundation of health care has arisen. Specialty care continues to be highly valued, but access to specialty services has become restricted by managed health care reimbursement systems. Primary care providers, such as family physicians, general internists, and pediatricians, are now often placed in the position of "gatekeepers" to referral or specialty care.

For most health care problems, the evolving system has served the patient well. While pharmaceutical and medical therapeutic approaches have advanced significantly over the last few decades, surgical diagnostic approaches and interventions similarly have increased in their sophistication and technological complexity. But the gatekeeper's breadth of knowledge of surgical conditions may affect the outcome of a patient's care. Not only physicians, but also physician assistants, nurse practitioners, and extended practice nurses may all be front-line or first-contact health care providers, but the extent of their surgical training may vary from years to weeks. Nevertheless, because surgical consultation is not always immediately available, the provider of first contact must be familiar with surgical problems. Such familiarity also helps when the primary caregiver and the surgeon communicate about the most appropriate option for a given problem in the unique context of the patient and his or her family. Both outcome and patient and professional satisfaction are improved by this kind of collaborative care.

This book is designed to be a rapid reference or refresher in surgery for primary care clinicians. By design, it certainly is not a textbook of surgery. Our goal is to offer guidance as to when to obtain a surgical consultation—"When to Call the Surgeon." Most chapters are coauthored by a surgeon and a primary care physician. This combination offers a balanced approach to surgical problems. Because the book was conceived to be an immediate resource for the primary care generalist, it was obvious to us that authorship by generalists as well as specialist surgeons would be essential in conveying a state-of-the-art initial approach to potential surgical issues for a variety of complaints and illnesses. Just as primary care providers vary in their training and continuing education about surgical approaches to common problems, so do they vary in their capability and desire to perform minor office procedures. This book, therefore, offers some guidance and tips on common procedures that are often performed in primary care offices. These tips may enhance the practice of the procedure-oriented primary care provider, or at least offer some basis for early patient education prior to a surgical consultation.

ROBERT A. KOZOL, M.D.
DAVID FROMM, M.D.
JOSEPH C. KONEN, M.D.

# Foreword

Primary care providers and surgeons interact frequently about patients' care. As a family physician, it is not uncommon for me to wonder about when to call the surgeon—do I bother them now? What is the urgency of this situation? Should I do a trial of therapy first? What should I do before I send them to the surgeon?

Once we have sent the patient to the surgeon, sometimes other questions arise. The patient or patient's family will often call and ask for our opinion on whether or not the surgery is necessary, or which type of surgery would be preferable. We may be in the position (primarily in health maintenance organizations) of approving or disapproving the surgery.

Surgical textbooks have often not been that useful to me. Yes, there are surgical textbooks in the office. Yes, I try to use them. But, they too often emphasize surgical technique, rather than the aspects of the cases that I need to know.

This textbook is designed to bring needed surgical information to primary care providers. How do surgeons think about the problems our patients have? What considerations go through their minds? The joint authorship of most of the chapters helps to provide the useful perspective of what primary care providers want to know from surgeons.

When I first received the galley proofs to read, I wondered about whether this would be a textbook to take home and read cover to cover, or whether it would be a textbook I would leave on the shelf in the office to use as a reference on a case-by-case basis. When I finished reading the book, I decided it was both. I truly enjoyed several of the chapters, which added to my depth of understanding of their topics. Other chapters, or subsections, provide knowledge on things I do not care to memorize, but will be useful for later referencing. It is easily divided by topic area, with clear bullet points summarizing when to refer. The short highlights also provide a useful reminder of the important issues from the chapter.

When to cut, when to wait, when to refer. Here it is.

MARJORIE A. BOWMAN, M.D., M.P.A.

# Contents

## Chapter 4

## Neck Pain and Sore Throat . . . . . . . . . . . . . . . . . . . . . . . . . . . . . . . . . . 36

WALTER SALWEN, MD, and LEE BEATTY, MD

## Chapter 5

## Airway Problems . . . . . . . . . . . . . . . . . . . . . . . . . . . . . . . . . . . . . . . . . . 44

MICHAEL DAHN, MD, PhD,
and LAWRENCE RAYMOND, MD, ScM

## Chapter 6

## Breast Problems . . . . . . . . . . . . . . . . . . . . . . . . . . . . . . . . . . . . . . . . . . 56

MARY ANN KOSIR, MD, RICHARD BLONDELL, MD,
and CHERYL GRIGORIAN, MD

# Headache

JOSEPH A. TRONCALE, MD,
and DANIEL B. MICHAEL, MD, PhD

Headache is one of the most common, most disabling, and, with the possible exception of chest pain, the most feared symptom experienced by patients. Those afflicted spend over 1 billion dollars per year on over-the-counter headache remedies. At the same time, headache is one of the least specific causes of pain and is, therefore, a difficult problem for the clinician. At least 40% of all individuals experience a headache yearly. Once a patient presents with the symptom of headache, logical clinical reasoning is essential to proper diagnosis and testing. It is important to decide reliably whether the presenting headache is benign or if there is a serious underlying cause. This chapter focuses on headaches that may require a surgeon's intervention, even though most headaches are benign, albeit painful. Tension, vascular disorders, and trauma are the most common causes of headaches, but in many cases the etiology of headache symptoms may be an enigma to primary care and specialty care providers alike.

Surgeons needed to assist primary care providers when confronted with a patient with headache may include neurologic surgeons (all head pain with or without neurologic symptoms); ophthalmologists (headache with eye findings); ear, nose, and throat specialists; head and neck surgeons; general and plastic surgeons (cutaneous and occasionally other head lesions, hypertension, and pheochromocytoma); and oral surgeons. Even a brief consultation between the primary care provider and the surgeon could facilitate further diagnostic workup and treatment. The neurosurgeon, for example, may help complete the workup (e.g., temporal artery or brain biopsy) and provide definitive care (critical care, intracranial pressure monitoring, and surgical intervention).

## Classification of Headaches

Headache is caused by irritation of the pain-sensitive structures of the head: skin, periosteum, dura, blood vessels, and sinuses. Headache symptoms may be categorized

TABLE 1–1

## Associated Signs and Symptoms Suggestive of Organic Headache

| Sign/Symptom | Suggested Disorders |
| --- | --- |
| Nausea and vomiting | Space-occupying lesion |
| | Migraine |
| Altered level of consciousness | Subarachnoid hemorrhage |
| | Meningitis |
| | Space-occupying lesion |
| Speech disturbance | Dominant hemispheric stroke |
| | Space-occupying lesion |
| Cranial nerve findings | II—Papilledema, hemorrhages, blindness, subarachnoid hemorrhage, space-occupying lesion, pituitary mass |
| | III—Palsy: expanding or ruptured p-com aneurysm |
| | IV—Diplopia: elevated intracranial pressure, space-occupying lesion |
| | V—Tic douloureux, petrous apexitis (Gradnego's) |
| | VII—Tic convulsif, cerebellopontine angle (CPA) mass |
| | VIII—CPA mass |
| | IX—Glossopharyngeal neuralgia |
| Motor or sensory findings | Hemiplegia, hemianesthesia—stroke, space-occupying lesion |
| Coordination problems | Hydrocephalus, posterior fossa mass |
| Hypertension | Stroke, elevated intracranial pressure |
| Bradycardia | Elevated intracranial pressure |
| Endocrinopathy | Pituitary mass |

p-com = posterior communicating.

into benign disorders and organic disorders. *Benign headache* does not mean that the pain is necessarily less severe than an organic headache, nor does it imply that the headache lacks an organic cause. "Benign" implies that the processes involved occur at the subtissue (molecular and subcellular) level rather than at the anatomic or cellular level as seen in tumors, hemorrhage, glaucoma, or infection. Benign headache is more common than organic, but the differential diagnosis of headache requires that organic factors be suspected in all cases.

A good history is helpful in delineating headache types, but the ubiquitous nature of headache may cause the cardinal symptoms of intensity, duration, and location to be less than helpful if one is not familiar with the nuances of the various headache syndromes. Although physicians are classically taught that the complaint of "the worst headache of my life" should cause one to consider a subarachnoid hemorrhage, statistically it is more likely that the patient has a migraine. Associated symptoms with headache may be helpful in diagnosis (Table 1–1). For instance, migraines are sometimes triggered by certain foods, activities, sleep patterns, and alcohol, and they sometimes are relieved by sleep and pregnancy. Some patients with headache, especially with migraine, have associated gastrointestinal symptoms such as nausea, vomiting, or diarrhea. Although classically described as unilateral, in fact only 60% of migraines fit this description.

The physical examination may be helpful in differentiating benign from organic headaches. Table 1–2 outlines findings with organic headache that might warrant surgical consultation.

The primary care provider may order numerous cranial and central nervous system imaging studies and other diagnostic tests when confronted with a headache patient. These tests include plain roentgenograms, computed tomography (CT) scans, magnetic resonance imaging (MRI), angiography, nuclear medicine studies, positron emission tomography (PET) scans, electroencephalograms (EEGs), and lumbar puncture. Some of these tests may be ordered based on the differential diagnosis arrived at after a complete history and physical and neurologic exam. Communication between the primary care provider and the appropriate surgical colleague may obviate costly, unnecessary studies.

• ▬
*Communication between the primary care provider and the appropriate surgical colleague may obviate costly, unnecessary studies.*

TABLE 1-2

## Causes of Organic Headache That May Require Surgical Intervention

| Classification | Examples of Findings |
| --- | --- |
| Congenital | Hydrocephalus |
| | Skull base malformations (may be present in adults) |
| Traumatic | Acute or chronic space-occupying lesions |
| | Foreign body |
| | Hydrocephalus |
| Vascular | Ischemic or hemorrhagic stroke |
| | Subarachnoid hemorrhage (aneurysm or AVM) |
| Inflammatory | Osteomyelitis |
| | Sinusitis |
| | Abscess |
| | Empyema |
| | Hydrocephalus |
| | Vasculitis (acute giant cell arteritis) |
| Neoplastic | Benign or malignant neoplasms of the head and its contents |
| Other | Psueudomotor cerebri |
| | Glaucoma |
| | Pheochromocytoma |
| | Surgically treated causes of hypertension |
| | Headache in the pediatric age group |

The International Headache Society classification codes 13 different types of headaches. Of these, surgeons would probably be consulted most often regarding four: glaucoma, neoplasms or infection, vascular disorders, and head trauma. The primary care provider, on the other hand, will most often encounter the other types, which include migraine, tension-type headaches and cluster headaches, headaches associated with substance abuse or withdrawal, headaches associated with infections in places other than the head, headaches associated with metabolic disorders, cranial neuralgias, headaches or facial pain associated with a disorder of the face or cranium such as a tooth abscess, and headaches due to minor blunt trauma.

Critical causes of acute headache, which may require prompt surgical consultation, include acute angle-closure glaucoma, acute sinusitis, tumors, temporal arteritis, cerebral vascular accidents, subarachnoid hemorrhage, malignant hypertension, meningitis requiring intracranial pressure monitoring, pheochromocytomas, complications of HIV, and trauma.

## Acute Angle-Closure Glaucoma

Persons with shallow anterior chambers of the eye are subject to a condition in which the normal fluid circulation in the eye is blocked. This condition is termed *acute angle-closure glaucoma*. This condition, which becomes more prevalent with increasing age, increases intraocular pressure and may cause eye pain; headache in or around the eye; a fixed, dilated pupil on the affected side; and blurry vision with corneal edema. Acute angle-closure glaucoma is an ophthalmologic emergency, as permanent blindness can ensue. If the diagnosis is suspected, intraocular pressure should be measured to confirm the diagnosis and treatment instituted as rapidly as possible. Ophthalmologic consultation should be obtained immediately if acute angle-closure glaucoma is suspected. If an ophthalmologist is unavailable immediately to perform an iridotomy, intraocular pressures may be improved with the use of acetazolamide (250 mg IV or 500 mg PO), parenteral osmotic diuretics such as 20% mannitol (250–500 mL IV over 2–3 hours), pilocarpine eye drops, and topical beta-blockers. Patients with shallow

*Ophthalmologic consultation should be obtained immediately if acute angle-closure glaucoma is suspected.*

anterior chambers who have an attack in one eye usually need prophylactic iridotomy on the unaffected eye to prevent a future attack.

## Acute Sinusitis and Other Head and Neck Conditions

*For patients with acute sinusitis, an otolaryngological consultation may be required to consider surgical drainage of the sinuses or any orbital or sphenoid involvement.*

Sinusitis may present with headache, fever, purulent nasal discharge, facial pain, tooth pain, and a variety of other symptoms. Acute sinusitis can be caused by *Streptococcus pneumoniae, Moraxella, Haemophilus influenzae,* and other organisms. In the intensive care unit, it is associated with prolonged nasal cannulation, and other, more virulent organisms, such as *Staphylococcus aureus,* may be involved. If there is intracranial extension, the diagnosis should be confirmed with plain films or CT scanning or both. An otolaryngologic consultation may be required to consider surgical drainage of the sinuses or any orbital or sphenoid involvement. Sinus infections may also extend into other structures such as adjacent bone, blood vessels, and nerves, so sinusitis complicated by extension causing epidural abscess, cranial nerve involvement, or other evidence of spread is a surgical emergency. The primary care provider should obtain laboratory studies including blood cultures prior to starting antibiotics if an abscess is suspected or identified.

Many other head and neck conditions associated with headache may require the intervention of an otolaryngologist or oral surgeon. These include mastoiditis, otitis media requiring myringotomy, head and neck cancers, and dental and retropharyngeal abscesses, among others. Thus, a complete exam including an oral survey is paramount.

## Brain Neoplasms

*Headaches that have changed in character, are rapidly worsening, awaken the patient at night, or are prominent upon rising in the morning suggest an intracranial neoplasm.*

It is beyond the scope of this text to cover the various types of brain neoplasms in detail. Suffice it to say that brain tumors may be histologically either benign or malignant and are usually classified by both cell type and location. Some so-called benign tumors may be lethal because of their location, and some malignant tumors, such as childhood astrocytomas of the cerebellum, may be cured.

Depending on their location, brain tumors usually do not cause neurologic symptoms until they obtain a mass of about 30 grams (Fig. 1–1). The advent of CT and MRI scanning has made earlier, more accurate diagnosis possible. Brain tumors that are expanding rapidly or are related to pain-sensitive intracranial structures are more frequently associated with headache. Headaches that have changed in character, are rapidly worsening, awaken the patient at night, or are prominent upon rising in the morn-

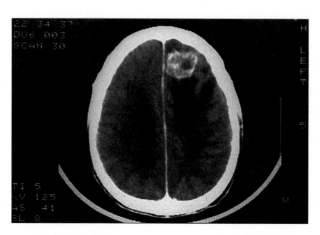

FIGURE 1–1
CT scan depicting a left frontal brain tumor.

ing suggest an intracranial neoplasm. These symptoms indicate CT or MRI imaging. Once identified, mass lesions in the cranium should receive neurosurgical consultation.

## Temporal Arteritis

Temporal arteritis should be considered as part of the differential diagnosis for older patients with headache. Associated symptoms include jaw claudication, visual symptoms, and temporal artery burning or pain. The sedimentation rate is usually elevated and surgical consultation may be indicated to obtain a temporal artery biopsy to confirm the diagnosis. If temporal arteritis is strongly suspected, steroid therapy to prevent blindness should not be delayed pending a biopsy, especially if there are visual symptoms.

*Steroid therapy should not be delayed pending a biopsy if temporal arteritis is strongly suspected.*

## Intracranial Hemorrhage

Classically, intracranial hemorrhage presents as the sudden onset of a severe, unremitting headache. The onset of the headache sometimes is associated with straining, strenuous activity, or sexual intercourse, but aneurysms are just as likely to rupture during sleep. Patients often describe headaches from intracranial hemorrhage as "the worst headache of my life." The patient may become stuporous or comatose. If there are additional neurologic findings or nuchal rigidity, immediate imaging studies of the brain are warranted. If the process involved is a leaking aneurysm or arteriovenous malformation, a neurosurgeon should be consulted to determine the proper intervention (Fig. 1–2) and the patient should be stabilized in a neurologic intensive care unit.

*Patients often describe headaches from intracranial hemorrhage as "the worst headache of my life."*

Hemorrhagic or ischemic strokes may also present with headache. The presence of hemiplegia or alteration of consciousness in these patients will alert the primary care provider to this diagnosis. Lumbar puncture may be helpful in diagnosing subarachnoid bleeding but should not be performed unless significantly increased intracranial pressure can be ruled out. Examination of the optic fundi for subhyaloid hemorrhages, and CT scanning or MRI exam for altered brain structure may be indicated. Patients who have had a documented subarachnoid hemorrhage should be admitted to a neurologic intensive care unit and given loading doses of anticonvulsants. Antiseizure medications also should be strongly considered for patients with an aneurysm, as seizure activity could both worsen the neurologic condition and predispose the patient to additional bleeding. Neurosurgical consultation should be obtained to determine if the aneurysm or arteriovenous malformation is amenable to surgical clips or ablation.

*Lumbar puncture may be helpful in diagnosing subarachnoid bleeding but should not be performed unless significantly increased intracranial pressure can be ruled out.*

**FIGURE 1–2**
Cerebral angiogram revealing an intracranial aneurysm.

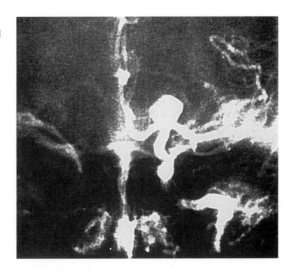

## Malignant Hypertension

*Malignant hypertension* is a medical emergency. It is defined by papilledema, often accompanied by retinal hemorrhages, in the presence of greatly elevated blood pressure, although the absolute degree of systolic or diastolic pressure elevation is not a criterion. Patients often have blood pressures exceeding 200/100 mm Hg. Symptoms may include headache, photophobia, blurry vision, focal neurologic deficits, alterations in consciousness, and seizure activity. Immediate lowering of blood pressure in a monitored unit is indicated while the cause for the blood pressure elevation is sought. The brain may suffer microscopic hemorrhages and other focal damage if the blood pressure is not corrected quickly. It is recommended that patients with suspected malignant hypertension should be admitted to an intensive care unit and begun on antihypertensive therapy such as sodium nitroprusside or a nitroglycerin drip to titrate the blood pressure to acceptable levels. If seizures occur, the patient should be given loading doses of an appropriate anticonvulsant.

Malignant hypertension with headache, palpitations, and diaphoresis suggests *pheochromocytoma*, a tumor of the adrenal medulla associated with excess serum catecholamine levels. Patients will often describe "spells" or episodes of headache and palpitations. These patients frequently are known to be hypertensive and to have poor blood pressure control despite multiple medications. Patients with suspected pheochromocytoma should be tested for levels of urinary catecholamine breakdown products (vanillylmandelic acid [VMA] and metanephrine). Testing of serum catecholamine is sometimes useful but less reliable. Other causes of malignant hypertension include renovascular disease, especially renal hypoperfusion as seen in renal artery stenosis, and abrupt withdrawal of antihypertensive medications, especially beta-blockers.

## Toxic Exposure

Many types of toxic exposures may cause headache. Some of the better known toxins include carbon monoxide, heavy metals, and certain drugs and foods. Patients with space heaters, gas kilns, and other open heaters are at especially high risk for carbon monoxide toxicity and should be warned to have carbon monoxide detectors in the house. Patients with carbon monoxide toxicity could present with shortness of breath, headache, confusion, and nausea. Cyanosis is seen more frequently than the supposedly classic "cherry red" skin. Immediate therapy with 100% oxygen at 10 L/min by a non-rebreather mask is the treatment of choice. Usually a thorough history of potential toxic exposures will suggest the correct diagnosis, but a high index of suspicion is required.

## Meningitis and Central Nervous System Infections

Meningeal infection leads to meningeal irritation, which causes headache. Multiple organisms may be associated with meningitis; the more virulent ones include *S. pneumoniae*, *H. influenzae*, and *Neiserria meningitidis*. Bacterial and viral meningitis are diagnosed with an examination of spinal fluid. Patients with headache, fever, nuchal rigidity, and mental status changes should be considered for spinal fluid examination. To guard against unanticipated brain herniation, patients with fever, headache, and any focal neurologic finding should have a CT scan of the head to rule out a brain abscess or other mass effect before a lumbar puncture is attempted. Occasionally, neurosurgical consultation is necessary to obtain intracranial pressure monitoring in patients with severe central nervous system (CNS) infections.

Individuals with HIV and headache require special consideration. HIV infection may cause encephalitis. Those with HIV often have unusual CNS infections, especially

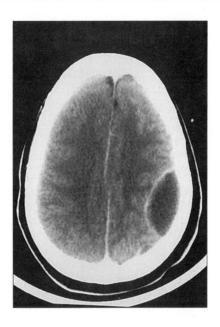

**FIGURE 1–3**
CT scan in a patient with a left sided subdural empyema.

cryptococcus and fungal organisms. Subdural empyema may present with symptoms of elevated intracranial pressure, including headache (Fig. 1–3). Other causes of headache in HIV include progressive multifocal leukoencephalopathy, generalized sepsis, and drug reactions.

## Trauma

### ACUTE HEMORRHAGE

Patients who have experienced head trauma are candidates for developing space-occupying lesions such as epidural or subdural hematomas. Head injury is the single most common cause of subarachnoid hemorrhage. Especially at risk are the elderly, who may fall and not remember because of poor memory, and substance abusers,

**FIGURE 1–4**
CT scan showing a chronic hematoma of the left hemisphere.

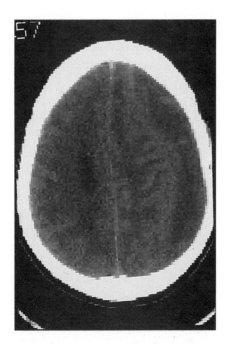

who have altered mental status from exogenous sources. Patients with chronic headache plus focal neurologic signs should have imaging studies to rule out chronic hematoma (Fig. 1–4). If diagnosed, immediate neurosurgical consultation is required. Patients with loss of consciousness, especially longer than 10 minutes, should have immediate CT scanning.

Iatrogenic headaches caused by spinal taps are fairly common, occurring in nearly a third of those who undergo the procedure. Sitting upright aggravates the headache and lying down alleviates the symptoms, which usually resolve in less than 48 hours. An epidural blood patch may be needed if the symptoms are prolonged.

## POSTCONCUSSIVE SYNDROME

Many patients who have suffered a blunt injury to the head have what is known as *postconcussive syndrome* or *postconcussive nervous instability*. These patients complain of headache, dizziness, disequilibrium, nausea, memory and personality changes, and other vague symptoms. The syndrome is well recognized by neurologists and neurosurgeons, but its exact cause is unclear. Research suggests that post-traumatic neuronal reorganization may contribute. The treatment is empiric and includes low-dose tricyclic antidepressants or low-dose benzodiazepines. The syndrome generally resolves over weeks to months, and neurosurgical consultation is not required in routine cases.

# *Conclusion*

The primary care provider will be able to diagnose and treat the vast majority of patients presenting with headache. Reassuring the patient that the headache is not due to a sinister organic cause is an important part of headache therapy. If a severe or unusual headache is encountered, prompt communication between the primary care provider and surgeon will improve cost-effective, quality patient care.

### *When to Call the Surgeon about Headache*

- Acute or chronic space-occupying lesions including tumors, hemorrhage, hydrocephalus, pseudotumor cerebri, etc.
- Infectious processes of the head (osteomyelitis, abscesses, chronic sinusitis, etc.)
- Inflammatory processes requiring tissue diagnosis (e.g., temporal arteritis)
- Acute glaucoma
- Pheochromocytoma or other surgically treated causes of hypertension
- Trauma to the central nervous system

## RECOMMENDED READING

Bartley, GB, and Liesegang, TJ (eds): Essentials of Ophthalmology. JB Lippincott, Philadelphia, 1992.

Isselbacher, KJ, et al (eds): Harrison's Principles of Internal Medicine. ed 13. McGraw-Hill, New York, 1994.

Olesen, JP, Tfelt-Hansen, and KMA Welch (eds): The Headaches. Raven Press, New York, 1993.

Rowland, LP (ed): Merritt's Textbook of Neurology. ed 9. Williams and Wilkins, Baltimore, 1995.

Schwartz, GR, et al (eds): Principles and Practice of Emergency Medicine. ed 3. Lea & Febiger, Philadelphia, 1993.

# Common Ear Disorders

## DON BURGIO, MD, and GEORGE YOO, MD

Otologic problems are very common, yet rarely life threatening. Most ear diseases are well managed by primary care providers alone, but some otologic problems require immediate consultation with an otolaryngologist, and others require a prompt referral. The key to making the correct diagnosis and appropriately treating and referring these patients is a complete otologic history and physical exam. When an otologic exam is combined with a history, a differential diagnosis can easily be obtained. Primary otologic symptoms include otalgia, otorrhea, tinnitus, vertigo and dizziness, hearing loss, and facial paralysis. An audiogram is another key feature of a thorough otologic evaluation. Specific features of the otologic evaluation will be discussed in this chapter. A primary care provider can use these features as aids in appropriately consulting an otolaryngologist.

## *Symptoms*

Most patients who present with a common otologic symptom will not have a dangerous problem, but certain clues can lead one to suspect a more serious process. These clues should lead a primary care provider to call an otolaryngologist in a timely manner or even urgently.

### OTALGIA

*Otalgia* is pain in the ear that can be direct or referred. Superficial cervical nerves and cranial nerves V, VII, IX, and X provide sensory innervation of the ear. Referred otalgia is mediated through cranial nerves V, IX, and X, which innervate the ear along with the temporomandibular joint (TMJ), pharynx, and larynx. Otalgia can accompany infections, such as otitis media and otitis externa, and tumors, such as cholesteatoma

**9**

*Otoscopic examination can reveal the etiology of most cases of otalgia.*

*If the temporomandibular joint is not tender and the patient is a smoker, the examiner should suspect a possible pharyngeal or laryngeal cancer.*

and external auditory canal cancers. Otoscopic examination can reveal the etiology of most cases of otalgia, such as otitis media and otitis externa. If otalgia is combined with fever, profuse granulation tissue in the external auditory canal, or mastoid swelling, it may suggest malignant otitis externa or coalescent mastoiditis with subperiosteal abscess.

When significant otalgia presents with a normal otologic examination, the examiner should aggressively try to identify the apparently hidden cause. The initial step would be to palpate the TMJ. Since this joint lies in very close proximity to the ear, many patients confuse TMJ pain with otalgia. If the joint is not tender and the patient is a smoker, one should suspect a possible pharyngeal or laryngeal cancer. Of patients presenting with advanced pharyngeal or laryngeal cancer, 20% to 40% complain of referred otalgia. Rarely otalgia will be caused by skull-base or parapharyngeal tumors.

### *When to Call the Surgeon/Otolaryngologist about Otalgia*

- Pain with a normal otoscopic exam and a nontender TMJ
- Persistent, profuse granulation in the external auditory canal
- Tenderness and swelling in the postauricular or mastoid area
- Cranial nerve dysfunction

## OTORRHEA

*When otorrhea is chronic and fails to respond to therapy, other disease processes should be considered.*

*Otorrhea* means fluid draining from the ear. Drainage can be caused by inflammation, infection, or tumors. Otorrhea typically occurs from infections in the external ear, the middle ear, or both. It can present acutely, lasting less than 3 weeks, or chronically, lasting more than 3 weeks. Patients who present with acute drainage and no other evidence of otologic complications can be treated expectantly with oral antibiotics and topical otologic drops that contain steroids and antibiotics. When otorrhea is chronic and fails to respond to therapy, however, the examiner should consider other disease processes, such as a cholesteatoma or chronic inflammation of the mastoid or middle-ear space. If there is no perforation in the tympanic membrane, and no granulation tissue or ulcerative lesions, then chronic otitis externa is present and one can continue to treat the patient with topical antibiotics and steroid solutions. If persistent granulation tissue or ulcerative lesions are present in the external auditory canal, however, one should be concerned about chronic granulomatous systemic diseases, infections, or possibly even a cancer (Fig. 2–1).

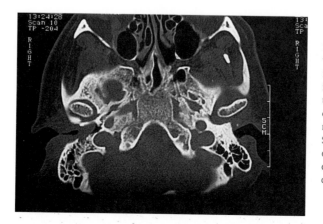

**FIGURE 2–1**

Right external auditory canal squamous cell carcinoma. This 60-year-old woman presented with right otorrhea, inflammation, and granulation tissue in the external auditory canal. This was treated with antibiotics and topical drops for 9 months. Then a right neck mass and facial paralysis developed. Subsequently, she was referred to an otolaryngologist, who performed a biopsy that revealed squamous cell carcinoma.

*When to Call the Surgeon/Otolaryngologist about Otorrhea*

- Suspicion of an acute intratemporal or intracranial complication
- Drainage that does not resolve with therapy
- Granulation tissue or ulcerative lesions in the external auditory canal

## TINNITUS

*Tinnitus* is the sensation of sound in the ear. Tinnitus alone is common and seldom a worrisome complaint. Most people will experience transient tinnitus at some point in their lives, either spontaneously or after exposure to loud noise. Often the cause is not identifiable and most patients with tinnitus will not have their lives disrupted by it.

Any patient who complains of persistent tinnitus should be screened and evaluated with an audiogram. Idiopathic tinnitus can be exacerbated by factors such as hypertension, stress, and many prescription and nonprescription drugs (including aspirin and nonsteroidal anti-inflammatory drugs [NSAIDs]). Therefore, patients who present with tinnitus should have these exacerbating factors treated or eliminated. Furthermore, underlying depression may increase the severity of tinnitus. Examiners should evaluate for a possibility of depression and pursue appropriate treatment.

Tinnitus is rarely the first symptom of a severe problem involving the middle ear, inner ear, or eighth cranial nerve, although some characteristic features can lead one to suspect a more serious problem. *Pulsatile tinnitus* is a beating or throbbing and is usually described as "hearing my heartbeat." The pulsatile nature of tinnitus can be caused by many common conditions, including conductive hearing loss and eustachian tube dysfunction; but more ominous causes, such as glomus tumor, carotid bruit, and dural fistula, should be ruled out. Lesions in the cerebellopontine angle (CPA), such as acoustic neuroma and meningioma, do not typically present with tinnitus alone. Occasionally patients with such lesions will present with unilateral tinnitus alone or with vertigo, hearing loss, and facial paralysis. Suspected lesions in the CPA and skull base should be evaluated further with a computed tomography (CT) scan, magnetic resonance imaging (MRI), or both.

*Pulsatile tinnitus is caused by many common conditions, but more ominous causes should be ruled out.*

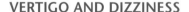

*When to Call the Surgeon/Otolaryngologist about Tinnitus*

- Severe and debilitating tinnitus
- Unilateral tinnitus
- Pulsatile tinnitus
- Tinnitus accompanied by unilateral hearing loss, vertigo, and facial paralysis
- Tinnitus with cranial nerve abnormalities

## VERTIGO AND DIZZINESS

*Vertigo* is a sensation of whirling or spinning. Dizziness, lightheadedness, disequilibrium, or feeling off balance are vague, nonrotary sensations often confused with vertigo that may overlap with it. All of these are common complaints of patients presenting to primary care practitioners. Dizziness, lightheadedness, disequilibrium, or feeling off balance may be caused by neurologic, vascular, or cardiac diseases.

Patients presenting with vertigo should have a full otologic, vestibular, and cranial nerve examination and a basic neurologic exam. An audiogram may also be indicated. The vestibular exam should consist of checking for nystagmus, performing a Dix-

Hallpike test,* gait testing, Romberg's test, and tandem Romberg's test; and checking the vestibular-ocular reflex and coordination.

The repetitive, jerky eye movements of nystagmus frequently represent a pathologic process, although a small amount of nystagmus normally is present in the peripheral gaze. Most nystagmus is related to a peripheral process, but vertical nystagmus is caused by a central process. Rotary nystagmus is characteristic of and diagnostic for benign positional vertigo.

The origin of vertigo can be peripheral (eighth cranial nerve, labyrinth) or central (intracranial). Vertigo is usually caused by a peripheral vestibular defect. At a minimum, those with persistent vertigo should receive a complete examination and audiogram. Central vertigo is associated with other neurologic findings. Common causes of central vertigo are multiple sclerosis, trauma, and tumors. Multiple sclerosis will present with vertigo or dizziness as the first symptom in 15% to 20% of cases. Ataxia, syncopal episodes, multiple falls, and drop attacks are rarely related to inner-ear pathology, and circulatory or neurologic causes, such as cerebellar hemorrhage, should be ruled out.

*If vertigo with fluid or infection in the middle ear persists, the labyrinthitis should be treated with antibiotics and placement of a pressure equalization tube.*

Benign positional vertigo, Ménière's disease, vestibular neuritis, complicated otitis media, and acoustic neuroma are some common otologic causes of vertigo and dizziness. Benign positional vertigo is characterized by sudden bouts of vertigo that are related to head position and last only a few minutes. Vertigo in Ménière's disease fluctuates and lasts for hours. Ménière's disease is also associated with fluctuating hearing loss. Vestibular neuritis is an inflammatory process of the vestibular nerve. Patients with this condition complain of vertigo and, rarely, hearing loss that lasts for days to weeks. Serous labyrinthitis is a complication of otitis media. If vertigo with fluid or infection in the middle ear persists, the labyrinthitis should be treated with antibiotics and placement of a pressure-equalization tube. An acoustic neuroma can present with vertigo and asymmetric hearing loss.

Dizziness associated with other otologic symptoms (hearing loss, tinnitus, aural fullness) requires evaluation by an otolaryngologist. When dizziness is severe and persistent, it is prudent to evaluate for and rule out nonotologic causes.

### When to Call the Surgeon/Otolaryngologist about Vertigo and Dizziness

- Severe and persistent vertigo when the cause is not apparent
- Dizziness associated with other otologic symptoms (hearing loss, tinnitus, aural fullness)
- Vertical nystagmus

## HEARING LOSS

*Hearing loss* is relatively common and can be caused by many different pathologic processes. Sound is transmitted to the oval window from the external auditory canal, tympanic membrane, and ossicles. In the cochlea, sound waves are converted by the sensory hair cells into electrical signals and transmitted by the cochlear nerve to be encoded by the brain. A perturbation along this pathway can cause a hearing loss. Any patient with a normal exam who complains of hearing loss should receive a complete audiometric assessment.

Typically hearing loss is either conductive or sensorineural. *Conductive hearing loss* is caused by abnormalities within the external auditory canal, tympanic membrane, or middle ear. It is important to ensure that the external auditory canal is not occluded with cerumen and that the tympanic membrane is intact and appears normal. The

---

*The Dix-Hallpike test is a positioning test for vertigo and nystagmus brought on by placing the patient in the head-hanging-left or head-hanging-right position.

most common causes of conductive hearing loss—middle-ear effusion and cerumen impaction—can be easily diagnosed with an otoscopic examination. Middle-ear effusion in children is due to eustachean tube dysfunction. The effusion need not be treated unless there is significant hearing loss (>30 dB), speech delay, or excessive absences from school. Placement of pressure-equalization tubes may be considered. Persistent middle-ear effusion in an adult requires evaluation of the nasopharynx to ensure that a nasopharyngeal carcinoma is not present. In an adult patient with a normal otoscopic examination and a conductive hearing loss, the examiner should suspect otosclerosis.

*Sensorineural hearing loss* is caused by alterations in the cochlea and eighth cranial nerve. Hearing loss that occurs in association with vertigo or facial paralysis implies inner-ear pathology and warrants further evaluation. Prevalent causes of sensorineural hearing loss include aging (presbycusis), noise exposure, trauma, and genetic predisposition. Presbycusis and noise-induced hearing loss are slowly progressive, occurring over many years. Acoustic trauma and temporal bone trauma can cause both transient and permanent hearing loss. Transient losses will usually resolve over days to weeks.

When sensorineural hearing loss is sudden, asymmetric, severe (>70 dB), and fluctuating, the patient should receive an aggressive evaluation. Sudden sensorineural hearing loss is an idiopathic entity, which might be caused by inner-ear vessel occlusion, autoimmune disease, or viral infection. It is usually moderate to severe and can be associated with vertigo. An expeditious assessment and treatment (systemic steroid therapy) can restore or halt the progression of sudden idiopathic sensorineural hearing loss.

*When sensorineural hearing loss is sudden, asymmetric, severe (>70 dB), and fluctuating, an aggressive evaluation should be performed.*

When a patient has asymmetric sensorineural hearing loss exceeding 15 dB, the possibility of a retrocochlear lesion or CPA tumor must be addressed. An auditory brainstem response test (ABR) or a $T_1$-weighted MRI with gadolinium can be obtained to exclude such lesions. Fluctuating sensorineural hearing loss, especially when accompanied by tinnitus, vertigo, or aural fullness, is usually due to Ménière's disease. Severe hearing loss can cause difficulty with normal daily activity, and the patient should be evaluated for hearing amplification and rehabilitation.

### When to Call the Surgeon/Otolaryngologist about Hearing Loss

- Sudden hearing loss
- Severe hearing loss
- Fluctuating hearing loss
- Persistent middle-ear effusion
- Conductive hearing loss without obvious cause
- Hearing loss with vertigo or facial paralysis

## FACIAL PARALYSIS

*Acute paralysis of the facial nerve* is a relatively common problem. When assessing facial paralysis, one should determine the time course of onset (sudden versus delayed), severity, completeness, and evidence of recovery. The most common causes of acute facial paralysis are idiopathic facial (Bell's) palsy, otitis media, trauma, and neoplasms. Relatively uncommon causes include herpes zoster oticus (Ramsay Hunt syndrome) and tumors of the skull base and facial nerve. Because facial paralysis without other neurologic findings is most commonly Bell's palsy, no further workup is necessary. Typically Bell's palsy presents as a sudden onset of complete facial paralysis that begins to improve in 2 to 3 weeks, with total recovery in 2 to 3 months. If facial paralysis is slow in onset and incomplete, and recovery is delayed, then the examiner should suspect a cause other than Bell's palsy.

*If facial paralysis is slow in onset and incomplete, and recovery is delayed, the examiner should suspect a cause other than Bell's palsy.*

When first evaluating a patient with acute facial paralysis, the examiner should rule out neoplasm in the parotid gland, Ramsay Hunt syndrome, otitis media, and a cerebral vascular accident. A neoplasm in the parotid gland can be detected by palpating the gland. Ramsay Hunt syndrome presents with intense pain and vesicles on the auricle, with possible dysfunction of other cranial nerves. An otoscopic examination can reveal whether acute otitis media is present, in which case the patient should be referred to an otolaryngologist immediately. Such a patient should undergo antibiotic therapy and placement of a pressure-equalization tube. If the paralysis does not affect the upper facial nerve branches, the possibility of a stroke must be excluded. The examiner should suspect a neoplasm of the facial nerve or acoustic neuroma if no recovery is demonstrable after 3 weeks. If there are other associated otologic symptoms, an acoustic neuroma should be suspected. A $T_1$-weighted, gadolinium-enhanced MRI is the preferred test to demonstrate a facial neuroma or acoustic neuroma. If facial paralysis is recurrent, one should suspect an acoustic neuroma, Guillain-Barré syndrome, or Lyme disease. If facial paralysis is bilateral, one should suspect Guillain-Barré syndrome, sarcoid, Lyme disease, or syphilis, and the appropriate laboratory tests should be ordered.

### When to Call the Surgeon/Otolaryngologist about Facial Paralysis

• Slow onset, slow recovery, or incomplete paralysis
• Bilateral or recurrent facial paralysis
• Vesicles and intense ear pain
• Mass in the parotid gland
• Associated otologic symptoms such as hearing loss, tinnitus, or vertigo
• Otitis media
• Sparing of upper facial nerve branches
• Trauma to the parotid gland or the temporal bone

## Audiometry

Standard *audiometry* consists of several tests. Pure-tone audiometry directly tests hearing at specified frequencies. The hearing loss will be separated into sensorineural, conductive, or mixed hearing loss (Figs. 2–2 and 2–3). Speech audiometry includes speech reception threshold (SRT) and the ability to discriminate speech (speech discrimination score [SDS]). Any patient who complains of a hearing loss should undergo audiometry.

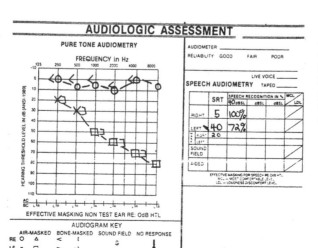

**FIGURE 2–2**
Audiogram of patient with unilateral sensory hearing loss. This 37-year-old healthy woman complained of hearing loss and tinnitus occurring over the past 6 months. This patient's symptoms warrant further evaluation to rule out an eighth-nerve lesion.

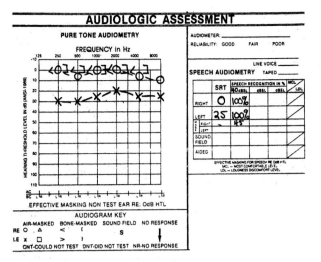

FIGURE 2–3

Audiogram of patient with unilateral conductive hearing loss. This 24-year-old man complained of aural fullness and hearing loss. This audiogram was obtained 4 weeks after an episode of otitis media. Otoscopy revealed amber fluid in the middle ear. His hearing loss is typical of that seen in patients with middle-ear effusion.

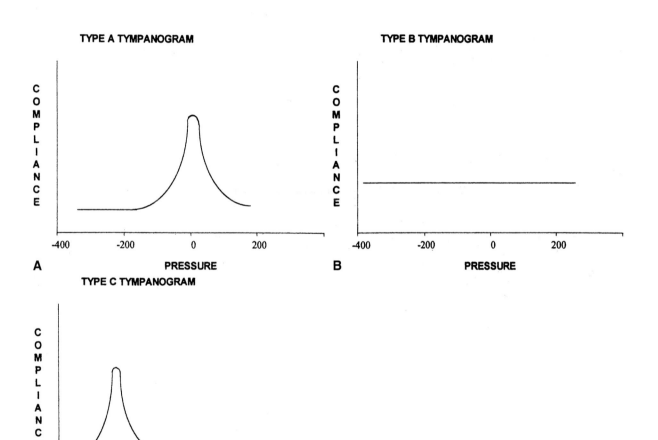

FIGURE 2–4

(A) Type A tympanogram. This indicates normal middle-ear aeration and pressure. Normal pressure varies from −150 mm Hg to +50 mm Hg. (B) Type B tympanogram. This 57-year-old woman had a history of intermittent otorrhea and hearing loss. Otoscopy revealed a 20% temporal mandibular perforation. Type B tympanograms also occur with middle-ear effusion. (C) Type C tympanogram. This 31-year-old man with a history of severe allergy and rhinitis complained of aural fullness and otalgia. Otoscopy revealed severe retraction of the TM without effusion. Type C indicates negative middle-ear pressure and eustachian tube dysfunction.

Differences in sensory hearing of more than 15 dB between ears should be further evaluated to rule out retrocochlear lesions. Conductive hearing loss greater than 20 dB also calls for further evaluation. Severe and profound hearing loss (>80 dB) warrants evaluation for cause and potential rehabilitation. Patients whose discrimination scores differ by 12% or more between ears also need further evaluation to rule out retrocochlear lesions.

*Tympanometry* evaluates middle-ear compliance (Fig. 2–4). Normal middle-ear pressures range from −150 to +50 mm Hg. Results of tympanometry should be correlated with otoscopic findings. Normal compliance (type A tympanogram) indicates normal middle-ear aeration and pressure but does not exclude ossicular chain problems. Fluid in the middle ear or a perforated tympanic membrane will yield a flat tympanogram (type B) and indicates no change in middle-ear compliance with pressure changes. A normal-appearing tympanogram with the peak shifted to the left (0 to −150) (type C) indicates negative middle-ear pressure. Severe negative pressure (less than −150 mm Hg) indicates prolonged eustachian tube dysfunction.

### *When to Call the Otolaryngologist about Audiogram Findings*

- Differences in sensory hearing between ears of more than 20 dB
- Discrimination scores differing by 12% or more between ears
- Conductive hearing loss greater than 20 dB
- Severe or profound hearing loss (>80 dB)
- Persistent type B or C tympanogram

## Specific Diseases

Some specific disease processes of the auricle, external, middle, and inner ear will require a referral. These include acute intracranial or intratemporal complications of otitis media, as well as malignancy, cholesteatoma, and severe or persistent infections. The acute intracranial complications of otitis media are epidural abscess, saggital sinus thrombophlebitis, subdural abscess, meningitis, brain abscess, and otitic hydrocephalus. The acute intratemporal complications are coalescent mastoiditis, subperiosteal abscess, petrositis, facial paralysis, and labyrinthitis.

### DISEASE OF THE AURICLE AND EXTERNAL AUDITORY CANAL

*Any lesion of the auricle that is ulcerative or changes in size or appearance should be biopsied.*

It is easy to examine the auricle. When a new lesion develops on the auricle, it could represent a squamous cell carcinoma, basal cell carcinoma, seborrheic dermatitis, or, rarely, a melanoma. Any lesion that is ulcerative or changes in size or appearance should be biopsied. Chondrodermatitis helicus (CDH) can be misdiagnosed for squamous cell or basal cell carcinoma. CDH forms a small (2–4 mm) nodular lesion on the superior rim of the helix that is extremely painful and tender. When an acutely tender nodular lesion presents on the superior rim of the helix, it can be watched to see if it regresses. If it does not, it should be biopsied to rule out malignancy. Infectious perichondritis, which presents as an extremely red and swollen auricle, should be treated with intravenous antibiotics. This aggressive treatment is warranted because the blood supply to the auricular cartilage could be compromised when the perichondrium is severely infected, which can lead to unpleasant cosmetic deformity later. A rare autoimmune disease called relapsing polychondritis should be considered when articular and nonarticular cartilage of the ear, nose, airway, or joints is involved. Classically, there is a beefy, red inflammation of the pinna, although the external auditory canal and the earlobes remain conspicuously normal. Relapsing polychrondritis should be referred for an immunologic workup.

Common diseases of the external auditory canal are acute otitis externa and chronic otitis externa. There can be mild to moderate inflammation from a chronically draining otitis media. Persistent drainage from the external ear with significant swelling or chronic granulation tissue or lesion could represent a granulomatous infection, a cancer, or a reaction to medication. Patients whose symptoms worsen with topical therapy using neomycin may have sensitivity to the antibiotic. Neomycin sensitivity typically presents with extreme redness and swelling in the external auditory canal and auricle. If symptoms persist for a long period and the auricle is swollen, the patient may have an exudative dermatitis—chronic skin inflammation from the infected, draining contents of the ear.

*Persistent drainage from the external ear with significant swelling or chronic granulation tissue or lesion could represent a granulomatous infection, a cancer, or a reaction to medication.*

### *When to Call the Surgeon/Otolaryngologist about External Ear Problems*

- Persistent or suspicious lesion on the auricle
- Granulation tissue in the external auditory canal
- Symptoms that persist or resist appropriate therapy
- Vertigo, hearing loss, or facial paralysis
- Auricular hematoma

## DISEASE OF THE MIDDLE EAR

The *middle ear* is an air-filled space between the tympanic membrane and the bone of the labyrinth. It communicates directly with the mastoid air cells and is aerated by the eustachian tube. The facial nerve courses through the temporal bone in close proximity to the middle ear. The hallmark symptoms of middle-ear disease include otalgia, otorrhea, hearing loss, and possible facial paralysis. Most middle-ear diseases are easily treated by standard therapy.

*Otitis media* is ubiquitous and easily treated. It can clinically present as acute, recurrent, serous, or chronic. Recurrent otitis media or persistent middle-ear fluid (serous otitis media) does not need further treatment unless, in the case of a child, his or her hearing loss exceeds 30 dB speech is delayed, or school attendance is seriously affected. Pressure-equalization tubes should be considered after an audiogram is obtained. *Chronic otitis media* is a perforated tympanic membrane with persistent drainage associated with cholesteatoma or chronic inflammation of the mastoid. Chronic otitis media that does not resolve with topical therapy and antibiotics should undergo surgical therapy.

*Mastoiditis* can be either acute or chronic. Acute mastoiditis associated with acute otitis media can be worrisome because of the potential for intratemporal and intracranial complications. Swelling, tenderness, and fluctuance in the postauricular area can represent a coalescent mastoiditis or subperiosteal abscess. Chronic mastoiditis is commonly associated with chronic otitis media. This requires antibiotics and surgical therapy. Prolonged negative middle-ear pressure associated with eustachian tube dysfunction can cause the formation of retraction pockets, atrophy of the tympanic membrane, and perforation.

*Swelling, tenderness, and fluctuance in the postauricular area can represent a coalescent mastoiditis or subperiosteal abscess.*

*Cholesteatoma* results when keratinizing epithelium migrates into or becomes trapped in the middle ear. Over time, squamous debris accumulates as a mass, and can cause bony erosion, hearing loss, and recurrent infection.

*Vascular lesions* in the middle-ear space will present as erythematous tumors or enlarged vessels behind the tympanic membrane. Common vascular lesions are glomus tympanum or jugulare, aberrant carotid artery, and arteriovenous (AV) malformation. Hemotympanum after a closed head injury can represent a skull base fracture or retrograde flow of epistaxis through the eustachian tube. All patients who present with hemotympanum after trauma should have a workup for a skull base fracture, including an audiogram and a CT scan of the temporal bones and skull base. One must carefully examine the facial nerve for paralysis.

### *When to Call the Surgeon/Otolaryngologist about Middle-Ear Problems*

- Suspected intracranial or intratemporal complication
- Otitis media with significant hearing loss or speech delay
- Formation of retraction pockets, atrophy of the tympanic membrane, or perforation
- Chronic otitis media that is not resolving with therapy
- Suspected vascular lesion
- Hemotympanum after trauma
- Suspected skull base or temporal bone fracture

## DISEASE OF THE INNER EAR

The *inner ear*, or labyrinth, consists of the cochlea, the semicircular canals, and the otolith organs, and is innervated by the vestibulocochlear or eighth cranial nerve. Any process involving the middle ear or mastoid can affect the inner ear. Patients with inner-ear disorders will usually present with hearing loss, vertigo, or facial weakness.

Common inner-ear disorders are vestibular neuritis, labyrinthitis, benign positional vertigo, Ménière's disease, and, rarely, acoustic neuromas. *Vestibular neuritis* is an inflammation (thought to be viral) of the vestibular part of the eighth nerve. It causes severe vertigo lasting from many hours to days. Recovery may be slow, and it may take several months for residual dizziness and unsteadiness to resolve. The cochlear branch of the eighth nerve can become involved, causing sensorineural hearing loss. Initial treatment of neuritis consists of steroids, an antiviral agent, and vestibular suppressants.

*Labyrinthitis* is an inflammatory process involving the inner ear. Bacterial labyrinthitis is associated with severe prolonged vertigo and sensorineural hearing loss. It is uncommon and usually occurs in conjunction with meningitis or otitis media. Toxic (serous) labyrinthitis from middle-ear effusion or infection and viral labyrinthitis may have more subtle symptoms such as mild dizziness with or without hearing loss. The underlying cause of labyrinthitis should be treated promptly.

*Benign positional vertigo (BPV)* is caused by dysfunction of the posterior semicircular canal and causes short-lived (seconds to minutes) rotary vertigo associated with changes in head position. BPV is one of the most common causes of vertigo. It is idiopathic and occasionally occurs after head trauma. Resolution is usually spontaneous, occurring over several days to months, but recurrences are common.

*Ménière's disease* is an idiopathic disorder of inner-ear fluid regulation. Hallmark symptoms include fluctuating sensorineural hearing loss, tinnitus, aural fullness, and episodic vertigo lasting hours. Series of attacks are usually separated by long remissions. Sometimes atypical variants occur in which patients do not experience all the symptoms.

Compression of the eighth nerve in the internal auditory canal (IAC) or CPA may cause dizziness, hearing loss, and tinnitus. Acoustic neuroma and meningioma are both common, benign neoplasms that cause these symptoms (Fig. 2–5). The facial nerve courses through the CPA, IAC, and the bone of the inner ear, but seldom has dysfunction due to these neoplasms. Unlike sudden facial paralysis, which is usually idiopathic,

•  ▬
*Unlike sudden facial paralysis, which is usually idiopathic, progressive facial weakness is more ominous and suggests a facial neuroma or other more aggressive process.*

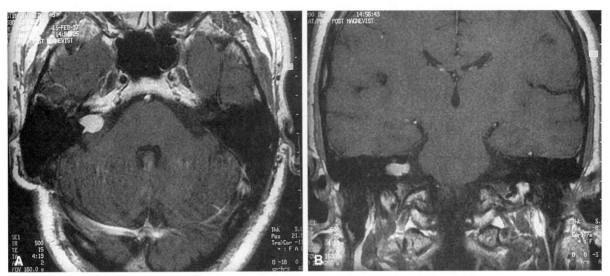

**FIGURE 2–5**

$T_1$-gadolinium-enhanced (*A*) axial section and (*B*) coronal section of right acoustic neuroma in a 41-year-old man with a 1-year history of hearing loss, tinnitus, and intermittent imbalance. The physical examination, including otoscopy, was normal. A neurologic exam revealed a left-beating horizontal nystagmus.

progressive facial weakness is more ominous and suggests a facial neuroma or another more aggressive process.

### When to Call the Surgeon/Otolaryngologist about Inner-Ear Problems

• Severe, prolonged vertigo
• Vertigo associated with otitis media
• Suspicion of a lesion affecting the eighth cranial nerve or CPA
• Facial weakness that is progressive and recovers slowly

# Chapter 3

# The Oral Cavity

JOHN G. SPANGLER, MD, MPH,
and PAUL LEE SALISBURY, III, DDS

Diseases of the oral cavity often call for an interface between medicine and dentistry. Soft-tissue oral lesions may also involve the head and neck, so that appropriate surgical consultations may involve not only dentists and oral surgeons but also otolaryngologists. The common developmental and acquired oral lesions are reviewed here.

## Developmental and Benign Conditions of Soft Tissues

Limitation of mobility of the anterior tip of the tongue due to a short lingual frenum is called *ankyloglossia*. This problem is uncommon and usually not severe enough to cause speech defects. If however by age 4 or 5 a child with this condition still has detrimental restriction of tongue function, the frenum can be cut to provide greater mobility. It is thought that this condition may be self-limiting because it is rarely seen in adults. The oral surgeon or otolaryngologist should be consulted in cases involving speech disorders.

*Fissured tongue* is fairly common, with an incidence of 2% to 5% of the population (Fig. 3–1). Fissured tongue is considered to have a significant hereditary component. Patients with this condition are usually asymptomatic but can experience burning sensations on the tongue. The dorsal surface of the tongue has multiple furrows that can be more than 5 mm deep. The condition is benign and does not need biopsy or treatment, although tongue hygiene may be more difficult.

*Geographic tongue (erythema migrans)* can occur concomitantly with fissured tongue or by itself and affects 1% to 3% of the population (see Fig. 3–1). Geographic tongue often brings patients to medical attention because of its striking clinical appearance. The classic presentation involves multiple, well-demarcated atrophic zones outlined by a curved, whitish, thickened border. The female-to-male ratio is 2:1, and the severity

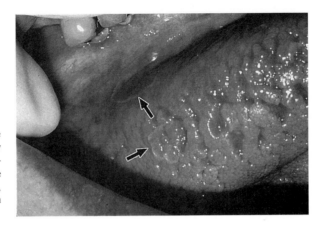

**FIGURE 3–1**
Fissured and geographic tongue in the same patient. Fissured tongue usually has multiple furrows 5 mm deep. Geographic tongue *(arrow)* shows multiple atrophic zones outlined by curved, whitish borders. See color photograph in Color Section 1.

in females may be related to hormonal levels. These lesions resolve and recur rapidly and seem to migrate over the anterior and lateral surfaces of the tongue. Histologically, geographic tongue resembles psoriasis, but there is no proven connection between the two conditions. The lesions are usually asymptomatic, but 10% of patients may have burning or irritation. Symptomatic patients can apply a topical corticosteroid several times a day in an attempt to reduce inflammation. There is no known malignant potential, and biopsies are useful mainly to reassure the patient that the condition is benign.

*Hairy tongue* is a remarkable condition seen in adults, which results from increased keratinization of the filiform papillae over the dorsal tongue surface (Fig. 3–2). Various causes have been suggested but none proved. The thick, matted surface becomes easily stained from food and bacteria accumulation. Tongue hygiene is impaired and the condition is unsightly but usually not symptomatic. Some patients complain of gagging. Biopsy is unnecessary for diagnosis, and there is no known treatment.

*Hairy leukoplakia* of the tongue (Fig. 3–3) is entirely different from hairy tongue and is seen in AIDS patients with low CD4 counts. This lesion is most often located on the lateral tongue border and is due to Epstein-Barr virus infection of the epithelium. A dentist or head and neck surgeon may be called for a biopsy, as with other types of leukoplakia (discussed later). The appearance of hairy leukoplakia is fairly distinctive to clinicians who have experience with AIDS patients. If HIV has been previously diagnosed, a biopsy is unnecessary because the lesion has no malignant potential. Any true leukoplakia (not candidiasis) over the lateral tongue border should be suspect, and the patient should be questioned and possibly tested for HIV.

*Oral varices*, or dilated veins, are seen in about two-thirds of adults over 60, but seldom in children. The most common ones occur on the undersurface of the tongue

*Any true leukoplakia over the lateral tongue border should lead to suspicion of HIV infection.*

**FIGURE 3–2**
Black hairy tongue, which is unsightly but usually asymptomatic, results from increased keratinization of the filiform papillae on the dorsal tongue. See Color Section 1.

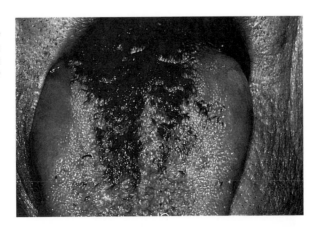

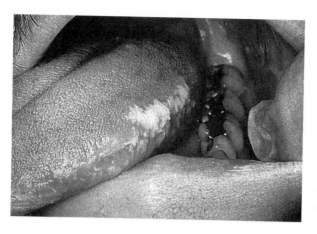

**FIGURE 3–3**
Hairy leukoplakia, seen in patients with HIV and low CD4 counts, is thought to be due to Epstein-Barr virus infection and occurs along the lateral edge of the tongue. See Color Section 1.

near the lateral borders and appear as multiple bluish nodules or cords. Sublingual varices are asymptomatic but can become thrombosed. On the lip or buccal mucosa, varices are usually solitary and firm to palpation. The dentist or oral surgeon does not need to be consulted unless the patient is symptomatic or the clinician is in doubt about the diagnosis. Because pigmented lesions in the oral cavity have several possible causes, both benign and malignant, such lesions should be documented in the medical record and accounted for either through clinical diagnosis or biopsy.

*Lingual thyroid* is ectopic thyroid tissue trapped between the foramen cecum and the epiglottis owing to failure of the primordial thyroid to completely descend into the neck. Lingual thyroid masses can be small and asymptomatic, or they can be very large, causing difficulty with swallowing and speech. The condition is diagnosable with a thyroid scan, but a biopsy of some type is necessary to rule out malignancy. Malignant transformation occurs in about 1% of cases, with men affected more often than women. Consequently, men over 30 with persistent lingual thyroid should have the mass excised. The otolaryngologist should be consulted for lingual thyroid.

*Microglossia* and *macroglossia* are very uncommon conditions that can occur as part of syndromes. Macroglossia also has metabolic and systemic causes. A speech pathologist should be consulted initially, and swallowing function should be evaluated. A surgeon would be needed only if symptoms could not be controlled by more conservative methods or if multispecialty assessment deemed that surgical management could enhance the long-term result.

There are numerous types of *developmental cysts*, but most are rare. One common type is found in the palate of newborn infants. These cysts are similar to gingival cysts of the newborn but they occur as single or multiple lesions at or around the midline, near the junction of hard and soft palate. Palatal cysts of the newborn quickly degenerate, and healing occurs within weeks following birth, so surgery is not required. Other developmental cysts can involve the lip, oral cavity, and neck; these occur along fusion lines, branchial clefts, and embryonic ducts. A mass eventually presents itself, and the patient will become symptomatic. An otolaryngologist or oral surgeon should be consulted to establish a diagnosis and recommend treatment.

*Mucoceles* are swellings of the lip resulting from trauma and spillage of mucus from an accessory salivary gland into the submucosal tissue (Fig. 3–4). Hundreds of mucous glands line the mouth. If a duct is blocked or severed, the gland may fail to drain properly and become infected. Mucoceles are typically superficial, fluctuant masses less than 5 mm in diameter, but they can feel somewhat indurated. Almost all are found on the lower lip. Periodic rupture with drainage is common, and this may lead to resolution. Many lesions, however, are chronic, and surgical removal of all the glands in the area is required. Recurrence following surgery is uncommon. Referral to the otolaryngologist or oral surgeon is appropriate.

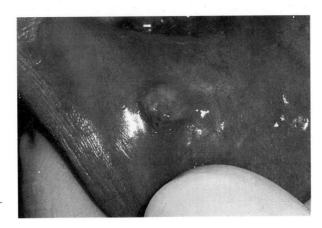

**FIGURE 3-4**
Mucocele of the lower lip (typical location). See Color Section 1.

# Orofacial Pain

## TEMPOROMANDIBULAR DISORDER

*Temporomandibular disorder (TMD)* is a general term that includes disorders of the temporomandibular joint (TMJ), the muscles of mastication, or both. The term is most often used to indicate pain in the face or joint area with associated symptoms. Associated symptoms include headaches, earaches, dizziness, muscle hypertrophy, and problems with dental occlusion; limited jaw opening or closed locking of the TMJ; and clicking or popping sounds in the joint. The pathology of TMD may involve dysfunction of the muscle, internal derangement of the joint, or a combination of effects. TMD symptoms can range from mild and clinically insignificant to severely painful and disabling. The female-to-male ratio is 2:1.

The level of controversy surrounding TMD is probably unsurpassed in clinical head and neck medicine. Generally accepted guidelines for scientifically based diagnosis and treatment of TMD are not available, owing in part to the variety of specialties involved in the care of these patients and the lack of meaningful research. New and inadequately tested approaches continue to be used.

The prevalence of self-reported TMD is thought to be between 5% and 15% of the population, with minimal gender differences and a peak prevalence between ages 20 and 40. Epidemiologic data indicate that signs and symptoms are self-limiting, with a lower prevalence in older age groups. Many symptomatic individuals do not seek treatment, and there are no data to help predict their long-term prognosis without intervention.

The history should include assessment of parafunctional habits such as grinding and systemic rheumatologic diseases that could cause or contribute to TMD. Psychosocial review can determine the extent to which pain and dysfunction have compromised quality of life and produced depression, anxiety, and dysphoria. Physical examination should assess the functional range of motion, occlusal status, the presence of joint and muscle tenderness and cutaneous hyperalgesia.

A variety of therapies seem to help TMD, and surgical intervention is rarely necessary. Initial management strategies of supportive care include patient education, exercise, stress management, and cessation of parafunctional habits. Control of pain with nonsteroidal anti-inflammatory drugs (NSAIDs) and opioids, physical therapy, and occlusal splint therapy are also important. These noninvasive, reversible treatment modalities have low morbidity and no potential to cause further degeneration or pathologic changes. General dentists, oral surgeons, prosthodontists, and orthodontists usually have had training in splint therapy. Unfortunately, some patients have persistent problems in spite of conservative therapy. If signs and symptoms do not remit, a stepwise

*Initial management strategies for TMD include supportive patient education, control of pain, physical therapy, and occlusal splint therapy.*

approach can be implemented, which includes supportive therapy as well as more aggressive treatment of the occlusion and temporomandibular joint. Finding a clinician to provide long-term care for TMD is more difficult, owing to the amount of time required for these patients and the chronic nature of this pain syndrome.

Surgery is indicated only for patients for whom conservative therapy has failed. These patients usually have disabling dysfunction, with or without severe pain. For internal derangements of the TMJ, the spectrum of surgical approaches includes arthrocentesis, arthroscopy, arthrotomy or arthroplasty, condylotomy, and orthognathic surgery. No randomized controlled studies have demonstrated the efficacy of any given surgical approach. While some patients benefit from surgery, others remain afflicted with the same or even worse symptoms.

Anxiety and depression are associated with TMD, either as contributing factors or as a result of the pain and dysfunction of the disorder. Psychological strategies used for other chronic pain conditions can be useful for TMD. Such strategies must be tailored to individual needs. They frequently include treatment with antidepressant medication.

## BURNING MOUTH SYNDROME

*Burning mouth syndrome (BMS)*, also known as *glossopyrosis* or *glossodynia*, is a chronic pain syndrome that affects about 2% of the population. Although usually seen in postmenopausal women, there is no proven link to hormone levels. Associated factors such as B-vitamin deficiencies, diabetes mellitus, iron and zinc deficiencies, hypothyroidism, and chronic gastric regurgitation are sometimes found, but most cases are idiopathic. The symptoms usually involve a burning sensation, and they occur on the anterior third of the tongue, the anterior palate, and the mucosal surfaces of the lips. All of these structures appear normal on clinical examination. BMS patients also frequently complain of dry mouth and altered taste, many experience depression and anxiety, and treatment with anxiolytic or antidepressant medications such as chlordiazepoxide and amitriptyline helps some of them. Reassurance that the patient does not have oral cancer is important. BMS seems to be self-limiting in some patients, with or without treatment, but others have symptoms indefinitely. This is not a surgical problem. A regional pain center might be the best place to refer these patients.

> •  ▬
> *BMS seems to be self-limiting in some patients, but others have symptoms indefinitely.*

# *Premalignant and Malignant Lesions*

*Leukoplakia* and *erythroplakia* (or *erythroplasia*) are two clinical entities widely considered to be premalignant (Fig. 3–5). The term *leukoplakia* refers to a white plaque on the oral mucosa that does not rub off and cannot be identified clinically as any other entity. Similarly, *erythroplakia* refers to a red mucosal plaque that cannot be identified as any other clinical entity. This red lesion is frequently associated with leukoplakia (*erythroleukoplakia*).

Leukoplakia is usually a hyperkeratotic response by the oral mucosa to chronic irritants such as cigarette smoking, chewing tobacco, repetitive oral trauma (e.g., pressure from dentures, habitual cheek biting) and long-term, excessive alcohol consumption. With a 3% to 6% malignant transformation rate, leukoplakia clearly has premalignant potential. Lesions occurring on the floor of the mouth, the ventrolateral aspect of the tongue, and the soft palate are at particularly high risk for malignant change.

> •  ▬
> *Leukoplakia occurring on the floor of the mouth, the ventrolateral aspect of the tongue, and the soft palate is at particularly high risk for malignant change.*

The presence of any degree of redness, or erythroplakia, within a white lesion greatly increases the likelihood of malignant progression. Homogeneous white leukoplakic lesions have a very low malignant transformation rate. Erythroplakia within a white lesion increases this rate up to 23%. Other features that increase the chance of malignant change of leukoplakic lesions include papillomatous features, the presence of leukoplakia in a non—tobacco user, and overlying candidal infection.

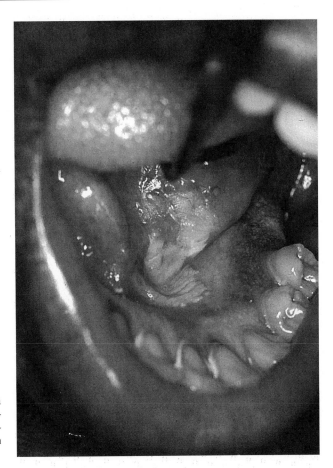

**FIGURE 3–5**
Leukoplakia and erythroplasia in a snuff dipper. Biopsy showed invasive squamous cell carcinoma, unsuccessfully treated by radiation therapy. See Color Section 1.

Clinically, leukoplakic lesions range from thin and almost nonpalpable to thick and dense. The color may vary from translucent white to gray, occasionally speckled with red. Most cases of leukoplakia occur on the tongue, mandibular alveolar ridge, or buccal mucosa. Less common but very important locations include the palate, maxillary alveolar ridge, and floor of the mouth.

The mean age of diagnosis of leukoplakia and erythroplakia is between 50 and 69 years, with fewer than 5% of cases occurring before age 30. With the increased use of chewing tobacco among younger age groups, however, this epidemiology may change. In the past most leukoplakia occurred among men, but this too is changing with increased alcohol and tobacco use among women.

The differential diagnosis of oral premalignant lesions includes lichen planus, which is frequently erosive and symptomatic, and oral hairy leukoplakia, a lingual manifestation of HIV disease felt to be related to Epstein-Barr virus. In addition, systemic lupus erythematosus (SLE), white sponge nevus, and hereditary keratosis may present with white, hyperkeratotic oral lesions.

Primary care providers should regularly examine the entire oral mucosa of patients at risk for premalignant and malignant oral lesions. These patients include heavy alcohol drinkers, cigarette smokers, and chewing tobacco users—especially those 40 years or older. Particular attention should be paid to the floor of the mouth, the ventrolateral aspects of the tongue, and the soft palate.

Any detected leukoplakic or erythroplakic lesions should be carefully investigated. Aside from alcohol and tobacco use, other useful historical clues include systemic illnesses (e.g., SLE) or risk factors for HIV. On physical exam, the primary care provider should evaluate whether other oral lesions exist, since multiple premalignant and malignant lesions can arise simultaneously (the "field cancerization" effect). Careful attention should be used in determining whether any degree of redness exists in detected lesions, and the location, size, and color of lesions should be documented explicitly.

After a careful examination, patients should be instructed to avoid all oral irritants for 2 weeks, and a follow-up appointment should be scheduled for that time to evaluate whether lesions have changed. Persistent leukoplakia without an obvious cause and all lesions with any redness should be referred for vigorous investigation by a surgeon with experience in the diagnosis and management of oral cancer.

Two screening modalities that can be used adjunctively in the evaluation of leukoplakic lesions are oral mucosa cytology scrapings and toluidine blue oral rinse. Although similar in technique to Papanicolaou smears for cervical dysplasia, oral mucosa cytology has not been prospectively evaluated for the diagnosis of oral cancer. Therefore this has not supplanted biopsy for suspicious lesions. Toluidine blue is a nucleic acid vital stain that is preferentially adsorbed by dysplastic tissue on the oral mucosa (Fig. 3–6). This stain test, which has not gained wide acceptance in primary care, is easily performed and interpreted and can direct attention to areas that should be biopsied. Again, this staining technique is not a substitute for careful examination and biopsy of potentially malignant lesions.

Many oral cancers are preceded by clinically detectable precancerous lesions. Early detection can reduce morbidity and mortality. Therefore regular and thorough oral cavity examinations of high-risk patients by primary care providers is prudent. The United States Preventive Services Task Force states, "Although direct evidence of a benefit is lacking, clinicians may wish to include an examination for cancerous or precancerous lesions of the oral cavity in the periodic health examination of persons who chew or smoke tobacco (or did so previously), older persons who drink regularly, and anyone with suspicious symptoms or lesions detected through self-examination." The American Cancer Society recommends a cancer checkup that includes a complete oral cavity examination every 3 years for persons over age 20 and annually for those over age 40.

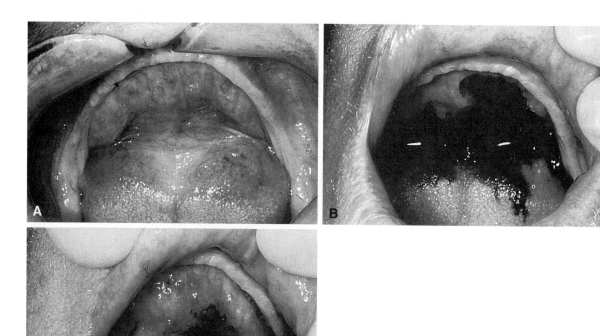

**FIGURE 3–6**
(*A*) Toluidine blue, a vital stain, can help identify where to biopsy a lesion, as in this patient with asymptomatic erythroplasia on the floor of the mouth. (*B*) After applying toluidine blue and (*C*) rinsing an area of intense uptake remained. Biopsy in this region revealed invasive squamous cell carcinoma. See Color Section 1.

Regardless of the interval or population in which one chooses to screen for oral cancer, examination of the oral cavity should be thorough. Since many cancers occur on the soft palate, the floor of the mouth, or the posterolateral aspects of the tongue, a proper oral cavity examination includes retraction of the tongue with gauze pads, use of a dental mirror, and digital palpation of the mouth and tongue with a gloved hand for masses. A headlamp or mirror allows both hands to be free for the examination. Lesions may be flat and superficial, exophytic, or ulcerative. Whenever a suspicious lesion is found, the patient should be referred to a head and neck surgeon with experience in diagnosis and treatment of oral cancers.

## AIDS-Related Oral Lesions

The oral cavity is one of the areas most frequently affected by HIV-related pathology. Oral manifestations of HIV include infections, inflammatory processes, and neoplasia. This section will focus on two common conditions: Kaposi's sarcoma and oral hairy leukoplakia.

### KAPOSI'S SARCOMA

A malignant tumor of probable lymphatic endothelial origin, *Kaposi's sarcoma (KS)* is by far the most common oral malignancy among patients with HIV disease (Fig. 3–7). Initially flat, violaceous, and asymptomatic, these lesions can appear anywhere in the oral cavity, but over 90% occur on the palate. KS can progress to become exophytic and ulcerated, secondarily infected, and increasingly painful, making adequate nutrition and oral hygiene difficult. When KS is noted in primary care patients with HIV, referral to an infectious disease specialist may be warranted, particularly if the diagnosis is in doubt. In addition, symptomatic KS should be referred either to an infectious disease specialist or to a radiation oncologist. Treatment options include low-dose radiation therapy and intralesional injection of vinblastine.

### ORAL HAIRY LEUKOPLAKIA

*Hairy leukoplakia* (see Fig. 3–3) of the oral cavity is a white, vertically fissured lesion occurring on the lateral aspects of the tongue, almost exclusively among patients with HIV. Its presence is associated with advanced immunosuppression. Although the lesion

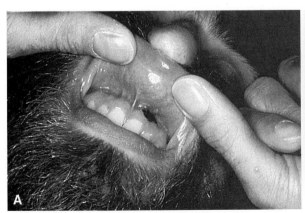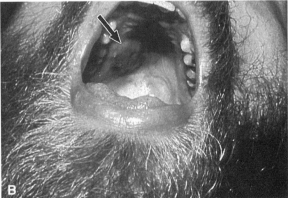

**FIGURE 3–7**

(*A*) Kaposi's sarcoma, the most common oral malignancy among patients with AIDS, appears as flat violaceous lesions on the oral mucosa. (*B*) The most common location is on the hard palate. See Color Section 1.

may become superinfected with *Candida albicans*, most authorities feel the disease is related to Epstein-Barr virus infection. Correct diagnosis depends on the appropriate clinical setting, histology, and HIV serology. Referral to a surgeon is necessary for biopsy only if the diagnosis is in doubt.

## Infections of the Oral Mucosa

### BACTERIAL OR FUNGAL INFECTIONS

A wide variety of organisms can infect the oral cavity, including fungi, bacteria, and viruses. This section will focus on common mucosal infections.

### Oral Candidiasis

Candida species are ubiquitous and frequently make up the normal flora of the human gastrointestinal and genital tracts. These organisms can cause many types of oral infections, of which thrush, denture stomatitis, and angular cheilitis are the most common.

### Thrush

*Thrush (pseudomembranous candidiasis)* is uncommon among healthy adults and is usually seen in infants, frail elderly patients, adults receiving antibiotics or inhaled or systemic corticosteroids, and adults who are immunocompromised in some manner (e.g., HIV infection, malignancy, chemotherapy). When present in HIV-positive individuals, it usually indicates that CD4 counts have fallen below $200/mm^3$.

Clinically, thrush appears as multiple creamy-white plaques on the tongue, throat, or buccal mucosa. If the plaques are scraped off, the underlying mucosa is usually red and painful. Most often, the diagnosis can be made by clinical appearance alone, but this can be augmented by potassium hydroxide smears, which reveal typical hyphae. Treatment with topical antifungal agents such as the imidazole derivatives (e.g., ketoconazole, fluconazole, and itraconazole) is usually effective, but resistance to these drugs has been reported. In addition, refractory cases are frequently seen among patients with advanced HIV disease. Such cases may require referral to an infectious disease specialist.

### Denture Stomatitis

*Denture stomatitis (chronic atrophic candidiasis)* is characterized by chronic inflammation and erythema in the areas of oral mucosa directly in contact with dentures. Although this condition may not be a true candidal infection (that is, the organism usually does not grow from tissue biopsy cultures), *candida* is frequently recovered in large numbers from the surfaces of the dentures that were in contact with inflamed mucosa. This condition is most often precipitated by continuous wearing of dentures at night. Treatment includes discontinuing denture wearing for short periods and disinfecting dentures with chlorhexidine or other antifungal agents.

### Angular Cheilitis

Resulting from a mixed infection of staphylococcus and candida, *angular cheilitis (perleche)* presents as inflammation, erythema, and exudative crusting and fissuring at the corners of the mouth (Fig. 3–8). Accentuated lip creases, most often caused by poorly fitting dentures, allow moisture to accumulate and macerate tissue. Vitamin $B_{12}$ and iron deficiencies, actinic keratosis, and basal cell and squamous cell carcinomas all can resemble angular cheilitis, however. Treatment consists of good oral hygiene, refitting dentures, and a course of topical antibiotics (mupirocin and antifungal creams). Be-

*Vitamin $B_{12}$ and iron deficiencies, actinic keratosis, and basal cell and squamous cell carcinomas can resemble angular cheilitis.*

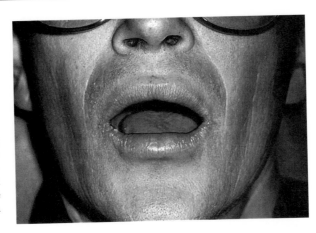

**FIGURE 3–8**
Angular cheilitis (perleche) is a mixed infection of *Staphylococcus* and *Candida* and presents as inflammation, erythema, and exudative crusting and tissue maceration at the corners of the mouth. Poorly fitting dentures are a frequent cause. See Color Section 1.

cause of possible confusion with malignant conditions, lesions that persist after initial therapy should be referred to a head and neck surgeon for biopsy.

## VIRAL INFECTIONS

### Herpangina

*Herpangina* is a vesicular exanthem of the soft palate that is most common in children between ages 2 and 10 and is accompanied by low-grade fever, malaise, and sore throat. Generally caused by Coxsackie group A viruses, lesions begin as multiple punctate macules on the soft palate, which vesiculate, leaving shallow yellow-white ulcers within 48 hours. Symptoms are usually mild, resolve within 7 days, and can be treated successfully with analgesics.

### Hand-Foot-Mouth Disease

*Hand-foot-mouth disease*, caused by Coxsackie virus A16, produces a vesicular eruption on the buccal mucosa and tongue (Fig. 3–9), with a similar eruption on the palms,

**FIGURE 3-9**
Hand-foot-mouth disease produces a vesicular eruption on the buccal mucosa and tongue, with similar vesicles on the palms, soles, and occasionally the genitals and buttocks. See Color Section 1.

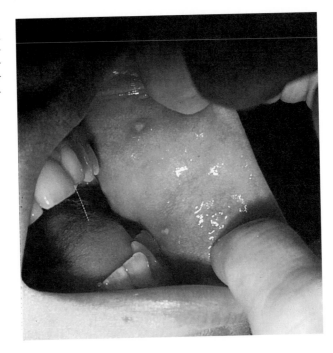

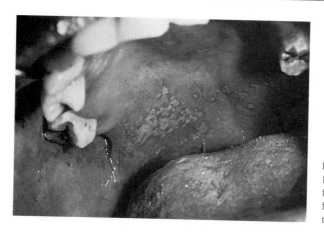

**FIGURE 3-10**
HSV I stomatitis during a primary infection. The patient also had malaise, fever, and vesicles scattered across the body. See Color Section 1.

soles, and occasionally the genitalia and buttocks. Usually, no more than 10 lesions are found in any given area, and 25% of cases have no cutaneous lesions. Fever is generally low grade. The condition resolves spontaneously within a few days and may be treated with analgesics or antipyretics.

## Herpes Simplex Virus (HSV) I and II

Infections by HSV I and II are frequently recurrent and can affect individuals of any age. Although HSV I tends to infect the mouth and face and HSV II tends to infect the genitalia, either virus can infect the other region. These disorders frequently occur in two distinct phases: primary infection and recurrent infection. In primary infection, the host lacks prior immunity to HSV and systemic signs and symptoms such as fever, malaise, and disseminated rash may occur. Primary HSV I tends to cause gingivostomatitis and ulcerations throughout the oral mucosa and on the lips (Fig. 3-10). Patients with this condition complain of severe pain at the sites of ulceration and often have fevers up to 102°F.

Recurrent HSV I infections usually cause vesicular eruptions on the outer lip (Fig. 3-11). Patients may notice a prodrome of tingling, burning, or itching 6 to 48 hours prior to the eruption, which appears as closely spaced vesicles. Pain is most severe for the first 2 days, and the vesicles gradually crust and resolve within 7 days. Eruptions of recurrent HSV I rarely occur inside the mouth (Fig. 3-12), except after oral surgery in which local anesthetic has been injected into the hard palate. In fact, most recurrent ulcerative lesions seen inside the mouth are not HSV but rather recurrent aphthous ulcers (see following section).

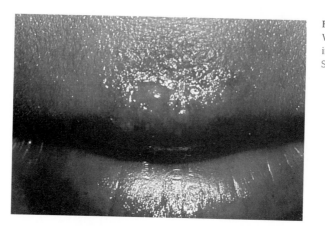

**FIGURE 3-11**
Vesicular eruption of recurrent HSV I infection on the outer lip. See Color Section 1.

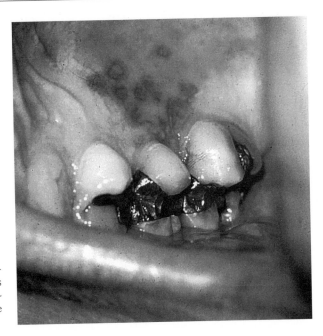

FIGURE 3–12
Recurrent, intraoral HSV I is not common. It starts out as vesicles and tends to occur on mucosa bound to underlying periosteum (e.g., the hard palate or gingiva). See Color Section 1.

## Ulcerative and Erosive Conditions of the Oral Cavity

Ulcers in the mouth have many causes, including physical injury to tissue, infections, and systemic processes. The cause of some recurrent ulcers (e.g., aphthous ulcers) is unknown. Oral ulcerations, particularly those that are persistent or severe or that have an uncertain diagnosis, may require referral to head and neck surgery, or oral surgeon for definitive identification and treatment. This section focuses on recurrent aphthous ulcerations and ulcerative conditions associated with systemic diseases.

### RECURRENT APHTHOUS ULCERATIONS

*Recurrent aphthous ulceration* of the oral cavity is a spectrum of conditions ranging from a few painful but infrequent ulcers to larger, severely painful, and persistent lesions. Lesions may appear anywhere within the oral cavity but most commonly affect the labial and buccal mucosa or the tongue. Milder forms of recurrent aphthae produce one to five ulcers that last less than 2 weeks. These lesions usually are a few millimeters in diameter but can range up to 1 cm. They appear as shallow ulcerations with a gray, white, or yellow center surrounded by a thin rim or erythema (Fig. 3–13). Scarring from these mild ulcers is uncommon. Conversely, major aphthae measure 1 cm or larger and may persist for 6 weeks or more. These lesions tend to be deeper, occur in larger numbers, and can cause scarring.

Although the etiology of aphthous ulcers has been investigated extensively, the cause remains elusive. The final common pathway involves the inflammatory response. Certain individuals with iron or vitamin $B_{12}$ deficiency seem to get aphthae more frequently than do other individuals. In addition, some women experience recurrences of their ulcerations during the luteal phase of their menstrual cycle. Viruses (especially HSV), bacteria (l-forms of streptococci), antigenic stimuli from food, psychological stress, and genetics have all been proposed as possible causes.

The differential diagnosis of recurrent aphthous ulceration includes infection with HSV, Behçet's disease, Crohn's disease and ulcerative colitis, and mucocutaneous ulcerative diseases such as erythema multiforme, lichen planus, pemphigoid, and pem-

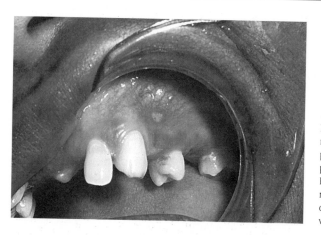

**FIGURE 3–13**
Recurrent aphthous ulcerations can range from one small lesion (as in this patient) to many large and extremely painful lesions. In contrast to recurrent HSV, aphthous ulcers tend to occur on mucosa not bound to underlying periosteum and are never preceded by vesicles. See Color Section 1.

phigus vulgaris. Unlike HSV, aphthous ulcerations are never initially vesicular and generally occur on the nonkeratinized mucosa of the tongue, the floor of the mouth, the soft palate, and buccal and labial mucosa. In contrast, recurrent HSV lesions, on the other hand, occur almost exclusively on keratinized mucosa bound to underlying periosteum, such as the hard palate or the gingiva. Behçet's disease can be virtually identical to major aphthae in appearance, but this uncommon disease usually involves the eyes, genitalia, neurologic system, and joints. Oral manifestations of Crohn's disease and ulcerative colitis also can look similar to aphthous ulcerations, but the patient with aphthae lacks gastrointestinal symptoms. Furthermore, biopsy of Crohn's oral ulcers will reveal the characteristic granulomatous inflammation. When the diagnosis of recurrent aphthous ulceration is in doubt, referral to an otolaryngologist for biopsy is warranted because of the significant therapeutic implications involved with these other conditions.

Without a clear-cut cause, treatment of recurrent aphthae is directed at symptomatic relief. Minor ulcerative eruptions can usually be handled by topical corticosteroid preparations (e.g., triamcinolone in an oral adhesive such as Orabase), topical film preparations (e.g., Zilactin), or local anesthetics such as viscous lidocaine. Laser ablation may also provide sustained pain relief. For longstanding, more severe lesions, systemic or intralesional corticosteroids may be beneficial. Because malignancy may present as a nonhealing ulcerative lesion, ulcers and erosions not responding to therapeutic measures within 2 weeks need definitive diagnosis. Primary care providers should refer such cases to an otolaryngologist, dentist, or oral surgeon for biopsy.

## BULLOUS DISEASES

Several bullous skin diseases can present with oral manifestations. *Pemphigus vulgaris* (Fig. 3–14) is an uncommon autoimmune disease that initially presents as oral erosions in most patients. These oral lesions are painful and make nutrition and oral hygiene difficult. Occasionally, the entire oral mucosa can be denuded. Pemphigus progresses to involve generalized cutaneous blisters that are initially flaccid but rapidly burst, leading to extensive fluid, electrolyte, and protein imbalances. Bacterial superinfection is typical and can be life threatening. Bullous pemphigoid is a more common disorder, primarily affecting the elderly. It is characterized by tense skin blisters and only rarely affects the oral cavity. Cicatricial pemphigoid is a bullous disease primarily affecting oral, nasal, and ocular mucosa (Fig. 3–15). Oral manifestations include erosions of the buccal mucosa, palate, and tongue; desquamative gingivitis is also common. Diagnosis of these conditions requires direct immunofluorescence studies of biopsy specimens in addition to routine H&E staining. Because of the potential for serious complications,

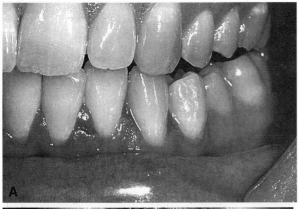

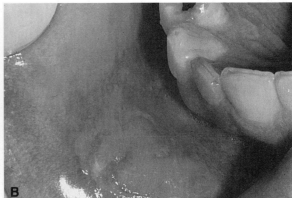

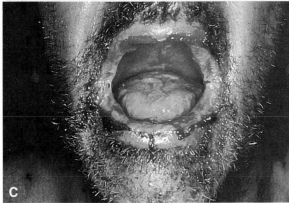

**FIGURE 3-14**
Pemphigus vulgaris is a life-threatening but uncommon autoimmune disease that can produce oral erosions and cutaneous bullae. (*A*) Smaller erosions may be barely perceptible, as in this 28-year-old woman with gingival lesions and one blister on her chest. (*B*) More extensive erosions can involve the gingiva and buccal mucosa. (*C*) Severe pemphigus vulgaris causes widespread oral erosions, cutaneous bullae, and extensive fluid, electrolyte, and protein imbalances. See Color Section 1.

patients with these disorders should be referred to dermatologists with experience in the diagnosis and management of bullous diseases.

## OTHER IMMUNODERMATOLOGIC DISEASES

Many other immunopathologic disorders involve the oral cavity. *Systemic lupus erythematosus (SLE)* can present with oral ulcerations, a sign heralding more severe disease (Fig. 3-16). Diagnosis is made by biopsy and by considering a collection of systemic

**FIGURE 3-15**
Cicatricial pemphigoid is a bullous disease affecting the oral, nasal, and ocular mucosa. Oral lesions produce sloughing of the gingival mucosa. See Color Section 1.

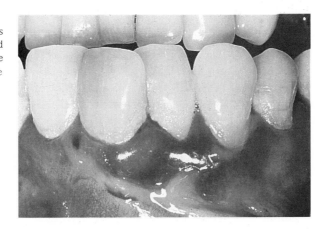

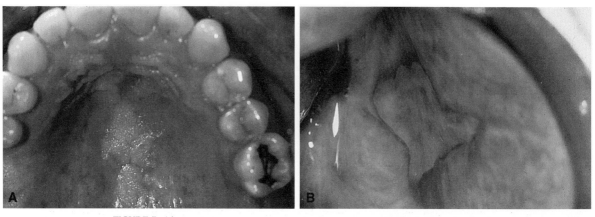

**FIGURE 3–16**
Systemic lupus erythematosus can cause oral ulcerations heralding more severe disease, as in these patients with (*A*) a hard palate ulcer, and (*B*) ulceration of the buccal mucosa. See Color Section 1.

signs and symptoms. *Lichen planus* is an idiopathic inflammatory condition of the skin, hair, nails, and mucous membranes (Fig. 3–17). Over half of patients with lichen planus will have oral lesions; in one quarter the only lesions are oral. Oral lesions usually appear as asymptomatic, white, reticular patterns on the bilateral buccal mucosa (Wickham's striae). More extensive disease may include painful oral ulcerations and erosions. Because lesions may mimic leukoplakia or oral cancer, patients should be referred to an oral surgeon, an otolaryngologist or dermatologist for definitive diagnosis.

The oral aphthae seen in patients with Behçet's disease are usually identical to those in patients with minor recurrent aphthous ulcers. Unlike recurrent aphthae, though, Behçet's disease involves multiple organ systems, including the eyes, central nervous system, skin, joints, and vasculature. Oral and genital aphthae in Behçet's disease begin as pustular vasculitic lesions, which quickly ulcerate. Milder mucosal lesions can be handled in the same manner as recurrent aphthous ulcers. Because systemic involvement can lead to complications and death, patients with Behçet's disease should be referred to a dermatologist or rheumatologist for comprehensive therapy.

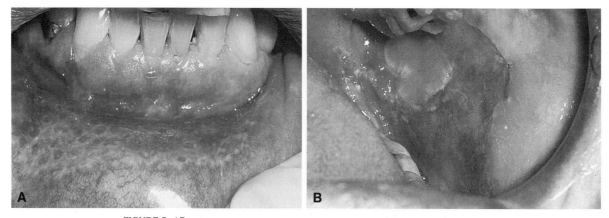

**FIGURE 3–17**
(*A*) Oral lichen planus usually produces a white reticular pattern on the labial or buccal mucosa. (*B*) More severe disease can produce painful ulcerations or erosions of the oral mucosa. See Color Section 1.

# Trauma

*Lacerations* of the gingiva and lip may accompany dental trauma and, if severe, may require surgical consultation. Gingival abrasion and superficial lip wounds will not usually require surgical closure. With facial lacerations involving the lip, particular attention has to be paid to the continuity of the vermillion border when suturing. If the lip is punctured by the teeth, radiographs should be obtained to be sure that no dental fragments are left in the lip. Infection from bacterial inoculation is a concern.

*Maxillofacial trauma* and jaw fractures are most often managed by one of three specialties: otolaryngology, plastic surgery, or oral surgery. Oral surgeons, having had dental training, are particularly knowledgeable about the alignment and occlusion of the teeth. Severe head and neck trauma with multiple fractures of the midface and mandible often require a team approach, utilizing several surgical specialists. Condylar fractures, for example, can be missed if the patient's occlusion is not checked by the appropriate specialist. Consequently patients from small communities are often transported to urban medical centers for management of maxillofacial trauma.

## When to Call the Surgeon about Diseases of the Oral Cavity

- Oral lesions suspicious for malignancy
- Recalcitrant TMD
- Developmental cysts (e.g., branchial cleft cysts)
- Chronic mucocele
- Leukoplakia and erythroplakia
- Oral ulcerations that do not heal within 2 weeks
- HIV-related oral lesions
- Oral or maxillofacial trauma

## RECOMMENDED READING

Johnson, JT, et al (eds): Infectious Diseases and Antimicrobial Therapy of the Ears, Nose and Throat. WB Saunders, Philadelphia, 1997.

Mashberg, A, and Samit, A: Early diagnosis of asymptomatic oral and oropharyngeal squamous cancer. CA Cancer J Clin 45:328–351, 1995.

National Institutes of Health Technology Assessment Conference Statement: Management of Temporomandibular Disorders, National Institutes of Health, April 29–May 1, 1996.

Neville, BW, et al (eds): Oral and Maxillofacial Pathology, ed 1. WB Saunders, Philadelphia, 1995.

Peterson, LJ, et al (eds): Contemporary Oral and Maxillofacial Surgery, ed 2. Mosby-Year Book, St. Louis, 1993.

Regezi, JA, and Sciubba, JJ (eds): Oral Pathology Clinical-Pathologic Correlations, ed 1. WB Saunders, Philadelphia, 1989.

Salisbury, PL, and Jorizzo, JL: Oral ulcers and erosions. Advances in Dermatology 8:31–30, 1993.

Silverman, S: Oral Cancer, 4th ed. B.C. Decker, Hamilton, Ontario, 1998.

Silverman, S, Jr (ed): Color Atlas of Oral Manifestations of AIDS, ed 2. CV Mosby, St. Louis, 1996.

United States Preventive Services Task Force: Guide to Clinical Preventive Services. Williams & Wilkins, Baltimore, 1996.

# Neck Pain and Sore Throat

WALTER SALWEN, MD,
and LEE BEATTY, MD

Many patients will present with complaints involving the neck and throat. The vast majority are due to benign, self-limiting conditions that require only reassurance or symptom-directed therapy. Recognition of conditions requiring surgical consultation depends on an accurate history and physical exam.

## History

Certain features of the head and neck exam deserve emphasis. Because of the neural complexity of the head and neck, many symptoms will be poorly localized. Therefore a complete exam must be carried out for all throat symptoms. Smoking or the heavy consumption of alcohol are unequivocally causative for most head and neck cancers, and the presence of either habit will direct proper symptom evaluation. Alcohol consumption may be described as "whisky equivalents" wherein 1 oz of hard liquor equals 4 oz wine or 12 oz of beer. The effects of smoking and alcohol on cancer risk are synergistic and not merely additive.

Duration and associated symptoms must be investigated because most inflammatory conditions are of recent onset and improve rapidly with medical treatment. It is important to note ear or periauricular discomfort. Although common in children, ear discomfort or pain in adults is unusual. The examiner must pay attention to the throat as well as the ear. Discomfort from lesions of the oral cavity via the lingual nerve, from the oropharynx (tongue, palate, or tonsil) via the glossopharyngeal nerve, or from the larynx or hypopharynx via the superior laryngeal nerve may all produce referred pain in the ipsilateral ear. In some patients blockage of the eustachian tube by a nasopharyngeal or tonsillar mass will produce secondary serous otitis media.

*Duration and associated symptoms must be pursued because most inflammatory conditions are of recent onset and improve rapidly with medical treatment.*

## Physical Exam

Physical examination of the patient with head and neck symptoms requires experience with the laryngeal mirror (indirect laryngoscopy) or flexible fiberoptic instrumentation. Both techniques provide excellent visualization of most of the throat. The flexible nasopharyngoscope provides a better view of the nasopharynx and in some individuals an improved view of the anterior commissure of the larynx. Most patients require no supplemental anesthetic. In patients with pronounced symptoms, caution should be taken when using topical spray anesthetics because obliteration of protective reflex mechanisms can produce airway problems. Neither examination technique is adequate to rule out malignancy. Two areas of poor visualization are the piriform sinuses (the pharynx lateral to each side of the larynx) and the postcricoid area (the mucosa posterior to the larynx). Rigid instrumentation in an operating room setting is necessary to evaluate these areas fully.

The presence of crypts in the tongue base and tonsils makes palpation essential because the normal surface may not reflect the presence of a deep invasive cancer producing only induration. The gag reflex can make this examination difficult for the patient and dangerous to the examiner if the patient is not cooperative. Palpation is critical in the evaluation of symptomatic patients and those presenting with neck masses. Melanoma is an increasing problem, so a thorough, compulsive skin exam is needed for all patients presenting with a neck mass.

## Voice Disturbances

Voice disturbances are common and usually not due to cancer. The high cure rates associated with early recognition of vocal cord cancer makes timely diagnosis a concern for all primary care providers. The voice is modulated at three anatomic levels. As speech is initiated, pitch and quality are altered by vocal cord mobility and contact between the opposing vocal cords. Any abnormality of the vocal cord such as edema or surface changes can produce voice alterations. The voice also can be affected by any structure beyond the vocal cords that modulates speech, such as the tongue or palate, or that inhibits swallowing, producing a wet or thicker voice.

Voice changes that persist beyond a few weeks are generally not due to self-limiting problems. A common cause of chronic voice changes is chronic inflammation of the vocal cord mucosa, commonly caused by smoking. If the vocal cord appearance does not suggest malignancy, the patient should attempt a 3- to 4-week trial of smoking cessation. Other common sources of chronic inflammation are associated with sinus drainage or gastroesophageal reflux. Both conditions are often linked with additional symptoms and respond well to medical therapy. Voice "abuse" or overuse is another common cause of voice changes and may be evident in the history. But for the patient who smokes or drinks alcohol, voice changes should not be ascribed to benign causes without a careful examination of the larynx and oropharynx.

*Voice changes that persist beyond a few weeks are generally not due to self-limiting problems.*

Cancer developing on the vocal cord produces early voice changes, which at first may wax and wane but do not improve to normal. The cancer generally develops in either the anterior third of the cord or the middle third. Voice alteration caused by a small lesion of the anterior commissure (where the two cords form a V) can be profound. This area can be particularly hard to see with a mirror, and flexible laryngoscopy is advisable if no other lesion is noted. If there is any question about the diagnosis of a vocal cord abnormality, a head and neck specialist should be consulted. Even a paralyzed vocal cord can be difficult to identify because of the mass action and rapidity of movement during phonation.

*If there is any question about the diagnosis of a vocal cord abnormality, a head and neck specialist should be consulted.*

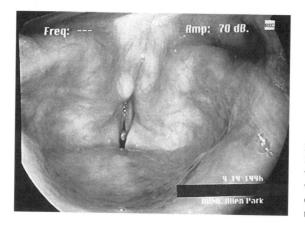

**FIGURE 4–1**
Plica ventricularis, excessive motion, and vocalization with the false cords. Here the view of the true cords is almost completely obscured by the false cords. See color photograph in Color Section 1.

## MUSCULOSKELETAL TENSION (SPASTIC DYSPHONIA)

Nonorganic causes account for a large percentage of problems presented to voice specialists. Musculoskeletal tension and emotional tension (the most common) produce excessive compensatory mechanisms of laryngeal muscles involved in voice production and result in mild to severe symptoms. Exam findings are often subtle and difficult for the nonspecialist to appreciate. A frequently recognized finding is vestibular-fold medialization or plica ventricularis (Fig. 4–1). In this condition the false cords (just above the true cords) move excessively and the true cords may be difficult to visualize. Treatment is directed toward the cause of the tension, and speech therapy should be initiated because the problem becomes cyclical.

## RHINITIS AND SINUSITIS

Persistent drainage of thick secretions leads to frequent coughing and throat clearing, with vocal cord irritation and edema. The patient may begin to use abnormal compensatory mechanisms that further aggravate the condition. The patient should avoid over-the-counter topical decongestants because dry, thicker secretions increase the dysphonia. Mucolytics such as guaifenesin may improve symptoms, as may increased water intake. Primary attention should be directed to the cause of the drainage by a thorough assessment of the sinonasal tract, including a history of allergies. Chronic sinusitis may require surgical consultation if severe and intractable because correctable anatomic causes may be contributory.

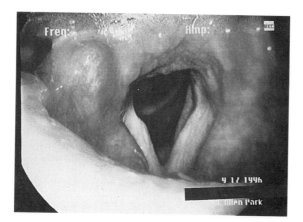

**FIGURE 4–2**
Reflux laryngitis. Thickened tissue and slight erythema over the arytenoid cartilages and posterior commissure. Erythema is not marked in this case. See Color Section 1.

# Color Plates 1–8

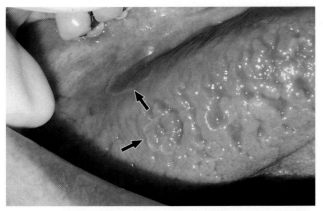

FIGURE 3–1
Fissured and geographic tongue in the same patient. Fissured tongue usually has multiple furrows 5 mm deep. Geographic tongue *(arrow)* shows multiple atrophic zones outlined by curved, whitish borders.

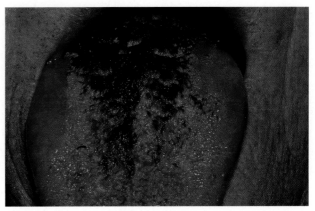

FIGURE 3–2
Black hairy tongue, which is unsightly but usually asymptomatic, results from increased keratinization of the filiform papillae on the dorsal tongue.

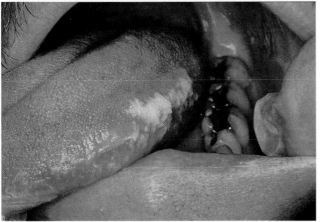

FIGURE 3–3
Hairy leukoplakia, seen in patients with HIV and low CD4 counts, is thought to be due to Epstein-Barr virus infection and occurs along the lateral edge of the tongue.

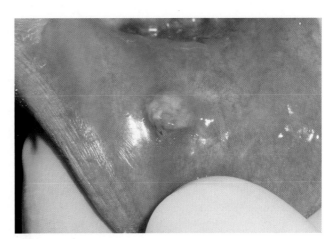

FIGURE 3–4
Mucocele of the lower lip (typical location).

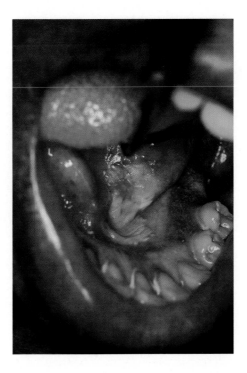

FIGURE 3–5
Leukoplakia and erythroplasia in a snuff dipper. Biopsy showed invasive squamous cell carcinoma, unsuccessfully treated by radiation therapy.

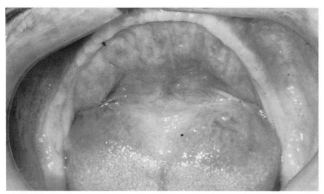

FIGURE 3–6A
Toluidine blue, a vital stain, can help identify where to biopsy a lesion, as in this patient with asymptomatic erythroplasia on the floor of the mouth.

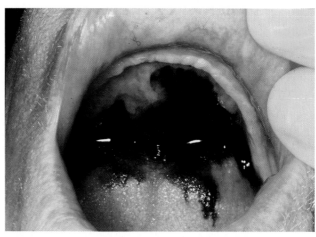

FIGURE 3–6B
After applying toluidine blue and rinsing,

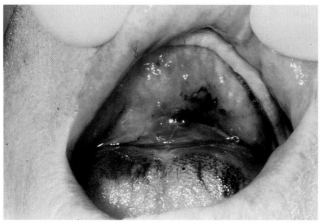

FIGURE 3–6C
an area of intense uptake remained. Biopsy in this region revealed invasive squamous cell carcinoma.

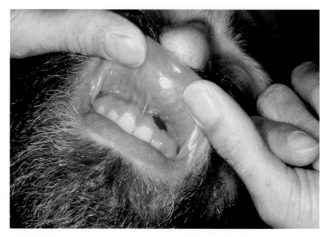

FIGURE 3–7A
Kaposi's sarcoma, the most common oral malignancy among patients with AIDS, appears as flat violaceous lesions on the oral mucosa.

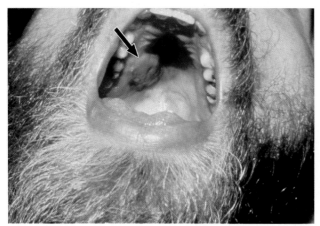

FIGURE 3–7B
The most common location is on the hard palate.

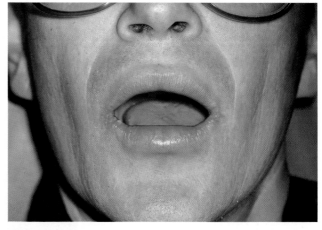

FIGURE 3–8
Angular cheilitis (perleche) is a mixed infection of *Staphylococcus* and *Candida* and presents as inflammation, erythema, and exudative crusting and tissue maceration at the corners of the mouth. Poorly fitting dentures are a frequent cause.

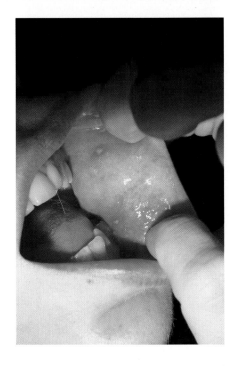

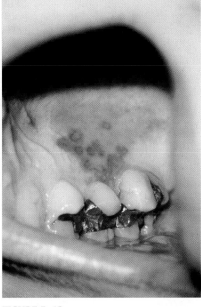

FIGURE 3-10
HSV I stomatitis during a primary infection. The patient also had malaise, fever, and vesicles scattered across the body.

FIGURE 3-9
Hand-foot-mouth disease produces a vesicular eruption on the buccal mucosa and tongue, with similar vesicles on the palms, soles, and occasionally the genitals and buttocks.

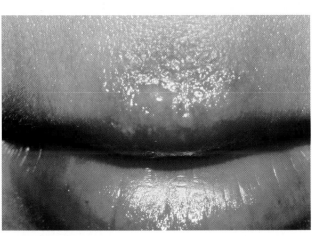

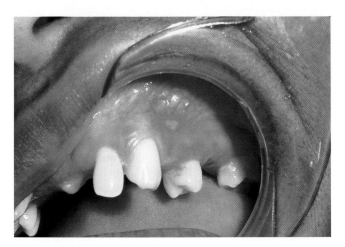

FIGURE 3-11
Vesicular eruption of recurrent HSV I infection on the outer lip.

FIGURE 3-12
Recurrent, intraoral HSV I is not common. It starts out as vesicles and tends to occur on mucosa bound to underlying periosteum (e.g., the hard palate or gingiva).

FIGURE 3-13
Recurrent aphthous ulcerations can range from one small lesion (as in this patient) to many large and extremely painful lesions. In contrast to recurrent HSV, aphthous ulcers tend to occur on mucosa not bound to underlying periosteum and are never preceded by vesicles.

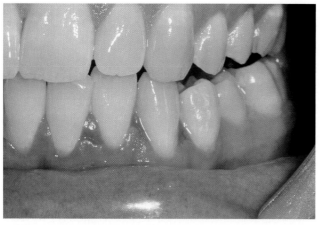

FIGURE 3–14A

Pemphigus vulgaris is a life-threatening but uncommon autoimmune disease that can produce oral erosions and cutaneous bullae. Smaller erosions may be barely perceptible, as in this 28-year-old woman with gingival lesions and one blister on her chest.

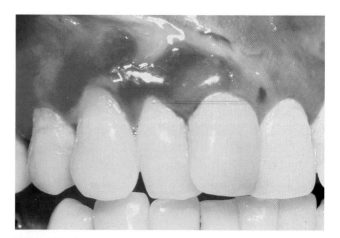

FIGURE 3–14B

More extensive erosions can involve the gingiva and buccal mucosa.

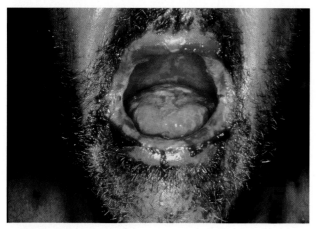

FIGURE 3–14C

Severe pemphigus vulgaris causes widespread oral erosions, cutaneous bullae, and extensive fluid, electrolyte, and protein imbalances.

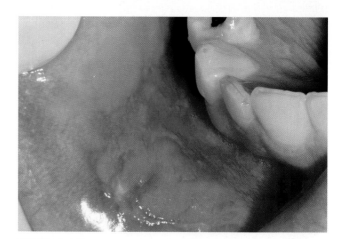

FIGURE 3–15

Cicatricial pemphigoid is a bullous disease affecting the oral, nasal, and ocular mucosa. Oral lesions produce sloughing of the gingival mucosa.

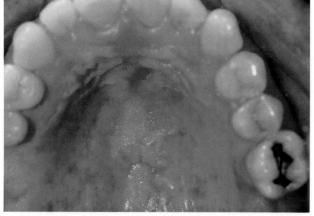

FIGURE 3–16A

Systemic lupus erythematosus can cause oral ulcerations heralding more severe disease, as in these patients with a hard palate ulcer, and

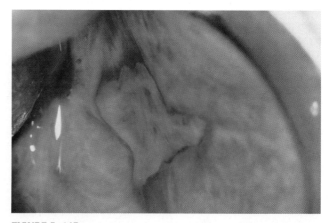

FIGURE 3–16B

ulceration of the buccal mucosa.

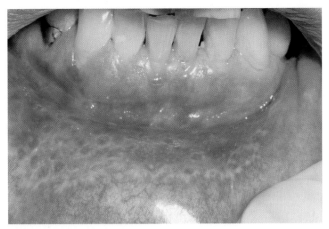

FIGURE 3–17A
Oral lichen planus usually produces a white reticular pattern on the labial or buccal mucosa.

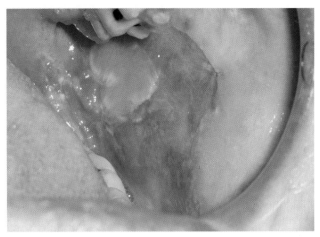

FIGURE 3–17B
More severe disease can produce painful ulcerations or erosions of the oral mucosa.

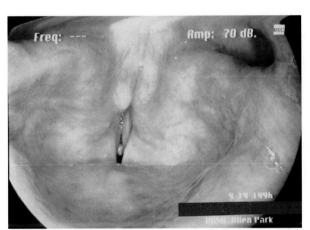

FIGURE 4–1
Plica ventricularis, excessive motion, and vocalization with the false cords. Here the view of the true cords is almost completely obscured by the false cords.

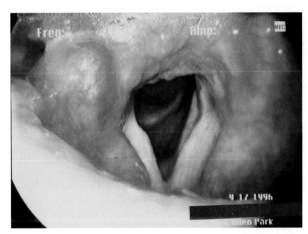

FIGURE 4–2
Reflux laryngitis. Thickened tissue and slight erythema over the arytenoid cartilages and posterior commissure. Erythema is not marked in this case.

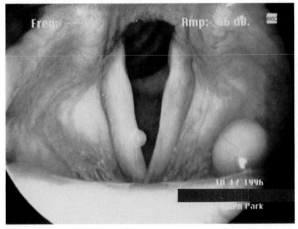

FIGURE 4–3
A benign-appearing right vocal cord nodule and left-sided benign-appearing epiglottic cyst.

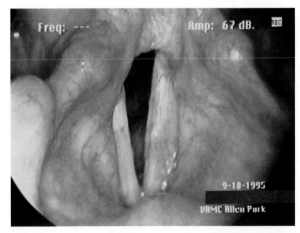

FIGURE 4–4
The view is not directly "en face," but slightly thickened and erythematous left vocal cord is visible. This patient complained of hoarseness. The diagnosis is extremely early cancer of the vocal cord.

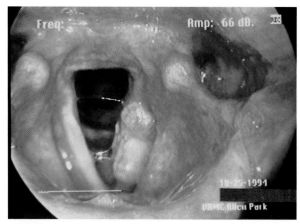

FIGURE 4–5
A more advanced cancer of the vocal cord.

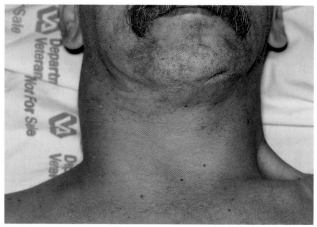

FIGURE 4–6
The neck appearance of a patient with a right parapharyngeal abscess.

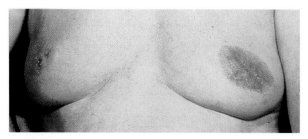

FIGURE 6–6A
Paget's disease of the nipple. The left breast has scaly, reddened, itchy skin of the areola and nipple, consistent with Paget's disease of the nipple.

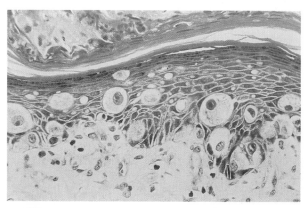

FIGURE 6–6B
Histologically, the skin contains cells with large nuclei. From Skarin, AT: Atlas of Diagnostic Oncology, ed 2. Mosby-Wolfe Limited, London, UK, 1991.

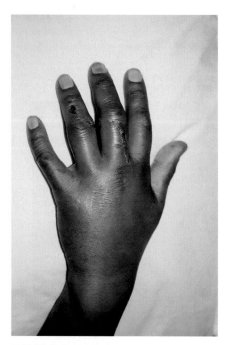

FIGURE 8–1
Cellulitis.

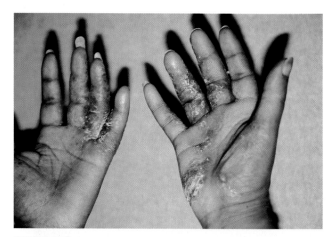

FIGURE 8–2
Herpes infection.

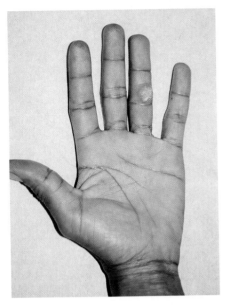

FIGURE 8–3
Viral wart.

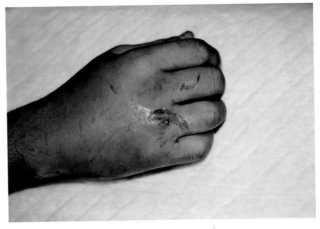

FIGURE 8–4
Human bite.

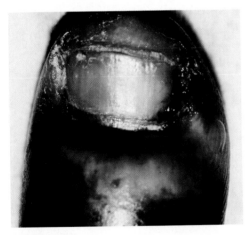

FIGURE 8–5
Paronychia.

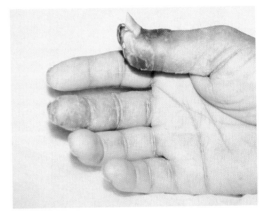

FIGURE 8–6
Untreated felon may lead to ischemia.

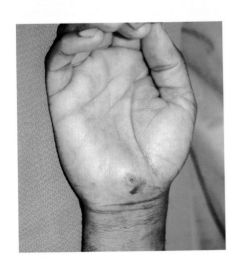

FIGURE 8–8
Palmar abscess.

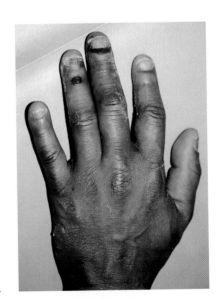

FIGURE 8–9
Subungual hematoma.

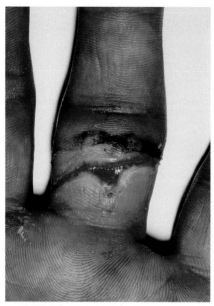

FIGURE 8-11
Ring avulsion injury.

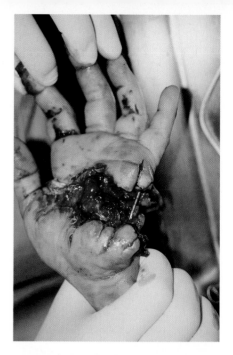

FIGURE 8-12
Crush injury.

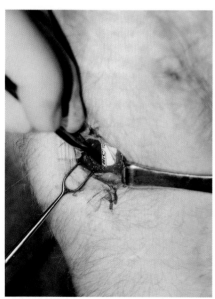

FIGURE 8-13
Foreign body.

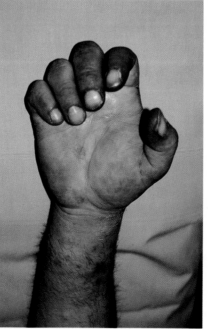

FIGURE 8-28
Ischemia of the hand from intra-arterial injection.

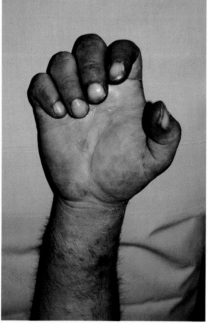

FIGURE 8-18
Frostbite.

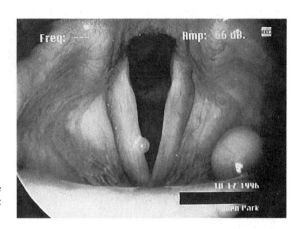

FIGURE 4–3
A benign-appearing right vocal cord nodule and left-sided benign-appearing epiglottic cyst. See Color Section 1.

## REFLUX LARYNGITIS

In a person who does not smoke or drink alcohol, voice changes associated with mild dysphagia or the sensation of a lump in the throat are suspicious for reflux laryngitis. Coexistent symptoms of gastroesophageal reflux further strengthen the suspicion. An exam might reveal bilateral arytenoid erythema and erythema of the posterior commissure but be otherwise unremarkable (Fig. 4–2). If the clinical picture is highly suggestive of gastroesophageal reflux, the patient should pursue an empiric course consisting of antacid or $H_2$-blocker therapy and avoidance of caffeine, cigarettes, and alcohol. Avoiding late meals may also be beneficial. Pro-motility agents may be added if antacid therapy is insufficient. Follow-up visualization of the larynx is indicated.

## VOCAL CORD ABNORMALITIES

An experienced laryngologist should examine visible vocal cord lesions. Many lesions require only nonoperative care, but the distinction between benign and early malignant lesions is not always obvious. The need for biopsy is best determined by the experienced eye (Figs. 4–3, 4–4, and 4–5).

### *When to Call the Surgeon about Voice Disturbances*

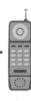

• Visible abnormality in examination of the throat

• Inability to examine the larynx or base of tongue

• Doubtful diagnosis or failure of the condition to improve with a 3- to 4-week course of medical therapy, speech therapy, or both

FIGURE 4–4
The view is not directly "en face," but slightly thickened and erythematous left vocal cord is visible. This patient complained of hoarseness. The diagnosis is extremely early cancer of the vocal cord. See Color Section 1.

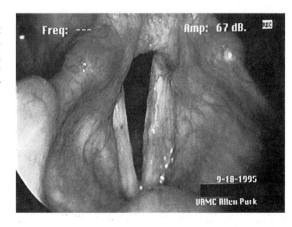

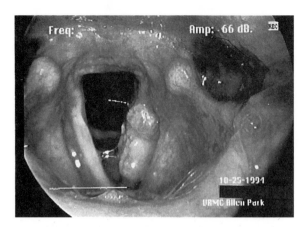

FIGURE 4–5
A more advanced cancer of the vocal cord. See Color Section 1.

## *Evaluation of the Sore Throat*

Discomfort in the throat may be caused by a myriad of conditions. The discomfort can range from very mild to severe (from tickling to incapacitating). When severe, it is usually associated with difficulty swallowing (dysphagia) or painful swallowing (odynophagia). Acute inflammatory conditions are well known to primary care providers and are only briefly described for completeness.

*Viral pharyngitis* causes an acute self-limiting illness characterized by fever, malaise, sore throat, petechia, and pharyngeal small-vessel enlargement. Resolution begins within 48 hours and treatment is nonspecific and symptom directed.

*Infectious mononucleosis* produces a similar clinical picture with fever, large and swollen tonsils (often with a dirty gray membrane), dysphagia, and odynophagia. There may be a skin rash and liver abnormalities. Rarely, tonsillar swelling can be so profound that the airway is compromised. A nasopharyngeal airway will bypass the obstruction. Short-term steroids may be of benefit, or in the extreme case a tracheotomy may be needed.

*Tonsillitis* presents with the symptom complex of sore throat, fever, painful and difficult swallowing, earache, headache and backache, and malaise. If inadequately treated or if treatment is delayed, the condition may evolve into *peritonsillar abscess*, which is indicated by worsening of symptoms and the development of drooling, trismus, or both. The physical examination reveals obvious unilateral swelling of the tonsil and palate, with deviation of the tonsil and uvula. Needle drainage of the abscess (Table 4–1) followed by prompt administration of antibiotics generally results in rapid recovery.

TABLE 4–1

### Technique of Aspirating a Peritonsillar Abscess

Equipment Required
   10% xylocaine spray
   1% xylocaine injectable
   Light (headlight or chair light and mirror)
   18- and 22-gauge and spinal needles and 10-cc syringe
Technique
   Spray soft palate with 10% xylocaine
   Inject 1–2 cc 1% xylocaine into soft palate at junction of soft palate and tonsil at upper pole
   Aspirate
   Culture if recurrent

*When to Call the Surgeon about Sore Throat*

- Need for needle aspiration (if primary care provider prefers)
- Recurrent peritonsillar abscess
- Failure to respond promptly to therapy
- History of more chronic symptoms suggesting malignancy

## Parapharyngeal Abscess

*Parapharyngeal abscess* is a complication of pharyngeal infection. It presents with sore throat, a toxic-appearing patient, and swelling in the neck, generally anterior to the sternocleidomastoid muscle (Fig. 4–6). The tonsil may or may not be acutely inflamed. *This kind of abscess requires surgical drainage through the neck.*

*Retropharyngeal abscess* may result from tonsillar infection or foreign body perforation. There is toxemia, pain, fever, dysphagia, and dyspnea if the airway is obstructed by marked anterior displacement of the posterior pharyngeal wall, a fluctuant pharyngeal mass, and pain on neck extension. *As for parapharyngeal abscess, this condition requires urgent surgical consultation for drainage under general anesthesia in an operating room.*

In summary, all retropharyngeal or parapharyngeal abscesses require urgent surgical consultation. Needle aspiration is *not* advised.

*All retropharyngeal or parapharyngeal abscesses require urgent surgical consultation. Needle aspiration is* not *advised.*

## Chronic Dysphagia

Chronic dysphagia or odynophagia lasting more than 1 month suggests malignancy. If the history and physical exam are unrevealing, direct laryngoscopy and esophagoscopy are indicated especially if associated with ear pain, weight loss, a neck mass, or hemoptysis. A barium swallow is generally obtained in patients with dysphagia, although the patient suffering from oropharyngeal dysphagia rather than an esophageal disorder may be unable to complete this test, or it may be falsely normal. A modified barium swallow using video fluoroscopy and small amounts of contrast of different consistencies improves diagnostic accuracy. This exam also allows a swallowing therapist to test different swallowing rehabilitation strategies and evaluate their efficacy. As already noted, gastroesophageal reflux can produce a sore throat and voice or vocal cord changes as well as mild dysphagia. Manofluorography is a sophisticated technique that measures pressure changes within the pharynx during a video swallow. It requires significant expertise and is more complicated than esophageal manometry and hence less available.

**FIGURE 4–6**
The neck appearance of a patient with a right parapharyngeal abscess. See Color Section 1.

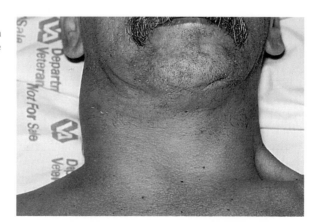

Myotomy for *cricopharyngeal spasm* (failure to relax the pharyngoesophageal sphincter) with or without a diverticulum may be performed on an outpatient basis or during a short hospital stay, but feeding by mouth is generally delayed 4 to 5 days if a diverticulum is removed.

## DOCUMENTED ASPIRATION

Surgical treatment of pulmonary aspiration ranges from endoscopic injection to medialize a paralyzed and abducted vocal cord to major surgery on the larynx. If aspiration is significant or if dysphagia is severe, an alternative means of nutrition such as gastrostomy should be considered. The patient should try swallowing rehabilitation prior to any irreversible surgery.

### When to Call the Surgeon about Abscess or Dysphagia

- Parapharyngeal or retropharyngeal abscess
- Foreign bodies lodged in the laryngopharynx or esophagus
- Documented cricopharyngeal spasm
- Suspicion of cancer

## *Evaluation of Neck Masses*

The evaluation of neck masses can be most vexing in the absence of other symptoms or physical signs. If present, associated symptoms should be the target of any investigation.

For clarity, neck masses will be grouped by location as submental, submandibular, upper jugular, midjugular, lower jugular, supraclavicular, and mid posterior. We will not discuss neck masses in the thyroid region because most solitary thyroid nodules should simply undergo fine-needle aspiration.

The differential diagnosis and evaluation of an otherwise asymptomatic patient with a neck mass begins with two historical features: the age of the patient and the duration of the mass. In patients aged from infancy to 15 years, about 85% of nonthyroidal neck masses are benign. Most of these are inflammatory, and the remainder have a congenital or developmental etiology. Inflammatory lesions are treated medically and developmental lesions are usually removed. Although neoplasia is uncommon, malignant neoplasms predominate over benign neoplasms in this age group. Supraclavicular and lower posterior neck lesions are more likely to be malignant, representing chiefly lymphoma or thyroid cancer. Patients aged 16 to 40 have a similar clinical picture, but even within the realm of neoplasm, benign lesions are more common than malignant ones. For patients over 40, neoplasm makes up approximately 80% of masses, of which about 80% are malignant. Of the malignant neck masses, 80% are metastatic, and 80% of metastatic lesions originate from primary sites above the clavicle. Thus most neck masses in adults need surgical attention.

Submental adenopathy should direct attention to the oral cavity, particularly the floor of the mouth and the undersurface of the tongue. If no lesions are present in the mouth by inspection or palpation, the presence of an inflammatory adenopathy is likely. Folliculitis barbae is a common cause of submental adenopathy (generally less than 1 cm) in African-American men.

Submandibular masses may represent enlarged lymph nodes or may reflect disease of the submandibular gland. A history of episodic enlargement, especially with a metallic or bitter taste, suggests intermittent ductal obstruction. A persistently enlarged, firm, or hard gland should be surgically removed if no stone in the duct can be removed

*Most neck masses in adults need surgical attention.*

intraorally. As in the submental area, a careful oral exam is warranted, as are intraoral x-rays of the floor of the mouth. Upper, middle, or lower jugular; supraclavicular; or posterior neck masses are almost always caused by enlarged nodes; in the adult over 40 years old these are usually malignant. Posterior cervical adenopathy affecting one or two nodes of less than 1 cm are generally benign and only require observation unless there are other indications of a malignant nature. A thorough history and physical exam remains the initial step with special attention to the caveats discussed previously.

Neck radiography or computed tomography (CT) is seldom helpful in the initial evaluation of neck masses. Almost all neck masses in adults will require (at a minimum) pathologic evaluation. Fine-needle aspiration cytology (FNAC) is a technique easily learned, and in the correct setting it may make more invasive procedures unnecessary. A "negative" FNAC result does not prove the absence of malignancy, however. It is most useful in the evaluation of supraclavicular adenopathy and can direct subsequent evaluation or therapy. It is usually unnecessary if a mucosal malignancy can be identified.

*A "negative" FNAC result does not prove the absence of malignancy.*

Inflammatory conditions such as acute and chronic infections of the skin, pharynx, or oral cavity commonly cause neck adenopathy. Surgical consultation should be sought for all neck masses in which no definite inflammatory cause can be found. It is also advised for inflammatory conditions, including those thought to be infectious, if they last more than a month into therapy. In addition, because of the high prevalence of mouth and neck cancers in adults with significant histories of smoking or alcohol use, such high-risk individuals who develop neck masses should also be referred to a surgeon for immediate consultation. Special consideration should also be given to those of Asian descent who develop upper neck masses, because this population has an increased risk of nasopharyngeal cancer.

### When to Call the Surgeon about Neck Masses

- All noninflammatory neck masses such as those not associated with acute skin, pharyngeal, or oral inflammation (or with chronic infections such as TB, mononucleosis)
- Inflammatory neck masses persisting longer than 1 month after treatment is begun
- All neck masses in smokers or drinkers, even if "acute" inflammation is suggested by history or exam
- Upper neck masses in patients of Asian descent

## RECOMMENDED READING

Becker, W (ed): Atlas of Ear, Nose and Throat Diseases, ed 2. WB Saunders, Philadelphia, 1984.

Gates, G (ed): Current Therapy in Otolaryngology Head and Neck Surgery, ed 5. CV Mosby, St. Louis, 1994.

Meyerhoff, WL, and Rice, DH: Otolaryngology–Head and Neck Surgery. WB Saunders, Philadelphia, 1992.

# Chapter

# 5

# Airway Problems

MICHAEL DAHN, MD, PhD,
and LAWRENCE RAYMOND, MD, ScM

Airway management is one of the most fundamental aspects of patient care. Suboptimal or delayed efforts to provide adequate ventilation for patients suffering from airway compromise will dramatically magnify the patient's severity of illness or precipitate sudden death. The causes of airway obstruction are legion. We do not intend to discuss all of them, but we will consider some relatively common diseases. Because the techniques for airway control are varied, it would be wise for the clinician to be aware of the different options used to manage airway problems in order to identify situations where selection of different maneuvers may be lifesaving. Each clinical circumstance in which the airway may be in jeopardy demands early planning and a willingness to alter the approach if progressive deterioration occurs.

## General Considerations

Typical signs and symptoms of patients who seek medical attention for airway disorders are indicated in Table 5–1. Most of the indicators are relatively nonspecific and may be observed in association with a variety of upper and lower airway disorders. With careful attention to the patient's presentation, however, the differential diagnosis may be focused significantly (Table 5–2), especially when the presentation is considered in conjunction with the history (e.g., duration of symptoms) and systemic signs (e.g., fever from an infectious cause).

For example, wheezing may arise from lower airway disease in the lung due to asthma, but it may be confused with mild stridor due to upper airway obstruction and heard best at the mouth. These two airway sounds may be further distinguished by timing their occurrence in the respiratory cycle. Stridor, which may also be described as a crowing or musical type of wheezing, is predominantly limited to the inspiratory phase of breathing and indicates laryngeal or tracheal obstruction. In contrast, wheezing associated with lower respiratory tract disorders is largely confined to the expiratory

TABLE 5–1

## Signs and Symptoms of Airway Obstruction

Dyspnea
Wheezing
Stridor
Dysphonia
Hoarseness
Accessory muscle use
Intercostal retractions
Paradoxical abdominal motion

phase of ventilation. Hoarseness and difficulty or inability to phonate helps to localize the pathology to the glottic region. Pain or sore throat frequently points to an inflammatory process involving the structures of the pharynx, larynx, or upper trachea. Conversely, painless obstruction is most likely caused by a neoplasm or foreign body. Disorders of the upper respiratory tract immediately require at least a consideration of the creation of a surgical airway, whereas lower tract disorders are almost exclusively managed through pharmacologic means in the acute phase.

Before implementing any therapeutic maneuvers, the primary examiner should attempt to establish a diagnosis. In addition to history and clinical observation, additional diagnostic studies are desirable, but patients who present with symptoms of significant upper airway obstruction must be managed expediently. An apparently elective situation may deteriorate precipitously with a progressive lesion or with minor airway manipulation. Patients who present with stridor typically have lost at least 50% of their upper airway diameter. Additionally, Pouseille's law states that flow is directly related to the radius of a lumen raised to the fourth power, so further reductions in luminal dimensions will have dramatically accelerated impact on respiratory ability. Thus, when the presenting sign is stridor, initial evaluation, including radiologic studies, should be performed in an area where continuous observation and urgent care is readily

*Patients with symptoms of significant upper airway obstruction should be managed expediently; those with stridor typically have lost at least 50% of their upper airway diameter.*

TABLE 5–2

## The Differential Diagnoses of Wheezing

*Upper (Extrathoracic) Respiratory Tract*
Angioneurotic edema
Foreign body
Goiter
Infection
Neuromuscular disease
Tracheal stenosis
Tumor
Vocal cord paralysis

*Lower Respiratory Tract*
Asthma
Aspiration
Bronchiolitis
Chronic obstructive pulmonary disease (COPD)
Foreign body
Adenopathy

*Systemic*
Acute respiratory distress syndrome (ARDS)
Congestive heart failure
Pulmonary embolism
Vasculitis

TABLE 5–3

## Ancillary Tests and Diagnostic Maneuvers That May Assist in the Diagnosis and Management of Acute Airway Disorders

Pulse oximetry
Arterial blood gas
Lateral neck and chest x-ray
Flow-volume spirometry (inspiratory/expiratory loops)
Direct and indirect laryngoscopy
Fiberoptic laryngoscopy/bronchoscopy
CT scanning of pharynx/larynx/trachea

---

● ▬▬▬

*Permitting a patient to be transferred to a remote diagnostic area unattended begs for a catastrophic outcome.*

available, such as the emergency room or the intensive care unit. Permitting a patient to be transferred to a remote diagnostic area unattended begs for a catastrophic outcome.

Ancillary tests to identify a specific disease entity are listed in Table 5–3. Pulse oximetry should be applied early to provide a continuous means of oxygenation assessment even during transport. Arterial blood gas values ($paO_2$ and $paCO_2$) provide additional information regarding the extent of ventilatory failure. Carbon dioxide retention should signal the need for more urgent intervention, as it indicates impending airway obstruction. Patients with an acute exacerbation of lower respiratory tract disease will often present with $CO_2$ retention; this situation must be discriminated from upper airway obstruction based on physical findings and history. A lateral soft-tissue x-ray will frequently provide valuable evidence of the acute upper airway process precipitating the patient's symptoms. Many inflammatory lesions such as those on the epiglottis may be identified on plain film (Fig. 5–1). Also, because the larynx in the adult and the cricoid cartilage in the child are the narrowest points of the airway, this

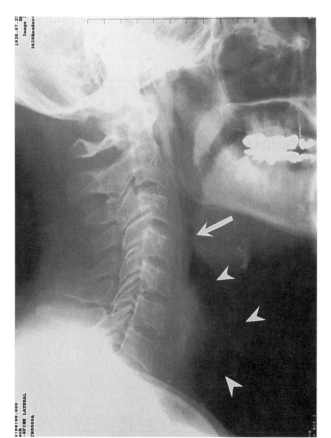

FIGURE 5–1
The airway silhouette in the neck may be demonstrated by a lateral soft-tissue x-ray *(arrowheads)*. The film defines the airway best if the patient is actively inhaling or exhaling. The epiglottis is best seen during expiration against pursed lips. In this film the epiglottis (arrow) is barely demonstrable, but in the presence of epiglottitis, the marked tissue edema can easily be seen protruding into the airway.

area is most frequently the stopping point of aspirated food and other foreign bodies, which will be visible on x-rays of the neck. Such foreign bodies can give rise to "sudden death" (so-called "café coronary syndrome"). Additionally, diagnostic information may be obtained from an anteroposterior chest x-ray that includes the neck and gives an additional silhouette view of the air column in the neck. As mentioned previously, because of the inherent instability of patients suffering from upper airway obstruction, these studies should generally be performed as portable studies in an acute care area.

Further management of these patients is dictated by the degree and rate of progression of respiratory distress and the best clinical assessment of the diagnosis. Under nonurgent conditions, the upper airway may be evaluated using spirometry to provide helpful diagnostic clues. Upper airway lesions exhibit characteristic flow volume loops depending on (1) location (extrathoracic versus intrathoracic) and (2) degree of fixation. Rigid, fixed obstructions such as firm tumors or fibrotic lesions tend to dampen both inspiratory and expiratory airway flow in the flow volume loop (Fig. 5–2A). If the lesion is extrathoracic but somewhat pliable and less fixed, a depressed (flattened) inspiratory flow and a relatively normal expiratory flow loop may be observed. This results from the tendency of the airway to collapse in response to a large negative inspiratory pressure. In contrast, intrathoracic lesions exhibit a predominant slowing of the expiratory flow loop because increased pleural pressure on expiration is transmitted to the involved airway wall, tending to worsen the degree of obstruction (Figure 5–2B). This assessment frequently can be performed in an outpatient office setting, but its performance should not delay more definitive diagnostic and management approaches under emergency conditions.

More specific diagnostic information frequently requires indirect or direct inspection of the pharynx and larynx. If time permits, it is highly desirable to involve a clinician who is experienced with these modalities because their use occasionally precipitates an airway crisis. Considerable judgment is required under these circumstances. For instance, direct laryngoscopy by the emergency room physician may permit the life-saving extraction of a foreign body, but manipulation of a markedly inflamed epiglottis may precipitate acute asphyxia. Such precautions are particularly important in the pediatric population because the small airway dimensions of young children magnify the impact of minor increases in pharyngeal and laryngeal edema. Computed tomography (CT) scanning is helpful in assessment and in planning the management of laryngeal injuries and upper respiratory tract tumors, but it must be used with great caution if significant respiratory distress is present.

If the potential exists for acute worsening of airway obstruction, especially during

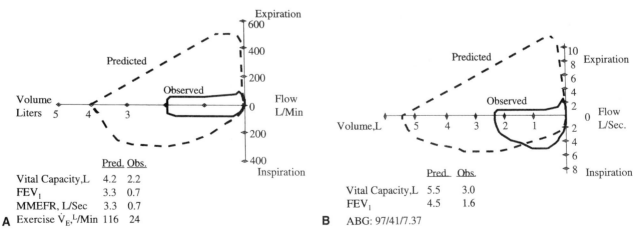

FIGURE 5–2

Flow volume loops are illustrated for two clinical conditions involving upper airway obstruction. (*A*) A fixed subglottic stenosis secondary to chronic tracheal intubation results in severe inspiratory *and* expiratory flow restriction compared to the predicted volume loop (- - - - -). (*B*) An intrathoracic tracheal malignancy shows impaired expiratory flow with a relatively normal inspiratory loop.

• ▬▬

*If the potential for acute
worsening of airway
obstruction exists, the means
to provide both endotracheal
intubation and a surgical
airway should always be
immediately accessible.*

airway manipulation, the means to provide both endotracheal intubation and a surgical airway should always be immediately accessible. Thorough preparation for such an eventuality, including the presence of an anesthesiologist and surgeon, will avoid confusion and delays in securing an airway. Diagnostic and therapeutic efforts should be coordinated in order to use these specialty services optimally.

# Disorders Associated with Airway Problems

## INFECTION AND INFLAMMATION

### Ludwig's Angina

Ludwig's angina, most commonly seen in young adults, is a rapidly spreading cellulitis involving the sublingual and submaxillary spaces, which include the regions between the inferior aspects of the tongue and the hyoid bone. The initiating factor is usually dental, such as a molar abscess, but intraoral injuries may become superinfected and progress in a similar fashion. Significant physical findings include tenderness of the floor of the mouth, edema of the suprahyoid region of the neck, and displacement of the tongue upward and posteriorly, thereby encroaching on the pharyngeal airway. Additionally, some patients present with marked trismus, making examination and airway access difficult. Antibiotic (penicillin) therapy is the mainstay of management, but in the presence of respiratory distress, airway control should be secured with nasotracheal intubation, cricothyroidotomy, or tracheostomy. Airway control should be very aggressive because compromise of the airway is the most frequent cause of death in this disorder.

### Retropharyngeal Infection

Infections involving the retropharyngeal space, which lies just anterior to the prevertebral space, can extend from the base of the skull down into the posterior mediastinum. Occasionally the lateral aspects of the pharynx also are involved. Characteristically, in addition to fever and respiratory distress, patients present with dysphagia. The major morbidity arises from the potential for airway obstruction and progression to mediastinitis. Most commonly, the disorder appears in children and stems from posterior pharyngeal trauma. Occasionally adults will present with vertebral osteomyelitis and a paraspinal as well as retropharyngeal abscess (see Chapter 4). The retropharyngeal space can be assessed on the lateral neck x-ray. Its normal anteroposterior distance is 1 to 7 mm at the level of C-2 and 9 to 22 mm at C-6. Enlargements of these dimensions usually indicate the need for surgical drainage. Borderline evaluations suggest the need for further study using CT scanning. Prior to drainage, it is important to exclude a vascular structure or aneurysm, which may be mistaken for an abscess. Finally, since the etiology of this process is bacterial, it requires parenteral antibiotic therapy (penicillin for *Bacteroides*, metronidazole for penicillin-allergic patients, or ceftriaxone for penicillin-resistant *Streptococcus pneumonia*).

### Acute Epiglottitis

*Acute epiglottitis* is a bacterial infection of the supraglottic structures in which the epiglottis is predominantly affected. Because of the regional tissue involvement, it is preferably called *supraglottitis* by many authorities. This entity is frequently confused with *laryngotracheitis* or *croup*, which involves the subglottic structures and generally has a benign, self-limited course (Table 5–4). Although epiglottitis most frequently affects children, its incidence is increasing in the adult population. Because of the smaller size of the pediatric airway, the risk of critical airway obstruction and the need for intubation or creation of a surgical airway is much greater in children. Adults can more frequently

**TABLE 5–4**

## Differentiating Characteristics of Laryngotracheitis ("Croup") and Epiglottitis

| Feature | Croup | Epiglottitis |
|---|---|---|
| Age | <3 years | >3 years and adults |
| Rate of onset | Days (in association with systemic viral syndrome) | Hours |
| Cough | Harsh | None |
| Speech | Hoarse | Muffled |
| Radiograph (plain film) | Narrowed subglottis | Enlarged epiglottis (thumb sign) |
| Cause | Viral | Bacterial (*Haemophilus influenzae, Streptococcus*) |
| Treatment | Humidification, bronchodilators, ? steroids | Airway control and antibiotics |

be managed without the need for invasive airway maneuvers. Patients usually appear toxic and are reluctant to assume a recumbent position. Lateral neck x-rays usually reveal a prominent epiglottis protruding into the airway, giving the appearance of a large thumb (thumb sign). Management includes antibiotics (ampicillin/chloramphenicol, second- or third-generation cephalosporins) and expeditious airway control with endotracheal intubation, cricothyroidotomy, or tracheostomy. This disorder is life threatening. Avoiding mortality from asphyxiation requires strict coordination between a clinician expert in intubation and a surgeon fully prepared for cricothyroidotomy or tracheostomy, preferably in the operating room.

*Avoiding mortality from asphyxiation requires strict coordination between a clinician expert in intubation and a surgeon fully prepared for cricothyroidotomy or tracheostomy, preferably in the operating room.*

### Diphtheria

Diphtheria, although quite uncommon, can progressively obstruct the airway. Its marked decline in incidence is ascribable to nearly universal diphtheria immunization in westernized cultures. Nevertheless, occasionally nonimmunized children or adults with a history of immunization develop pharyngeal/laryngeal diphtheria. The disorder is caused by *Corynebacterium diphtheriae* and is slowly progressive, presenting with hoarseness and sore throat. Examination reveals tightly adherent grayish membranes involving the tonsils, pharynx, and larynx. In the presence of respiratory distress, airway control is best obtained through elective tracheostomy. Attempts at endotracheal intubation may be complicated by disruption of these membranes, resulting in acute airway obstruction. Additional therapies consist of diphtheria antitoxin administration and intravenous antibiotics (penicillin or erythromycin).

### Allergic or Hereditary Angioedema

Patients may be afflicted with recurrent episodes of edema involving the face, upper airway, and other tissue regions, stemming from a known or unknown allergy. The process may progress quite rapidly and demand immediate intubation in response to marked respiratory compromise. Cricothyroidotomy should be performed promptly if intubation attempts are unsuccessful. Supplemental therapy consists of antihistamines, epinephrine, and steroids.

## FOREIGN BODY ASPIRATION

Foreign body aspiration occurs in a variety of populations, such as (1) small children who have a predilection for mouthing toys or ingesting food fragments that are too large, (2) individuals with a depressed level of consciousness due to organic brain disease or use of alcohol or sedatives, or (3) patients suffering from degenerative neurologic diseases, particularly if the cranial nerves are involved. Sometimes aspiration is simply a sporadic event. The event itself is signaled by the abrupt onset of coughing, gagging, hoarseness, and stridor. Because most foreign bodies lodge at the level of the larynx, dysphonia commonly accompanies the onset of symptoms.

The extent of respiratory distress depends on the degree of upper airway obstruction. Mild obstruction allows time for a systematic workup of the patient, culminating in direct laryngoscopy and foreign body extraction. Complete loss of the airway is associated with cyanosis and the universal sign of severe distress, clutching of the neck. This condition requires immediate therapeutic action if the patient is unable to cough and quickly expel the foreign body. There are three approaches for resolving this crisis: (1) a finger sweep into the patient's larynx in an attempt to dislodge or remove the foreign body, (2) three or four sharp knocks between the patient's shoulder blades, or (3) the Heimlich maneuver. Currently, the Heimlich maneuver is the primary basic life support maneuver recommended for adults by the American Heart Association. Back blows and chest thrusts instead of the Heimlich maneuver are recommended for infants, to avoid the potential for intra-abdominal injury. Finger sweeps may be performed after the tongue and jaw have been grasped and lifted anteriorly to open the airway, but this maneuver should be performed only in unconscious patients. Failure of these maneuvers requires immediate airway access via needle tracheal puncture or cricothyroidotomy. Intermediate levels of respiratory distress must be judged individually as to their urgency. Direct examination of the airway by an experienced examiner, such as a general or head and neck surgeon, could be both diagnostic and therapeutic. It is important to note that adult patients may present with a history compatible with a foreign body aspiration only to have a neoplastic lesion discovered. This unexpected situation may require the skillful placement of an endotracheal tube or surgical airway, reaffirming the need for the performance of direct laryngoscopy by an expert examiner.

*• ▬*

*Back blows and chest thrusts are recommended for infants instead of the Heimlich maneuver.*

## OBSTRUCTING TUMORS

The most common neoplastic obstruction of the upper airway results from the extension of a carcinoma of the larynx to the subglottic larynx. Fortunately, these tumors usually grow slowly and symptoms of stridor and dyspnea are preceded by a lengthy history of hoarseness. Thus, the history is strongly suggestive of the diagnosis.

Depending on the degree of obstruction, symptomatic patients may not be easily treated by endotracheal intubation because of the obstructing nature of the lesion and its vascularity. Management options include endoscopic (laser) treatment, tracheostomy below the obstructing lesion, or intubation, if possible, followed by later definitive therapy. Some authorities have recommended the avoidance of early tracheostomy, which is associated with an increased infection rate and an increased incidence of local tumor recurrence following a definitive laryngectomy. Transendoscopic tumor ablation using laser therapy to establish an airway has gained in popularity; this approach avoids early tracheostomy. Thus, early laryngoscopic evaluation by a specialist is required to develop a thoughtful plan that will minimize local morbidity for the patient.

Substernal goiter may present with acute-onset respiratory distress and may even mimic asthma. A soft-tissue mass that deviates the trachea on chest x-ray suggests this diagnosis.

## ACUTE FACIAL AND LARYNGEAL TRAUMA

Patients presenting with major head and neck trauma are in immediate peril from the disruption of air flow and secondary aspiration. Additionally, the examiner must always be vigilant for additional injuries that are not obvious. Conditions such as flail chest, lung contusion, hemothorax, or pneumothorax will worsen respiratory difficulties. Presenting symptoms may therefore be quite difficult to interpret, and the examiner must always maintain a high threshold of suspicion for associated injuries. Also, the potential for cervical spine injuries must be considered and evaluated early in the patient's course.

Facial injuries are commonly associated with nasal, oral, and mandibular injuries with aspiration of blood and teeth and disruption of the tongue support mechanism (mandibular fracture). Management may consist of simply clearing the oral airway of tissue debris and placing a nasal or oral airway. Control of severe epistaxis should be performed with the help of a specialist in head and neck surgery. Supplemental oxygen by mouth or nasal cannula should be applied early while a rapid radiographic assessment of the cervical spine and a clinical evaluation for the existence of a basilar skull fracture (raccoon eyes, rhinorrhea, midface instability) is performed to assess the risk of intubation if airway control cannot be obtained otherwise. Suspicion of a basilar skull fracture speaks against the use of nasotracheal intubation. The inability to exclude a cervical spine fracture supports the use of endotracheal intubation with in-line stabilization or proceeding directly to a cricothyroidotomy. Percutaneous cricothyroid needle puncture, using a 14-gauge needle or larger, remains a temporizing option used in preparation for surgical cricothyroidotomy.

*Suspicion of a basilar skull fracture speaks against nasotracheal intubation.*

*Percutaneous cricothyroid needle puncture, using a 14-gauge needle or larger, remains a temporizing option.*

When the clinical circumstances include the possibility of laryngeal trauma, such as following a steering wheel impact, careful attention must be given to the patient's history and physical findings to exclude that possibility. Hoarseness, dysphagia, laryngeal pain and tenderness, and local hematoma suggest the need for further evaluation of the larynx. To preserve the airway, emergent measures must also include resuscitation, stabilization of the cervical spine, and a systematic search for other organ injuries. If a laryngeal injury is suspected in the presence of an unstable airway, the preferred management is probably a tracheostomy rather than endotracheal intubation or cricothyroidotomy, if possible. This will avoid further disruption of laryngeal structures requiring subsequent repairs. Proper assessment of the larynx may require fiberoptic laryngoscopy and laryngeal CT scanning in order to detect mucosal laceration, laryngeal fractures, and dislocations. This form of evaluation demands the attention of an otolaryngologist.

## AIRWAY BURNS

Injury to the airway following entrapment in a fire may result from either thermal responses or chemical exposure of the respiratory mucosa to noxious elements. Asphyxia and respiratory failure secondary to chemical exposure (such as cyanide or carbon monoxide) are probably the most common causes of death associated with a thermal event. Evidence of thermal injury to the airway is suggested by facial burns and the presence of carbonaceous material in the pharynx, but the need for airway control is best suggested by clinical indicators including (1) physical findings of drooling, hoarseness, and stridor, and (2) the presence of hypoxemia, tachycardia, and tachypnea. If an inhalation injury is suspected based on these indicators, further evaluation by bronchoscopy may be warranted to assess the extent of injury. Bronchoscopy is best accomplished by a surgeon who also has the expertise to create a surgical airway as obstructive symptoms evolve.

*Asphyxia and respiratory failure secondary to chemical exposure are the most common causes of death associated with a thermal event.*

## Airway Access

Table 5–5 lists the various approaches that may be used to relieve upper airway obstruction. In the unconscious patient, airway function can generally be improved simply

**TABLE 5-5**

### Methods Used to Gain Access to or Assist in Maintaining Patency of the Airway

Posterior head tilt/chin lift or jaw thrust maneuver
Oral/nasal airways
Oral or nasal endotracheal intubation
Fiberoptic bronchoscope-assisted endotracheal intubation
Retrograde tracheal intubation
Translaryngeal needle ventilation
Cricothyroidotomy
Tracheostomy

by distracting the mandible to a more anterior position. This is accomplished with a posterior head tilt and chin lift or jaw thrust maneuver. If the integrity of the cervical spine is in question, the head tilt maneuver must be omitted.

Placement of a pharyngeal airway helps to maintain a patent airway and facilitates evacuation of respiratory secretions. Oral airways should be used only in patients with an impaired level of consciousness who exhibit a depressed gag reflex. In awake patients, their use will be complicated by gagging and retching, leading to vomiting and possible aspiration. Nasal airways induce less gagging and may be used in either conscious or unconscious patients. Their use should be temporary, however, since they engender nasal mucosal injury, sinusitis, and otitis.

If endotracheal intubation is required, either a transoral or transnasal route may be used. Success in the outcome of either of these approaches depends on familiarity with the proposed method, careful patient preparation, and availability of an alternate plan if the intubation attempts fail. Successful intubation requires technical proficiency and a recognition of the relative contraindications to the different approaches. Oral intubation is preferred in the apneic patient and can be performed more rapidly in a crisis. It also is less traumatic to the mucosal surfaces, a factor that may be significant in patients with a bleeding diathesis. Nasotracheal intubation provides airway access in patients with trismus, oral trauma, decerebrate rigidity, and obstructing lesions of the mouth. Because nasal tubes are smaller, however, airway hygiene is more difficult and they are best placed in a patient with spontaneous respiratory activity. Preparation of the awake patient includes topical anesthesia, preoxygenation, and possible sedation, muscle paralysis, or both. It is important to recognize, however, that these maneuvers increase the aspiration potential and also may convert a patient with a spontaneous respiratory effort who might be difficult to intubate into a patient who now exhibits respiratory arrest and still may be equally difficult to intubate. Thus, the use of pharmacologic agents to assist with airway control is fraught with great risk. The responsible clinician should always be prepared to implement an alternate plan if multiple intubation attempts fail, particularly if upper airway obstruction prevents tube passage.

Additional approaches to consider include fiberoptic, bronchoscope-guided nasotracheal intubation and retrograde transtracheal-guidewire-assisted intubation. These methods are only for nonapneic patients, however, who can be maintained for up to 5 to 10 minutes prior to successful completion. If the situation is critical and the patient is *in extremis*, this delay in obtaining a definitive airway is intolerable.

For immediate tracheal access, cricothyroidotomy is recommended if intubation efforts fail. As a temporizing maneuver under critical circumstances, needle cricothyroidotomy can be employed. A 14-gauge or larger needle is used to puncture the cricothyroid membrane. The needle hub may be connected to the barrel of a 3 mL syringe, which is then attached to an adapter from a 7.5 mm endotracheal tube. Providing intermittent high-pressure oxygen through this assembly can sustain a patient for 30 to 45 minutes while preparations for a cricothyroidotomy are made.

*The responsible clinician should always be prepared to implement an alternative plan if multiple intubation attempts fail.*

# Surgical Airway Access

## CRICOTHYROIDOTOMY

Cricothyroidotomy has been recommended for surgical emergency airway access because of its increased safety and speed compared to tracheostomy. Its potential for bleeding and encroachment on the mediastinum is much less than for tracheostomy. Cricothyroidotomy can potentially be performed by any primary care provider, with a relatively low morbidity rate. The indications for cricothyroidotomy include any airway-obstructing lesion that cannot be circumvented by translaryngeal endotracheal intubation. This includes both the anatomic disorders reviewed earlier and functional disorders such as trismus. Patients with apparent upper airway obstruction who present in extreme respiratory distress and cyanosis and fail a single attempt at intubation should undergo an immediate cricothyroidotomy as a life-saving maneuver. Delays caused by repeated attempts at intubation lead to a high morbidity and mortality rate. Some authorities have strongly recommended cricothyroidotomy in the presence of a cervical spine fracture. This injury is generally considered a relative indication for the procedure because endotracheal intubation can be accomplished with in-line stabilization.

The procedure of cricothyroidotomy is illustrated in Fig. 5–3. The cricothyroid membrane, which averages 9 mm in the cephalad-caudad dimension and 30 mm in the left-to-right dimension, is easily palpable in most subjects. This membrane is much

*Patients with apparent upper airway obstruction who present in extreme respiratory distress and cyanosis and fail a single attempt at intubation should undergo an immediate cricothyroidotomy.*

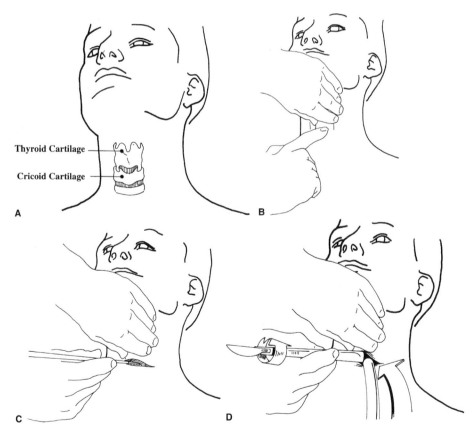

**FIGURE 5–3**
Cricothyroidotomy can be performed entirely with a single instrument—a knife blade. This sequence depicts the procedure. (*A*) The cricothyroid membrane is the preferred site of emergency airway access. (*B*) The thyroid cartilage is stabilized with one hand and the site of incision is palpated. (*C*) A transverse or vertical skin incision is carried down through the cricothyroid membranes. (*D*) The back end of the knife may be used to spread the cricothyroid space in order to introduce a tracheal tube.

smaller in children, particularly in those below the age of 10 to 12 years, and the procedure is not recommended in this patient population. Various authorities have recommended either a vertical or transverse skin incision, followed by a transverse incision through the laryngeal membrane. The use of a transverse skin incision has been criticized because it occasionally results in anterior jugular vein injury if taken too far laterally under duress. Once the airway is entered, the cricothyroid space may be spread with the knife handle or a specialized spreading device to permit the introduction of a tracheal tube. A 6-mm tracheal tube is frequently recommended for ease of placement and to avoid excessive distraction of the laryngeal cartilages by larger tubes.

Complications associated with cricothyroidotomy include subglottic stenosis (1%–4%), voice changes (15%), misplaced cannulas, and local wound problems (bleeding, infection). The most feared complication, subglottic stenosis, appears to occur most frequently in the presence of laryngeal inflammation, such as may occur following extended periods of translaryngeal intubation (7–10 days). Despite the low incidence of subglottic stenosis, cricothyroidotomy is recommended only as an emergency measure because of its seriousness. Although potentially any clinician can perform this procedure, the incidence of cannula malplacement has been reported to be as high as 67% in the hands of nonsurgeons. Such an event could result in sudden death due to unrelieved upper airway obstruction, suggesting that the procedure is preferably performed by a surgeon.

## TRACHEOSTOMY

Tracheostomy is used to provide airway access in a fashion similar to that provided by cricothyroidotomy except that instead of traversing the cricothyroid membrane, the tracheal tube is usually placed just below the second tracheal ring. The incidence of laryngeal injury is thus substantially lower. Tracheostomy is a more difficult procedure to perform, however, and is associated with two to five times the complication rate when performed during an emergency. Thus, under urgent conditions cricothyroidotomy is preferred. Occasionally, the presence of a subglottic tumor or thyroid-cartilage fracture can make an emergent tracheostomy the preferred approach because of the specific location of the pathology involved, but these circumstances are quite uncommon.

Tracheostomy is most commonly indicated for long-term mechanical ventilation, facilitation of airway hygiene, and relief of chronic upper airway obstruction that is not remediable by other means. Also, a cricothyroidotomy is usually converted to a tracheostomy if the expected duration of ventilation is prolonged, in order to minimize the incidence of voice dysfunction and subglottic stenosis. The most common indicator for tracheostomy is for the conversion of translaryngeal airway cannulation in patients intubated for mechanical ventilation. Complications associated with translaryngeal intubation that may be attenuated or eliminated by tracheostomy include oral or nasal tube discomfort, tube kinking or displacement, sinusitis, laryngeal dysfunction, and stenosis. Furthermore, management of bronchial secretions is usually much easier with a tracheostomy than with a translaryngeal tube. The recommended timing for this conversion to tracheostomy has been extensively debated without a clear resolution. Supporters for early conversion (7 days) suggest that patient comfort and the laryngeal complication rate are improved. Advocates of delayed tracheostomy (14–21 days) state that unnecessary procedures will be avoided, thereby reducing local wound complications (i.e., infection, postoperative hemorrhage, etc.). Most authorities have adopted an intermediate approach based upon their knowledge of the disease process being managed. If the patient is expected to be intubated much longer than 7 days, a tracheostomy is recommended early. However, if the patient's course cannot be predicted easily, it is acceptable to delay the decision until the need for tracheostomy becomes more evident.

### *When to Call the Surgeon about Airway Problems*

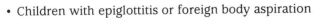

- Children with epiglottitis or foreign body aspiration
- Oropharyngeal infections or inflammatory lesions (e.g., retropharyngeal or peritonsillar abscess, epiglottitis with stridor, allergic angioedema with threatened airway)
- Patients with facial or laryngeal trauma or skull fracture
- Upper airway tumors
- Persisting stridor at any age
- Airway burns
- Acute airway obstruction due to aspiration of foreign bodies
- Head and neck anatomy suggesting difficult intubation
- Diagnostic or clinical findings provide evidence for an obstructive upper airway lesion

## RECOMMENDED READING

Ballenger, JJ, and Snow, JB (eds): Otorhinolaryngology: Head and Neck Surgery. Williams and Wilkins, Baltimore, 1996.

Boster, SR, and Martinez, SA: Acute upper airway obstruction in the adult. Postgrad Med 72:50–59, 1982.

Cohean, R, et al: Percutaneous dilatational tracheostomy. Arch Surg 131:265–271, 1996.

Darley, R, et al (eds): The airway: emergency management. Mosby-Year Book, St. Louis, 1992.

Guidelines for cardiopulmonary resuscitation and emergency cardiac care. JAMA 268:2135–2302, 1992.

Heffner, JE: Airway management in the critically ill patient. Crit Care Clin 6:533–550, 1990.

Heffner, JE (ed): Airway management in the critically ill patient. Clinics in Chest Medicine 12(3):1991.

Hollingsworth, HM: Wheezing and stridor. Clinics in Chest Medicine 8:231–240, 1987.

Miller, RD, and Hyatt, RE: Obstructing lesions of the larynx and trachea: clinical and physiologic characteristics. Mayo Clinic Proceedings 44:145–161, 1969.

Scott, PMJ: All that wheezes is not asthma. Brit J Clin Pract 49:43–44, 1995.

Shaefer, SD, and Close, LG: Acute management of laryngeal trauma. Ann Otol Rhinol Laryngol 98:98–104, 1989.

Shapskay, SM, et al: Obstructing tumors of the subglottic larynx and cervical trachea: Airway management and treatment. Ann Otol Rhinol Laryngol 97:487–492, 1989.

Weese, GL, et al: Bedside tracheostomy in the intensive care unit. Arch Surg 131:552–555, 1996.

# Chapter 6

# Breast Problems

MARY ANN KOSIR, MD,
RICHARD BLONDELL, MD,
and CHERYL GRIGORIAN, MD

## The Basics

Considerable resources are expended to detect and treat breast cancer. The expected new cases of breast cancer are 180,000 per year in the United States. The expected deaths from breast cancer are 45,000 per year. It is the most common cancer in women in the United States (excluding skin cancer) and follows lung cancer as the second most common cause of cancer death. Although the mortality statistics have been stable for 50 years, evidence now suggests that screening by mammography coupled with physical examination can decrease mortality by 30%. Currently, breast self-exam, practitioner exams, and mammography are the standard methods of detection and follow-up of breast cancer. In 7% to 10% of cases of a palpable cancer, however, the mammogram is negative, so a good history and physical exam are still the cornerstones of breast care. New developments for identifying individuals at increased risk include genetic testing for inherited genes implicated in breast cancer. Biomarkers and radio-pharmaceutical agents are being developed as diagnostic tools for breast cancer.

### HISTORY AND PHYSICAL EXAM

#### Elements of the History

Questions about the specific breast complaint should address the duration and description of symptoms and factors that affect the symptoms. Important background information includes timing of symptoms with the menstrual cycle, parity, use of hormonal preparations, nipple discharge, and other medical and surgical history, especially of the breasts. Questions should address the presence of risk factors (Table 6–1), even though about 75% of breast cancer cases involve women with no risk factors. If a patient

**TABLE 6-1**

### Risk Factors (and Relative Risk Factors) for Breast Cancer

First-degree relatives with breast cancer (mother, sister, daughter)
Other relatives with breast cancer (aunt, grandmother, other)
Personal history of breast cancer (risk increased 3-4 times)
Benign breast diseases such as sclerosing adenosis, multiple (peripheral) intraductal papillomas, and
   atypical ductal hyperplasia
First child after age 30
Nulliparity
Early menarche (before age 12)
Late menopause (after age 55)
Increasing age (risk increases with age)
Female gender (female:male ratio is 100:1 for breast cancer)
Exposure to radiation (e.g., irradiation of thymus, fluoroscopic exams, treatment of lymphoma)

has had biopsies of the breast, copies of the pathology and surgical reports may be important.

### Elements of the Physical Exam

Begin with the patient seated upright (Fig. 6-1). Examine the breasts for symmetry and direction of the nipples while her arms are raised and when her hands are placed on the hips. Pay attention to signs of dimpling, indicating a breast condition that is pulling on the suspensory ligaments of the breast, as in breast cancer. Make note of skin thickening, redness, asymmetry of the breasts or nipples, or scaling of the nipple and areola. Although palpation for axillary lymphadenopathy can be performed while the patient is supine, it may be easier to perform the axillary examination while the patient is sitting.

Breast palpation should be done with the patient supine. Occasionally, also palpating the breasts with the patient sitting upright may better define a breast problem. All areas of each breast should be palpated systematically, including the tail of Spence. Check for nipple discharge by gently pushing on the areola-nipple complex with two fingers.

FIGURE 6-1
Key aspects of the breast examination. (*A*) Examine the breasts and nipples for symmetry and dimpling while the patient is sitting, (*B*) with arms above the head, and (*C*) with arms on the hips. (*D*) Examine the axilla in the sitting position. (*E*) Palpate the breast and axilla, noting areas of tenderness, asymmetry, palpable masses, and nipple discharge. Measure the size of masses and determine mobility and shape, noting location and depth.

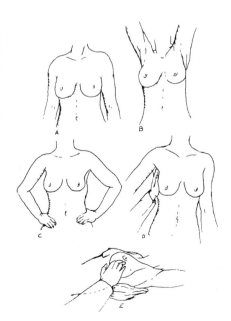

## BREAST IMAGING

### When to Order Mammography

There are two types of mammograms: screening and diagnostic. The purpose of a *screening mammogram* is to detect early breast cancer in generally asymptomatic women. The screening mammogram consists of two standard views only: the medio-lateral oblique (MLO) view, and the craniocaudal (CC) view. The presence of a radiologist on site is generally not required. The purpose of a *diagnostic mammogram* is to evaluate a breast symptom or follow a mammographic abnormality such as a mammographic mass, calcification, or asymmetric density thought to be benign. For women with implants or previous lumpectomy for cancer, special views are also required. Under these circumstances, a radiologist should be present to direct the exam.

Screening mammography can detect breast cancers that are smaller and at an earlier stage than can be detected by palpation alone, reducing breast cancer mortality in women between the ages of 50 and 69. There has been controversy between the recommendations of the American Cancer Society, the National Cancer Institute (NCI), and the U.S. Preventive Services Task Force (Table 6–2) as to how early to begin mammography screening. However, all major groups agree that women between the ages of 50 and 69 should receive a mammogram every 1 to 2 years and that judgment should be guided by the presence of risk factors, personal history of multiple benign breast problems, and life expectancy in the face of a negative physical exam. In addition, a dialogue with the patient is essential so that her wishes can be respected, should she request mammography. In early 1997, The American Cancer Society strongly advised yearly mammograms for women between 40 and 50 years of age. It is expected that the NCI will also support this new recommendation.

### When to Order Breast Ultrasonography

The main indications for breast ultrasonography are the following:

1. Mammographic evidence of a nonpalpable mass, in order to differentiate a cyst from a solid mass. Depending on the density of the breast, however, a mass demonstrated on mammography that is not seen by ultrasonography should be considered a solid mass.

2. The initial evaluation of a palpable mass in a woman under 30 years of age.

3. Evaluation of a palpable mass in a woman over 30 years of age with a negative mammogram.

4. Evaluation of an area of mammographic asymmetric density when a focal abnormality is suspected as the cause.

TABLE 6–2

| Recommendations for Screening Mammography | | | |
|---|---|---|---|
| Age | American Cancer Society | National Cancer Institute | U.S. Preventive Services Task Force |
| >50 yr | Yearly | Yearly | Every 1–2 years, depending on risk, clinical findings, previous radiologic exams*; for those with a reasonable life expectancy; no evidence of benefit otherwise over age 75 |
| 40–49 yr | Yearly | Yearly | Same as above |
| <40 yr | Baseline films between ages 35 and 40, frequency then based on risk factors | Depends on risk factors | Same as above |

*An example of radiologic findings is microcalcifications that are judged "probably benign." These should be followed with serial mammograms for up to 2 years to determine that they are stable.

Breast ultrasonography is *not* suited for breast cancer screening because it cannot reliably depict microcalcifications, which are the most important sign of ductal carcinoma.

Breast ultrasonography can accurately classify some solid lesions as benign, allowing imaging as follow-up rather than biopsy. Breast ultrasonography is also useful in performing a core biopsy of a breast mass. Stavrof and colleagues reported that in 750 breast nodules examined by ultrasonography that were also sampled by core biopsy, 123 of 125 were correctly classified as indeterminate or malignant (98.5% positive predictive value). Their negative predictive value was 99.5%. The radiologist should obtain at least five core samples while viewing the process under real-time ultrasonography to demonstrate that the core needle goes through the lesion, ensuring diagnostic adequacy. Solid masses larger than 10 mm in diameter can be sampled with ultrasound-guided core biopsy and can delineate benign disease that does not require further surgical treatment. In the cases of complicated cystic structures, ultrasound-guided aspiration should be performed.

*Ultrasonography is not suited for breast cancer screening because it cannot reliably depict microcalcifications.*

### Stereotactic Biopsy

The technique of stereotactic biopsy is used to sample abnormalities seen on mammography. These include microcalcifications, lesions not well seen on ultrasonography, and lesions seen in only one view by mammography. Core needle biopsies are obtained using a specialized mammographic unit. At least 5 samples from masses and 10 samples from microcalcifications should be obtained to ensure an adequate sample. If microcalcifications are seen, not all should be removed. Microcalcifications may be located in only a fraction of a cancerous tumor, yet they may represent the only way to identify the malignancy visually. An alternative is to place a small titanium clip at the time of stereotactic biopsy, as a marker. If the diagnosis is cancer, then the remaining microcalcifications or the clip can be localized by guide wire for excisional biopsy or even lumpectomy.

### Magnetic Resonance Imaging

Magnetic resonance imaging (MRI) is not routinely used due to its low specificity and high cost. The basic principle of enhancement of breast tissue with contrast is that enhancement is a reflection of the inherent blood supply. Therefore, many benign lesions and normal breast tissue in young women will exhibit enhancement. Research is studying the rate of enhancement of normal and benign tissue versus carcinoma. The current indications for MRI include:

1. To evaluate implant integrity.
2. To search for breast carcinoma in patients with biopsy-proven breast adenocarcinoma from a supraclavicular or axillary node, without a palpable breast mass and without evidence of a malignancy on mammography.
3. To evaluate chest wall masses seen on mammography in only one view or to assess chest wall recurrence of breast cancer.
4. To examine a patient who is at high risk for breast cancer for whom other imaging is limited, or to detect a recurrence at a lumpectomy site with equivocal mammographic findings.

MRI is not a substitute for mammography but rather a specialized examination usually recommended by the radiologist for specific indications.

## Clinical Problems

### PALPABLE BREAST MASS

Breast masses, whether palpable or not, occur in all age groups and need explanation. A complete history regarding risk factors for breast disease and physical examination of the breasts is essential. In a woman younger than 35, a palpable mass is more likely to be fibroadenoma, cyst, lipoma, or asymmetric fibroglandular tissue rather than breast cancer, but risk factors may influence the differential diagnosis. As age increases, the risk of cancer in a newly identified breast mass increases.

The palpable mass should be measured by caliper or ruler. Its shape, mobility, and texture should be noted. Likewise, associated skin changes or tenderness are important.

Imaging should be done by mammography (where appropriate for age). In addition to the palpable mass, there may be other nonpalpable abnormalities seen only on mammography, including satellite lesions. There may also be abnormalities in the contralateral breast that are not detectable on clinical examination. If the mass is not seen well on the mammogram, then an ultrasound should be performed. The ultrasound may determine whether the mass is solid or cystic. In a woman under 30 years of age with a palpable breast abnormality, an ultrasound should be obtained initially, because dense glandular tissue makes interpretation of mammograms difficult.

The next step is tissue diagnosis of the mass. A symptomatic simple cyst can be aspirated in the office. This may require ultrasound guidance. If it recurs, an excisional biopsy is recommended. Often the aspiration of a cyst will relieve pressure symptoms. If the cyst fluid is not clear yellow or the typical green-brown fluid, then it should be submitted for cytology—especially if bloody.

Fine-needle aspiration (FNA) is indicated for a palpable mass (Fig. 6–2). The FNA can be performed without a prior ultrasound or mammogram if the mass is easily palpated and able to be held during the FNA. Three findings are possible:

- a cancer,
- a fibroadenoma or fibrocystic breast disease, or
- cells that do not support either diagnosis.

A *fibroadenoma* can be followed, with reexamination, imaging, or both in a year because of the low potential risk of breast cancer (less than 0.1%). If there are no changes, it can be observed. If it increases in size, it becomes symptomatic, or if the patient prefers, then it should be removed. About one-third of fibroadenomas involute with menopause and become coarsely calcified on the mammogram. The exception is

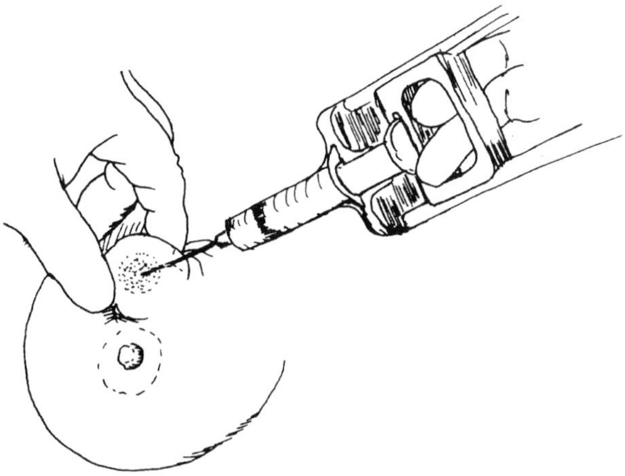

*In a woman under 30 years of age with a palpable breast abnormality, an ultrasound should be obtained initially.*

*Fine-needle aspiration (FNA) is indicated for a palpable mass.*

FIGURE 6–2

Technique of fine-needle aspiration (FNA). The mass should be immobilized with the fingers of one hand while the FNA is performed with the other hand. After preparing the skin, using sterile gloves, infiltrate the skin and anticipated needle tract with 1% xylocaine. Keep the mass immobile with one hand. With the other hand, aspirate the mass using continuous suction once the skin is entered by the needle (usually 21 gauge). Move the needle around in several directions while maintaining suction. When the needle is removed, place the specimen onto a slide or container as instructed by the pathologist. Separate the needle from the syringe, draw in air, and reattach the needle, pushing out remaining material from the hub of the needle.

the juvenile fibroadenoma, found in young girls after puberty; these should be removed because they can grow to great size and compress surrounding normal, developing breast tissue.

All cytologic diagnoses that are cellular, without a definite diagnosis, should lead to a core needle biopsy or excision of the palpable mass. Whenever an FNA result indicates inadequate sample for a diagnosis, a core needle biopsy should be performed to determine the tissue diagnosis rather than repeating the FNA.

### *When to Call the Surgeon about a Breast Mass*

- A tissue diagnosis must be made.
- Fine-needle aspiration is nondiagnostic or shows cells that are not clearly benign.
- A breast cyst recurs, or a mass remains after cyst aspiration.
- The breast examination demonstrates asymmetry, but not a well-defined area.
- The patient requests excision of a mass.
- There is a new mass after the start of hormone replacement therapy or during pregnancy.
- There is dimpling on the breast exam.
- The skin of the areola and nipple is abnormal.
- The skin of the breast is thickened, reddened, or both, resembling an orange peel.
- A tissue diagnosis of cancer has been established.

## ABNORMAL MAMMOGRAM

Table 6–3 describes abnormal mammographic findings of breast cancer, which include microcalcifications and breast masses that are not palpable. To reduce confusion that arises from the inconsistent use of descriptive terms, the American College of Radiology (ACR) has proposed reorganization of reports as well as a dictionary of terms that will be adopted by all radiologists. The basic format of the breast imaging report should include the following: pertinent clinical history and physical exam findings, type of

**TABLE 6–3**

### Mammographic Findings of Breast Cancer*

Mass
    Spiculated mass most often seen in invasive ductal carcinoma
    Circumscribed mass most often seen in well-defined ductal carcinoma
Calcification(s)
    Microcalcifications (clustered and heterogeneous) commonly seen in intraductal carcinoma
Asymmetric density
    Asymmetric density most often seen with infiltrating lobular carcinoma
Architectural distortion
Skin thickening
Skin retraction
Nipple retraction
Enlarged lymph nodes

*Lobular carcinoma in situ (LCIS) is usually not seen on mammography. It is most often an incidental pathologic finding. LCIS is not cancer, but rather, a marker for the increased risk of breast cancer bilaterally.

study, whether a previous examination is to be compared to the current examination, and a general summary of the distribution of breast tissue (provided as an indicator of the expected sensitivity of the examination, because dense breast tissue limits mammographic sensitivity). Next, a description of the findings, such as specifics for masses, calcifications, or asymmetric density, is included. Interpreting the report and making the referral is based on the ACR classification (0–5). The assessment of the findings should fit the following categories:

ACR 0: Needs additional evaluation; incomplete.

ACR 1: Negative. Follow screening recommendations.

ACR 2: Stable benign. Follow radiologic recommendations or follow screening recommendations.

ACR 3: Probably benign. Short-interval follow-up is suggested. Follow radiologic recommendations. Risk of cancer less than 3%. Findings may be described as a small benign-appearing nodule, multiple groups of coarse microcalcifications, or a slightly increased number of calcifications. The radiologist anticipates no change on subsequent studies. If changes occur, refer to a surgeon. If there are risk factors for breast cancer, some examiners refer patients to a surgeon earlier for an opinion.

ACR 4: Moderately suspicious. Has a 20% to 30% chance of breast cancer. Refer to a surgeon for tissue diagnosis.

ACR 5: Highly suspicious. Has at least an 80% chance of breast cancer. Refer to a surgeon for tissue diagnosis.

*Obtain a surgical opinion for patients with moderately suspicious and highly suspicious lesions on mammogram (ACR 4 and 5).*

It is important to obtain a surgical opinion for patients with moderately suspicious and highly suspicious lesions on mammogram (ACR 4 and 5). The repertoire of further diagnostic tests used by the general surgeon include needle-localized biopsy, stereotactic biopsy, and ultrasound-guided core biopsy. The choice of diagnostic tests affects the surgical options possible. For example, stereotactic biopsy (where available) of a nonpalpable suspicious mass (Fig. 6–3) can simplify the care of a patient with cancer. When the diagnosis of cancer is made by this method, the definitive cancer surgery (lumpectomy with radiation therapy and axillary dissection versus modified radial mastectomy) can be considered by the surgeon and patient. On the other hand, as already

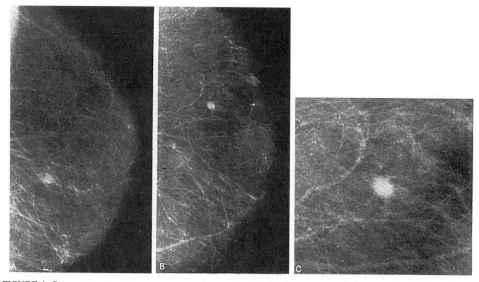

**FIGURE 6–3**
Abnormal mammogram: invasive ductal carcinoma. On (*A*) lateral and (*B*) craniocaudal views, a nonpalpable, spiculated mass is present more posteriorly in the lower outer quadrant of the breast. A magnified view in (*C*) shows the ill-defined edges of this mass. On pathologic exam it was found to be an infiltrating ductal carcinoma.

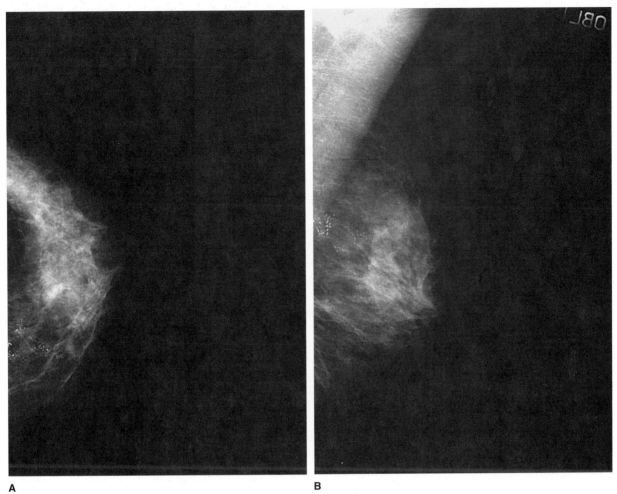

**A**  **B**

**FIGURE 6–4**
Abnormal mammogram: ductal carcinoma in situ. On two views, the left breast of this 38-year-old woman shows microcalcifications in a linear arrangement in the upper inner quadrant of the breast. She underwent a needle-localized biopsy, which showed ductal carcinoma in situ.

mentioned, for suspicious microcalcifications (Fig. 6–4), the stereotactic biopsy must leave some microcalcifications behind. If not, further surgical excision by lumpectomy would not be possible, since the area could not be localized. Under some circumstances, the needle-localized biopsy can achieve negative margins, hence lumpectomy, without the need for further surgery of the breast itself.

In another circumstance, a core-needle biopsy may be done despite an FNA showing cancer if neoadjuvant chemotherapy (i.e., chemotherapy before cancer surgery) is being considered. Neoadjuvant chemotherapy is used in large masses (>5 cm) where breast conservation surgery could be considered if the cancer shrinks. Again, the surgeon should coordinate this.

In cases of inflammatory breast carcinoma, a skin biopsy may be required within the area of any possible surgical excision. Again, chemotherapy and radiation therapy will be given prior to any surgery, and these steps require coordination among clinicians.

### *When to Call the Surgeon about an Abnormal Mammogram*

- ACR classification of 4 or 5
- ACR classification of 3 and a breast mass (palpable or nonpalpable) that requires tissue diagnosis

- Any ACR classification and a family history of breast cancer or ovarian cancer
- Any change in mammogram regarding microcalcifications, asymmetry, or masses

## BREAST PAIN

*Breast pain should not be dismissed without clinical examination and complementary imaging.*

Breast pain is a difficult problem because the symptom is subjective and individuals tolerate a wide range of pain. Nevertheless, the presence of breast cancer must be considered. Breast pain should not be dismissed as a cyclical premenstrual symptom without clinical examination and complementary imaging. Any palpable abnormalities should be evaluated as previously described.

After appropriate evaluation for any palpable lesions or abnormalities on imaging studies, other causes of breast pain should be considered. The problem may be related to the use of hormone replacement therapy, and the patient should then receive a lower dose. Other sources of exogenous estrogen, such as dietary sources and topical agents, should also be identified. Nonhormonal treatment options are available for those with vasomotor symptoms of the perimenopause. A properly fitting bra may alleviate pain, especially with cyclical swelling, when even a different size or style may help. An athletic bra may provide better support with less movement of the breasts, especially for active patients. Some work situations require repeated pressure against the anterior chest (and breasts). A change of job duties, even temporarily, may indicate if this is the cause of the pain. Danazol (danocrine) is indicated for fibrocystic disease when conservative measures fail to relieve symptoms. Some clinicians have used bromocriptine or tamoxifen. Some patients find relief with nonsteroidal anti-inflammatory agents. While the patient tries these measures, there should always be attention to the detection of cancer in the breast. Some imaging studies may need to be repeated at intervals. It is no longer acceptable to assume a noncancer diagnosis in the presence of breast pain.

### *When to Call the Surgeon about Breast Pain*

- Any mammographic or palpable abnormalities are present.
- A second opinion is desired.

## NIPPLE DISCHARGE

*Bloody discharge is commonly associated with an intraductal papilloma.*

The history and physical should include questions about whether the discharge occurs spontaneously (higher risk) or after manipulation (lower risk). In addition, the character of the nipple discharge should be noted. Bloody discharge is commonly associated with an intraductal papilloma. Nipple discharge that is bloody, coming from either a single duct or both, is of concern.

The examination should document the quadrant or location of the discharge. Radial palpation of the breast, "milking" toward the nipple, will identify which duct is involved (Fig. 6–5). If the findings suggest cancer, the fluid should be sent for cytologic examination. Some examiners prefer to spread the sample on a glass slide, and others prefer to place it on a frosted surface of the slide without further spreading. Usually a fixative is applied immediately. Check with the pathologist who will receive the specimen.

Mammography is indicated in women over 35 years of age who experience nipple discharge. Even though the cytology and mammogram are negative, referral to a surgeon is indicated whenever a patient wishes to undergo excision of the duct. Further workup may be performed, such as a ductogram, where the discharging duct is can-

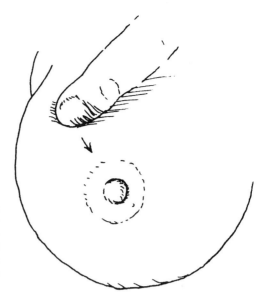

**FIGURE 6-5**
Technique of radial palpation for nipple discharge. During the breast examination, look for nipple discharge by palpating toward the nipple along a ductal system (like the spokes of a wheel). This helps identify any discharge and the duct involved. A ductogram and excisional biopsy of the duct can be performed.

nulated and dye is injected into it. The filling defects within the dye-filled duct are nonspecific; they can represent hyperplasia of the ductal cells or cancer. Nevertheless, this study may assist the surgeon in determining the extent of dissection of the duct.

For bilateral discharge, it is important to consider galactorrhea and an endocrine evaluation. In patients who have not breastfed in the previous year, bilateral discharge is abnormal. Hyperprolactinemia is responsible for most bilateral breast discharge and may be associated with amenorrhea or oligomenorrhea. The hyperprolactinemia may be due to several etiologies: Stimulation of the sensory nerves of the breast by trauma, scars, cancers, herpes zoster, or nipple manipulation by loose-fitting clothes or sexual foreplay can increase prolactin. Drugs that increase pituitary prolactin release are oral contraceptives, alpha-methyldopa, reserpine, tricyclic antidepressants, phenothiazines, and butyrophenones (haloperidol). Some diseases increase prolactin; these include disease of the hypothalamus or pituitary stalk, such as neurosarcoidosis; prolactin-secreting neoplasms, such as pituitary adenomas; and diseases associated with primary hypothyroidism and renal failure. Extremely elevated serum prolactin levels (>200 ng/mL) are usually due to a prolactin-secreting pituitary adenoma. MRI of the brain is the imaging study of choice for diagnosis. If the prolactin level is less than 50 ng/mL, a nonadenoma cause of nipple discharge is likely. If the level is between 50 and 200 ng/mL, patient counseling and repeated serial prolactin levels are recommended.

### When to Call the Surgeon about Nipple Discharge

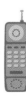

- The discharge is bloody, it comes from a single duct, or both.
- Abnormal cells are present on cytologic examination of the discharge.
- The patient requests excision of a duct with discharge.
- The patient has a pituitary adenoma and hyperprolactinemia (refer to neurosurgeon).

## NIPPLE ITCHING

The most important diagnosis to consider for the complaint of nipple itching is Paget's disease of the nipple, which is caused by intraductal carcinoma of the large subareolar

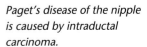

*Paget's disease of the nipple is caused by intraductal carcinoma.*

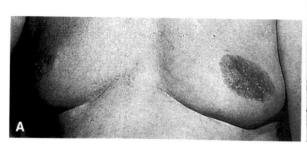
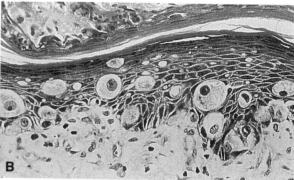

**FIGURE 6–6**
Paget's disease of the nipple. (*A*) The left breast has scaly, reddened, itchy skin of the areola and nipple, consistent with Paget's disease of the nipple. (*B*) Histologically, the skin contains cells with large nuclei. From Skarin, AT: Atlas of Diagnostic Oncology, ed 2. Mosby-Wolfe Limited, London, UK, 1991. See color photographs in Color Section 1.

ducts, with involvement of the nipple and areola (Fig. 6–6). A complete history and physical exam of the breasts, coupled with mammography (for women >30 years of age) should be performed. The scaling area of involvement may include not only the nipple itself, but also the areola, because the ducts can open in the areola.

Refer to a surgeon because a biopsy of the skin of the areola-nipple complex may be indicated.

### When to Call the Surgeon about Nipple Itching

- The itching is associated with scaling of the skin of the areola, the nipple, or both.
- There is an abnormal mammogram or palpable abnormality as well as nipple itching.

## ERYTHEMA AND PAIN OF THE BREAST

Breast abscess, mastitis and inflammatory breast carcinoma should be considered in women who present with breast erythema and pain. Breast abscess commonly occurs in younger women who are lactating. If there is no fever, leukocytosis or fluctuance, a trial of antibiotics alone is acceptable. If the mastitis does not respond to a short course of antibiotics, however, surgical treatment is indicated. Surgical drainage of the abscess is needed along with antibiotics to prevent breast destruction and to control the infection, so referral to a surgeon is indicated.

If significant inflammation of the skin lasts longer than several weeks, inflammatory breast carcinoma must be considered. Physical findings of thickened skin (*peau d'orange*) may also point to inflammatory breast cancer. A mammogram and referral to a surgeon are imperative.

### When to Call the Surgeon about Erythema and Pain of the Breast

- There is associated fever and leukocytosis requiring incision and drainage of the breast abscess in the operating room.
- There is a question of inflammatory breast carcinoma with or without mammographic or palpable abnormality.

## FAMILY HISTORY OF BREAST CANCER

With the availability of genetic testing and greater acceptance of prophylactic mastectomy based on genetic markers of risk, genetic counseling is indicated for people with a family history of breast cancer even without breast cancer symptoms. It is estimated that 10% to 15% of breast cancers are due to inherited factors. However, as research shows more mutations of these genetic markers, the assessment of risk may become more difficult. Although an individual may be negative for known genetic markers of breast cancer, new markers are under development. Referral to a genetic counselor or multidisciplinary breast center is indicated for patients at high risk for breast cancer because the criteria for testing and risk assessment are defined based on current knowledge. As new developments occur, these criteria will no doubt change.

Some authorities suggest imaging well before the usual age that breast cancer has appeared in a patient's family, especially in her mother. Ten years before the age of occurrence of cancer in a woman's premenopausal mother is not too early to begin genetic testing and screening for breast cancer.

### *When to Call the Surgeon about Family History of Breast Cancer*

- The patient requests prophylactic mastectomies.
- First-degree relatives have breast or ovarian cancer or both.
- Breast cancer occurred in relatives who were under 50 years of age.

## *Summary*

Each breast complaint requires a specific determination for cause. One of the aims of the evaluation is to determine the presence of carcinoma. Surgical treatment of certain benign conditions, as well as cancer, is appropriate.

Until other diagnostic tools are available, the history and physical examination, coupled with mammography, remain the primary means of screening for and finding breast cancer.

### *When to Call the Surgeon about Breast Disorders*

- Breast mass
- Abnormal mammogram
- Breast pain
- Nipple discharge or itching
- Erythema of the breast skin
- Breast abscess

### RECOMMENDED READING

Bassett, L: Breast Imaging. Current Status and Future Directions. Radiologic Clinics of North America 30:1–286, 1992.

Bassett, L, et al: Stereotactic core-needle biopsy of the breast: A report of the Joint Task Force of the American College of Radiology, American College of Surgeons, and College of American Pathologists. CA, A Cancer Journal for Clinicians 47:171–190, 1992.

Blondell, RD: Selected disorders of the endocrine and metabolic system. In Taylor, RB (ed): Family Medicine, Principles and Practice, ed 4. Springer-Verlag, New York, 1994, pp. 989–996.

Cady, B, et al: Evaluation of common breast problems: Guidance for primary care providers. CA, A Cancer Journal for Clinicians 48:49–63, 1998.

Eberlein, TJ: Current management of carcinoma of the breast. Ann Surg 220:121–136, 1994.

Harris, JR, et al (eds): Breast Diseases, ed 2. JB Lippincott Company, Philadelphia, 1991.

Hoskins, KF, et al: Assessment and counseling for women with a family history of breast cancer: A guide for clinicians. JAMA 273:577–585, 1995.

Jackson, VP: Breast imaging. Radiologic Clinics of North America 33:1027–1289, 1995.

Stavrof, AT, et al: Solid breast nodules: Use of sonography to distinguish between benign and malignant lesions. Radiol 196:123–134, 1995.

Taubes, G: The breast-screening brawl. Science 275:1056–1059, 1997.

Wells, SA, Young VL, Andriole, DA (eds): Atlas of Breast Surgery. Mosby-Yearbook, Inc., St. Louis, 1994.

# Chest Pain

JAMES TYBURSKI, MD,
and LAWRENCE RAYMOND, MD, ScM

As one of the most common reasons for seeing the doctor, chest pain has implications that range from life-threatening to trivial. It is never trivial to the one in pain, however. There are few instances of chest pain that do not warrant some medical contact, if only for reassurance.

## Coronary Artery Disease

Atherosclerotic cardiovascular disease and its risk factors are so common in developed countries that coronary insufficiency must be seriously considered in any patient who complains of chest pain. Even in the *absence* of chest discomfort, this condition should be included in the differential diagnosis of many sudden illnesses, since about 20% of myocardial infarctions are silent. Specific therapy that can improve both the immediate and long-term outcomes of many patients is often available. Risk stratification of all patients with myocardial ischemia has been greatly improved by the addition of blood tests for cardiac troponins T and I. These indicators offer promise for improving the precision of therapeutic choices for subsets of these patients.

*About 20% of myocardial infarctions may be silent.*

Patients with symptomatic coronary artery disease present most commonly with chest pain. In cases of either angina pectoris or myocardial infarction, the pain is typical in character and location. The character of the pain is usually aching or described as a tightness or heaviness. The pain is usually substernal or left anterior and may radiate down the anteromedial aspect of the left arm. With angina, the episode may be brought on by exertion or stress and may be relieved with rest or nitroglycerin. Each episode of angina typically lasts 1 to 10 minutes. With myocardial infarction, the pain is unremitting and may be accompanied by diaphoresis, nausea, and vomiting.

The primary provider caring for a patient with unstable angina or myocardial infarction must quickly decide which form of therapy is optimal, available, and acceptable to the patient and family. The logistics of such therapy can be improved by minimizing

TABLE 7–1

## Contraindications to Thrombolytic Therapy

Unstable hypertension (200/120)
Suspected dissecting aneurysm
Intracranial tumor or vascular malformation
Major bleeding, surgery, or trauma within past 3 months
Bleeding diathesis
Pregnancy
Stroke within past 6 months

the denial phase, which sometimes causes serious delay. One may recall patients like the senior congressman at home with angina, waiting for a return call from his physician, who was attending Sunday morning services. The congressman collapsed by the phone and could not be resuscitated. A short ride to the hospital could have saved his life, as it might the lives of many other patients, half of whom who delay their care by 2 to 6 hours. All patients who have coronary risk factors should, of course, be helped to modify the ones they can modify and be treated for the treatable ones. Should they not also be coached on how to react to the early phase of myocardial ischemia, just as diligently as we counsel patients to recognize early breast or skin cancer?

Among the current treatment options, several require advanced diagnostic and interventional procedures or surgical approaches not readily available to all patients. For example, emergency percutaneous transluminal coronary angioplasty (PTCA) may not be an option in about 80% of hospitals. In those hospitals, urgent use of thrombolytic agents will be the best treatment for those without contraindications (Table 7–1). Thrombolysis can be offered with the assurance that it is highly likely to improve survival and cardiac function.

In some locations and for all patients in whom thrombolysis is contraindicated, transfer to a facility where PTCA is available deserves serious consideration. The further delay associated with such transfers may compromise the patient's outcome, however. (Death or serious complications occur early in over 20% of patients ineligible for reperfusion therapy.) Although it is urgent to recognize and treat those who stand to benefit from such measures, it is also necessary to identify those who may not need such interventions, such as patients in Killip Class I (Table 7–2), especially in the absence of recurrent angina or other peri-infarction instability.

For more seriously ill patients in institutions where PTCA is available, the choices of therapy include PTCA (with or without stenting), thrombolytic agents, and coronary artery bypass grafting (CABG). Substantial controversy exists over the choice between PTCA and thrombolysis as primary therapy, where both are options. Nine large studies suggest that thrombolytic therapy given within 12 hours of the onset of symptoms will save 20 to 40 lives per 1000 patients treated. The *ideal* candidate is one with anterior

TABLE 7–2

## Killip Classification of Patients with Acute Myocardial Infarction

| Class | Definition | Patients with Acute Myocardial Infarction Admitted to CCU in This Category (%) |
|---|---|---|
| Class I | Absence of rales and absence of S3 | 30–40 |
| Class II | Rales over 50% or less of the lung fields or the presence of S3 | 30–50 |
| Class III | Rales over more than 50% of the lung fields (frequently pulmonary edema) | 5–10 |
| Class IV | Shock | 10 |

ST-segment elevations or bundle-branch block, who is 55 to 75 years old. Evidence of improved outlook also extends to other age groups and sites of infarction and is not erased by effects of blood pressure and Killip Classes III or IV. PTCA has not been as extensively studied and may be viewed as a secondary procedure for patients in whom thrombolytic therapy is contraindicated or does not restore perfusion. It should be emphasized that local considerations may alter the relative merits of thrombolysis versus PTCA, since success with any intervention requires a critical mass of performance experience.

When is CABG necessary? For the 5% to 10% of patients in Killip Class IV, it may be a life-saving measure. In preparation for CABG, pulmonary artery catheterization and intra-aortic balloon counterpulsation may optimize treatment of patients in shock. In other patients whose critical lesions are demonstrated angiographically after the failure of thrombolytic agents, if angioplasty or stenting are not deemed optimal approaches, then early CABG may be the preferred treatment, especially in those with diabetes. The role of "surgical standby" for the less invasive procedures will vary from one institution to another. The need for close cooperation between primary care providers, cardiologists, and thoracic surgeons is obvious, although the primary provider generally consults first with cardiology.

# Noncoronary Cardiovascular Causes of Chest Pain

Many cardiovascular conditions other than coronary insufficiency can cause chest pain. Those that may require surgical intervention are aortic dissection, pericarditis with pericardial tamponade or constriction, and pulmonary emboli.

## AORTIC DISSECTION

Dissecting aortic aneurysm is a medical-surgical emergency in every sense of the word, since its correct diagnosis and management are truly life-saving. The pathophysiology of aortic dissection is a rent in the intima of the aorta with dissection of blood into the media. This "false lumen" may propagate either proximally or distally from the initial site (Fig. 7–1).

The symptoms from a dissection are due to the dissection itself, ischemia of organs whose blood supply is compromised by occlusion of aortic branches, and compression of periaortic structures. The chest pain in patients with dissecting aneurysm is classically described as quite severe, unrelenting, and having an unusual, tearing quality with radiation to the interscapular region or elsewhere in the back. If dissection is proximal,

**FIGURE 7–1**
Proximal aortic dissection. Note the true and false lumen in the ascending aorta.

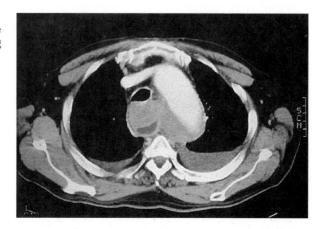

aortic valve regurgitation and pericardial tamponade, with their associated signs and symptoms, can result. Distal involvement may present as a loss of peripheral pulses, acute asymmetry in blood pressures, bowel ischemia, and renal failure. Ischemia to the central nervous system may be secondary to cerebral vessel involvement or ischemia to the spinal cord. Dysphagia, changes in voice, and Horner's syndrome can be present due to compression of adjacent neural structures.

Chest radiographs may show a widened mediastinum or a left-sided pleural effusion. The electrocardiogram is often nondiagnostic. Transthoracic ultrasound imaging may be diagnostic, although in some instances the transesophageal technique may be necessary. Aortography has been the gold standard diagnostic test to confirm the diagnosis, but is being challenged by MRI, which, if available, visualizes the dissection well and does not involve the use of intravascular radiologic dyes.

*A surgeon should be consulted in all cases of aortic dissection, as changing conditions may necessitate emergent surgery.*

A surgeon should be consulted in all cases of aortic dissection, even if the initial plan is for medical management, because changing conditions may necessitate emergent surgery. Absolute indications for surgical repair include ischemia of vital organs, severe aortic valve regurgitation, cardiac tamponade, and severe, continued pain (a sign of continued propagation). Surgical consultations should not delay the initiation of medical control of blood pressure and cardiac contractility.

### *When to Call the Surgeon about Aortic Dissection*

- Always when the diagnosis is seriously considered (suspicion often based on history and findings on chest x-ray)
- Especially with proximal dissection, organ ischemia, or evidence of continued propagation

## PERICARDITIS

Most patients with acute pericarditis have a self-limited illness, often of viral etiology. The classic presentation features severe, pleuritic substernal discomfort relieved by leaning forward. Examination often finds a three-component friction rub, sometimes accompanied by a separate pleural rub. Surgical input becomes important when pericarditis leads to pericardial tamponade or constrictive pericarditis.

### *Pericardial Tamponade*

Cardiac tamponade occurs when a pericardial effusion becomes large enough to compromise cardiac function. The rate of accumulation of fluid greatly influences the amount that causes hemodynamic changes. A modest effusion (150–200 mL) will cause symptoms if it occurs acutely, as in trauma, whereas an effusion of more than 1200 mL may be relatively asymptomatic if it accumulates slowly, as in uremia. The final common pathway is increasing pericardial pressure, which decreases ventricular filling, progressing to right atrial and right ventricular diastolic collapse.

The signs of cardiac tamponade can include the well-known triad of distant heart sounds, distended neck veins, and hypotension. In many instances, however, the signs are not as clear and more like congestive heart failure. The presence of pulsus paradoxus (a drop in blood pressure with inspiration that exceeds the normal 6 to 10 mm Hg) is strongly suggestive of pericardial tamponade. Paradoxical pulses may also be present in severe asthma and other forms of obstructive lung disease, however, so the finding must be interpreted with caution.

The electrocardiogram (ECG) may show low-amplitude QRS complexes and electrical alterans. A pulmonary artery catheter will reveal equalization of right-atrial, right-ventricular, and pulmonary-artery diastolic pressures; all are elevated in most circumstances. Echocardiography has become the method of choice in diagnosing cardiac tamponade. It is reliable, widely available, and noninvasive. It not only can establish the presence of a pericardial effusion, but it also can assess the presence of septal shift and diastolic collapse of the right atrium and ventricle.

The treatment of pericarditis is medical, but if an effusion is present or develops, a patient must be observed for signs of tamponade. Serial echocardiography, along with venous and arterial pressure monitoring, is warranted with increasing or large effusions. If the condition progresses to cardiac tamponade, then removal of the pericardial fluid becomes critical. Pericardiocentesis can be employed in the acute setting and is both diagnostic and therapeutic. It is done quite safely and effectively under echocardiographic guidance. A catheter may be left in place to drain further fluid.

Many times, however, a surgical pericardial window via either the subxiphoid or transthoracic approach is necessary if long-term drainage is required or adequate drainage cannot be performed via pericardiocentesis. Great care must be exercised on induction of general anesthesia in such patients, as all cardiac depressants should be avoided. The pericardial window has the advantage of providing more reliable long-term drainage of the pericardial space and allows for collection of tissue samples (e.g., pericardium) for diagnosis. A drain may be left in the pericardial sac or a chest tube (if the transthoracic approach is employed) may drain any additional effusion.

Surgical consultation should be sought for any patient with an enlarging pericardial effusion so that the patient can be properly evaluated by the surgeon before clinical tamponade is evident. The greater the hemodynamic instability of the patient, the greater the risk of pericardial manipulation, particularly because cardiac depressive drugs must be avoided.

## CONSTRICTIVE PERICARDITIS

One of the long-term sequelae of a bout of pericarditis is the formation of constricting scar tissue surrounding the heart. The pericardial space is obliterated in the formation of a thick, adherent scar. These patients present with signs of general malaise, mild dysphagia, and often congestive hepatomegaly and ascites. Careful evaluation of ECG, echocardiography, and cardiac catheterization is needed to distinguish this from other cardiomyopathies. The distinction is important because constrictive pericarditis is treatable by surgical removal of the pericardium. The earlier the diagnosis, the better the chances for a more complete resection without damage to the myocardium, which occurs when extensive scarring and calcification invade deeply into the myocardium (Fig. 7–2). A surgeon should be consulted when the diagnosis of constrictive pericarditis is made, for definitive treatment of the condition.

*Constrictive pericarditis is treatable by surgical removal of the pericardium.*

FIGURE 7–2
Pericarditis with calcifications. Note the calcification on the distended pericardium.

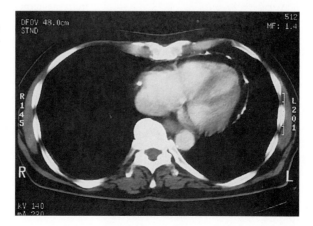

*When to Call the Surgeon about Pericarditis*

• When a large effusion is not responding to medical therapy

• For any traumatic pericardial effusion

• At the earliest sign (clinical or echocardiographic) of tamponade

• When a tissue specimen (e.g., pericardium) is needed for culture or other diagnostic purposes

• For constrictive pericarditis

## PULMONARY EMBOLISM AND DEEP VENOUS THROMBOSIS

Pulmonary embolism (PE) and the closely associated condition of deep venous thrombosis (DVT) are prominent causes of preventable morbidity and mortality. Although the vast majority of patients with these conditions are treated medically with anticoagulants or thrombolytic therapy, some specific conditions warrant surgical intervention.

Surgical procedures in PE treatment include placement of a vena caval filter, ligation of the vena cava, and pulmonary embolectomy. The placement of a vena caval filter is by far the most common surgical procedure performed for PE/DVT. This involves the placement (usually percutaneously) via the jugular or femoral veins of a wire filter that allows continued venous flow and catches all but very small (<2 mm) emboli. The most commonly used filter is the Titanium Greenfield Vena Cava Filter. This is the most widely evaluated filter and has been shown to be more than 95% effective at preventing pulmonary emboli.

*Indications for a vena caval filter include a patient with a known DVT and a contraindication to anticoagulation.*

The indications for the placement of a vena caval filter include a patient with a known DVT and a contraindication to anticoagulation, a patient who develops a complication from anticoagulants, and a patient who develops a PE while receiving adequate medical therapy. Relative indications for a filter include a pre-existing cardiopulmonary disease and a DVT in a patient who would not survive a PE—even a relatively minor one—or a massive PE in a patient who would not survive a recurrent embolism. Somewhat more controversial is its use as a prophylactic measure in a multiple-trauma patient at high risk of developing a DVT (with obvious contraindications to anticoagulants).

Surgical ligation of the vena cava, which causes lower-extremity swelling and requires surgical access to the retroperitoneum, is largely of historical interest in the face

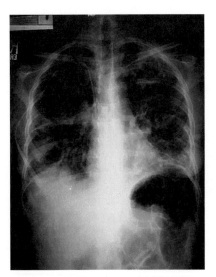

FIGURE 7–3
Septic pulmonary emboli. Note the multiple bullous lesions from long-term septic emboli.

of vena cava filters. It is indicated, however, in the unusual circumstances of life-threatening septic emboli originating from a pelvic source that are not responding to anticoagulants or antibiotics (Fig. 7–3). In this setting, elimination of all infected emboli is indicated.

Pulmonary embolectomy has been used as a life-saving procedure in the patient in shock who is not responsive to pharmaceutical therapy. It is obviously very invasive and requires complete cardiopulmonary bypass capabilities. It has had limited success in some cases, and it has been supplanted in some centers by the use of invasive radiological techniques using local thrombolytic or mechanical extraction procedures.

### *When to Call the Surgeon about DVT/PE*

- Failure, contraindication, or complication of anticoagulation therapy
- Septic emboli not responding to medical therapy
- Consideration of pulmonary embolectomy for a patient in shock

## Traumatic Causes of Chest Pain

A patient with blunt thoracic trauma and chest pain may have a myriad of injuries, ranging from benign to life-threatening. In general, it is prudent to seek surgical consultation in any chest trauma with significant pain or tenderness.

## RIB FRACTURES

The diagnosis of rib fractures is a clinical one. X-ray findings are of minor importance when compared to the clinical pulmonary status of the patient. The inability to maintain oxygenation and (much more commonly) ventilation is of far greater concern. A patient with a severe chest-wall contusion who cannot take a deep breath and cough is at high risk of subsequent pneumonia, whether or not there is radiographic evidence of a rib fracture. Indeed, many chest radiographs do not reveal rib fractures that are proven on autopsy. Rib radiographs provide no additional information and should be condemned as time consuming and expensive.

The clinical ability to ventilate is the key factor in deciding treatment. If a patient can demonstrate a good cough and the ability to breath deeply, then oral analgesia (non-narcotic) may be the only treatment necessary. However, if the patient's ability to ventilate is compromised significantly, then local or regional pain relief is needed in the form of intercostal nerve blocks, thoracic epidural catheter placements, or both. These patients must undergo vigorous pulmonary toilet during the period of pain relief to clear secretions and eliminate atelectasis. Systemic narcotics, with their respiratory depressive effects, should be avoided.

A *flail chest* is defined as a section of chest wall in which at least three consecutive ribs are each broken in two places, resulting in a free-floating segment of chest wall. Again, the major consideration is the ability to ventilate and oxygenate, not the number of rib fractures. Pain control and respiratory support should be initiated as early as indicated.

*Pulmonary contusion*, the bruising of lung parenchyma, is a major sequela of blunt thoracic trauma. It usually occurs in high-energy trauma, such as automobile accidents or a fall from height. It is usually associated with rib fractures, but not necessarily so, especially in the pediatric population, who have very elastic chest walls. It presents as a high A-a oxygen difference in a trauma patient with a chest radiograph demonstrating a hazy density. A useful early indicator of the severity of the contusion is the $PaO_2/FIO_2$ ratio. Many patients with an initial ratio less than 300 will require intubation.

*Rib radiographs provide no additional information and should be condemned as time consuming and expensive.*

## TRAUMATIC RUPTURE OF THE AORTA

Blunt trauma associated with a significant energy transfer may result in a traumatic rupture of the aorta. The rupture most commonly occurs in the descending thoracic aorta just distal to the takeoff of the left subclavian artery. Most of these patients die before they reach the hospital. Those who arrive alive have a contained rupture, which is at risk to rupture freely at any time.

Patients often complain of chest and intrascapular pain. Physical signs of a thoracic aorta rupture include pulse deficits, upper extremity hypertension, and a precordial systolic murmur. The chest radiograph may be normal or may reveal any combination of a widened mediastinum, obscuring of the aortic knob, depression of the left mainstem bronchus, or deviation of the esophagus (nasogastric [NG] tube) to the right. A hemothorax is indicative of a free rupture into the pleural space. The diagnosis is confirmed by aortogram and the treatment is surgical repair. During the time the patient is being stabilized, it is important (as in an aortal dissection) to monitor the arterial blood pressure and not allow the patient to be hypertensive.

Surgical consultation should be obtained in all multiple trauma patients, especially when the diagnosis of traumatic rupture of the aorta is being considered. The decision for transfer or treatment will depend on the level of expertise and facilities available locally.

*When to Call the Surgeon about Blunt Thoracic Trauma*

- Any chest trauma with significant pain or tenderness
- A patient with a rib fracture and poor pulmonary toilet
- A patient with a flail chest segment
- A patient with a pulmonary contusion
- When the diagnosis of traumatic rupture of the aorta is being considered
- A patient with traumatic pneumothorax or hemothorax

## *Pneumothorax*

The introduction of air into the pleural space causes pleuritic chest pain, loss of lung volume, and impairment in pulmonary function. The degree of clinical significance is dependent on the extent of lung collapse and the amount of pulmonary reserve (Fig. 7–4).

Pneumothoraces can be divided into three categories: spontaneous, traumatic, and

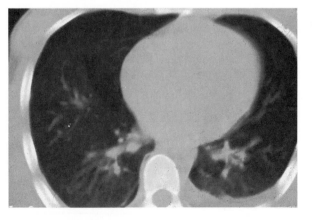

FIGURE 7–4
CT scan of single right-sided pneumothorax.

tension pneumothoraces. A *spontaneous pneumothorax*, as the name implies, occurs without an identifiable inciting event. Patients often have a history of underlying lung disease or cigarette smoking. The patient presents with pleuritic chest pain and varying degrees of shortness of breath. A small spontaneous pneumothorax in a stable patient without respiratory distress may be observed, with the possible employment of supplemental oxygenation to hasten the reabsorption of the pleural air. If the pneumothorax is larger, then simple aspiration can be employed, but if the patient is in respiratory distress, the pneumothorax enlarges, or the pneumothorax reoccurs following the above measures, then a tube thoracostomy should be performed.

If a chest tube is inserted, any air leak must be closely monitored, because this is an important factor in avoiding reoccurrence once the tube is removed. If this is a recurrent episode, then a sclerosing agent should be administered via the chest tube to help avoid future recurrences. If there is a large air leak, and particularly if the lung does not expand with tube thoracostomy, the patient should be evaluated for thoracoscopy, as bleb resection and pleural abrasion are quite effective as definitive treatment.

*Traumatic pneumothoraces* can be the result of either blunt trauma, penetrating trauma, or barotrauma. Small pneumothoraces secondary to blunt trauma can be observed in controlled, monitored conditions, but tube thoracostomy is employed much more aggressively than with spontaneous pneumothoraces because of the unpredictable nature of the injuries and the concurrent condition of hemothorax. A surgeon should be consulted in all cases of traumatic pneumothorax or hemothorax because these conditions can rapidly deteriorate into life-threatening symptoms. A high-output chest tube or a large air leak may signify significant vascular injury or tracheal bronchial disruption. Significant exceptions to the axiom that traumatic pneumothoraces require a chest tube are those that are secondary to a central line placement or a thoracentesis. These iatrogenic pneumothoraces generally have a benign course and can be treated with conservative measures.

> • **▬▬**
> *A surgeon should be consulted in all cases of traumatic pneumothorax or hemothorax, which can rapidly deteriorate into life-threatening symptoms.*

A *tension pneumothorax* occurs when the pleural pressures become positive enough to cause a shift of the mediastinum. This combination severely compromises cardiac output and can rapidly cause profound hypotension and death. Tension pneumothorax occurs almost exclusively in patients on positive pressure ventilation. Signs of this condition are clinical hypotension, absent breath sounds, hyperresonance by percussion, distention of neck veins, and shift of the trachea from the midline. Treatment is immediate decompression using a large-bore IV catheter followed by tube thoracostomy. Because of the propensity for simple pneumothoraces to become tension pneumothoraces in patients undergoing positive pressure ventilation, no pneumothorax, regardless of size, can go untreated in patients on mechanical ventilatory support. *All* pneumothoraces in patients on positive pressure ventilation *need* tube thoracostomy treatment.

> • **▬▬**
> *All pneumothoraces in patients on positive pressure ventilation need tube thoracostomy treatment.*

## Traumatic Hemothorax

The presence of blood in the pleural space is common to thoracic trauma. As with pneumothoraces, some small hemothoraces secondary to blunt trauma in hemodynamically stable patients may be observed. In general, hemothoraces secondary to penetrating trauma should be treated with tube thoracostomy. As with the pneumothoraces, an exception is the rare hemothorax or hydrothorax that occurs after the placement of a cervical venous catheter. These can often be treated with removal of the catheter, careful observation, and radiographic studies. Occasionally, however, the injury to large intrathoracic vessels can be catastrophic, with a massive hemothorax. If chest pain develops after the placement of a central venous catheter or during the infusion of IV fluids, the catheter should be evaluated and the infusion stopped. A surgeon should be consulted to evaluate virtually all traumatic hemothoraces or hydrothoraces.

## EMPYEMA

*Empyema* is the presence of purulent material in the pleural space. This can be due to a multitude of causes, but trauma, lung abscess, and progression of a parapneumonic effusion are the most common. Effective antibiotic treatment for lung abscesses and adequate drainage of traumatic hemothoraces or pneumothoraces are of paramount importance in prevention. A tube thoracostomy should be placed once the diagnosis of empyema has been reached (usually by thoracentesis). Empyemas often become loculated rather quickly. Computed tomography (CT) scanning can be very valuable in defining the anatomy of the empyema and in guiding the placement of a chest tube for drainage. If these measures do not work alone with the administration of proper antibiotics, an open drainage or decortication may be indicated. Surgical consultation should be sought immediately once the diagnosis of empyema is made.

### *When to Call the Surgeon about Pneumothorax, Hemothorax, or Empyema*

- For spontaneous pneumothoraces not responding to tube thoracostomy or with a persistent or large air leak
- For traumatic pneumothorax or hemothorax, especially secondary to penetrating trauma
- For chest pain or hydrothorax or hemothorax associated with a central venous catheter
- Once the diagnosis of empyema is made

## *Esophageal Diseases*

### ACHALASIA

*Achalasia* is characterized by the failure of the lower esophageal sphincter to relax, resulting in marked abnormalities in esophageal function. Chest pain along with dysphagia and regurgitation of undigested food are the classic triad of symptoms. The markedly dilated esophagus may be visible on chest x-ray, particularly if there is an air-fluid level in the mediastinum. Diagnosis is confirmed with an esophagram. Medical treatment is generally not effective. Either endoscopic balloon dilation of the lower esophageal sphincter or surgical division of the muscles of the distal esophagus is required. The balloon dilation method is generally effective, but it usually requires repeated sessions and poses the risk of perforation. If balloon dilation fails or if a perforation occurs, surgical consult should be obtained.

### REFLUX ESOPHAGITIS

*Reflux esophagitis*, the reflux of acidic gastric contents into the esophagus, is also a cause of noncardiac chest pain. The treatment is generally medical, but mechanical strictures, Barrett's esophagus (metaplasia of the distal esophagus), or dysplasia of the esophagus may warrant a surgical antireflux procedure. Dysplasia is especially worrisome, as moderate to severe dysplasia may be indicative of invasive cancer; resection may be indicated.

### ESOPHAGEAL PERFORATION

Esophageal perforation is a condition treatable with acceptable morbidity if it is recognized and treated promptly, but delays in diagnosis and initiation of treatment can be devastating. Perforation is classified as iatrogenic, spontaneous (usually related to vomiting), traumatic, or secondary to intrinsic esophageal disease (usually from transluminal carcinoma).

Chest pain, usually closely related to the level of the perforation, is a consistent finding. Nausea and vomiting with hematemesis are not uncommon. Perforation into the pleural cavity causes pleural effusion and significant respiratory symptoms. Early signs of sepsis, such as tachycardia and hypotension, are common. Physical signs of mediastinal air by auscultation include crackling with each heart beat, known as Hamman's crunch. A chest x-ray with mediastinal air and pleural effusion with a suggestive history is highly indicative of esophageal perforation. A high amylase content in the pleural effusion confirms the diagnosis. Any patient suspected of esophageal perforation should have an esophagram to confirm the diagnosis and delineate the site of perforation, which greatly influences the treatment options. The initial esophagram should be performed with diatrizoate meglumine (Gastrografin). If this is negative, then barium should be used. Barium has a higher sensitivity, but is more irritating if introduced into the mediastinum. Surgical consultation should be sought for a patient with a pleural effusion or pneumomediastinum or both in the context of recent esophageal instrumentation, ingestion of a foreign body or caustic substance, vomiting or retching, or known esophageal disease with chest pain. Early surgery can be very effective in reducing long-term morbidity. Broad spectrum antibiotics also should be administered early in the treatment plan while surgery is being contemplated.

### When to Call the Surgeon about Esophageal Disease

- Achalasia not responding to endoscopic dilation
- Reflux esophagitis not responding to medical therapy
- Reflux esophagitis with Barrett's esophagitis containing dysplasia of mucosa
- Whenever perforation is being considered (postesophagoscopy or suspected "spontaneous" perforation after vomiting).
- A diagnosis of esophageal cancer is made

## RECOMMENDED READING

Braunwald, E: Pericardial disease. In Isselbacher, KJ, et al (eds): Harrison's Principles of Internal Medicine. McGraw-Hill, New York, 1994, p. 1094–1101.

Collins, R, et al: Aspirin, heparin, and fibrinolytic therapy in suspected acute myocardial infarction. N Engl J Med 336:847–860, 1997.

Northfield, TC: Oxygen therapy for spontaneous pneumothorax. Br Med J 4:86, 1971.

Peterson, ED, et al: Risk stratification after myocardial infarction. Ann Int Med 126:561–582, 1997.

Simoons, ML: Myocardial revascularization—bypass surgery or angioplasty? N Engl J Med 335:275–276, 1996.

Skinner, DB: Perforation of the esophagus: Spontaneous (Boerhaave's syndrome), traumatic, and following esophagoscopy. In Sabiston DC (ed.): Textbook of Surgery. WB Saunders, Philadelphia, 1991, p. 701–704.

Wilson, RF, Steiger Z: Thoracic trauma: Chest wall and lung. In Wilson, RF, Walt, AJ (eds.): Management of Trauma: Pitfalls and Practice. Williams & Wilkins, Baltimore, 1996, p. 314–342.

# Hand Problems

CHENICHERI BALAKRISHNAN, MD,
and MARK P. KNUDSON, MD, MSPH

Throughout history the hand has distinguished man from most other animals, allowing humans to explore the environment and put thought into action. Unfortunately, disorders of the hand are very common. Approximately a third of all industrial accidents and a third of the patients presenting to the emergency room have disorders involving the hand. Assessment of hand disorders requires understanding of hand anatomy, understanding of common conditions of the hand, and integration of the individual patient's history and physical examination. Disorders of the hand are of great significance to the patient. Restoration of grasp, power and precision, pinch, tactile sensation, and normal appearance are the goals in treating hand disorders.

## *Diagnosis of Hand Disorders*

A history of hand disorders should include the patient's age and occupation, and documentation of the dominant hand. Elicit the mechanism of injury, where the injury happened, and any history of previous injuries. Inquire about the patient's perception of pain, sensory loss, and loss of hand function.

Physical examination of the hand must be methodical. Inspection of the skin may reveal unsuspected injury or confirm the extent of a known injury. Malalignment of hand structures may be evident with observation. The integrity of tendons, muscles, and ligaments can be checked by examining both active and passive range of motion of the joints of the hand and wrist.

Some tendons, such as the flexor digitorum profundus (FDP) and the flexor digitorum superficialis (FDS) require special attention. Stabilize the middle phalanx to test the FDP and its ability to flex the distal phalanx at the distal interphalangeal joint (DIP). Immobilize the distal phalanx of the surrounding digits to test the FDS with flexion of the middle phalanx at the proximal interphalangeal joint (PIP). (*Note*: the

FDP can flex the PIP also but cannot contract one digit independent of the surrounding digits.)

The motor and sensory function of the three main nerves should be evaluated to determine the nerves' integrity. On the dorsal aspect of the hand, the radial nerve innervates the thumb, the proximal aspect of the index finger and middle finger, and the radial aspect of the ring finger. The median nerve innervates the volar aspect of the thumb, index finger, middle finger, and radial half of the ring finger. The ulnar nerve innervates the little finger and the ulnar half of the ring finger.

Sensory integrity may be examined by testing two-point discrimination with a paper clip or caliper. The normal sensory two-point discrimination is up to 4 mm over the volar surface of the fingertips. All neurologic examinations and range of movements of joints should be documented before using local anesthetic agents; postponing these examinations until after the use of anesthesia is a common medicolegal error.

Additional testing should be based on the history and physical examination findings. Other useful tests might include x-rays to detect bony derangement and significant soft tissue swelling, complete blood count to investigate for infectious complications, and bone scanning to detect occult fracture or osteomyelitis.

*All neurologic examinations and range of movements of joints should be documented before using local anesthetic agents.*

## *Infectious Disorders*

### CELLULITIS

*Cellulitis* of the hand or fingers may be associated with both major and minor trauma (Fig. 8–1). Most cellulitis can be treated conservatively with elevation and antibiotics. If there are any associated systemic signs or symptoms such as fever, lymphangitis, or an elevated white cell count, or if infection has caused dysfunction or deformity, these patients should be admitted to the hospital for observation and intravenous antibiotics appropriate to the type of infection. Although *Staphylococcus* and *Streptococcus* are the organisms most commonly isolated from hand infections, attention to risks of specific infections as described later allows for more appropriate choice of antibiotics. In the patient without other risk factors, amoxicillin/clavulenate, oral cephalosporins, or ciprofloxacin is appropriate.

**FIGURE 8–1**
Cellulitis. See color photograph in Color Section 1.

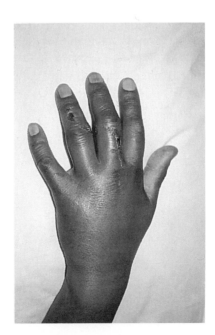

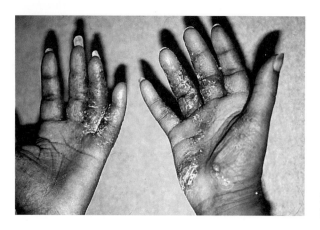

FIGURE 8–2
Herpes infection. See Color Section 1.

## VIRAL INFECTIONS

The most common viral infections in the hand are herpes (Fig. 8–2), warts (*verruca vulgaris*) (Fig. 8–3), and *molluscum contagiosum*. *Herpes* manifests as painful, grouped blisters on an erythematous base, with or without regional lymphadenopathy. Pain is usually out of proportion to physical findings. Incision and drainage should be avoided to prevent secondary infection. Oral acyclovir may be helpful if used early in the course of disease.

*Warts* are common in children and are frequently multiple. Ablation with various chemicals, electrodesiccation, or cryotherapy with liquid nitrogen may be helpful if the warts do not resolve spontaneously. Most warts in children, however, will resolve in 3 to 6 months without therapy.

*Molluscum contagiosum* is the third most common viral infection involving the hand. It can appear, as small, flesh-colored papules distributed on the trunk and extremities. The papules eventually umbilicate. Treatment options include observation, debridement with a scalpel or curette, or ablation, as with warts.

•  ▬▬

*Most warts in children will resolve in 3 to 6 months without therapy.*

## AQUATIC INFECTIONS

Infections that develop in wounds sustained in an aquatic environment may be complicated by the gram-negative rod *Aeromonas hydrophilia*. These infections are often resistant to penicillin and cephalosporin but sometimes respond to quinolones or trimethoprim/sulfa. Saltwater injuries are sometimes associated with *Vibrio vulnificus*,

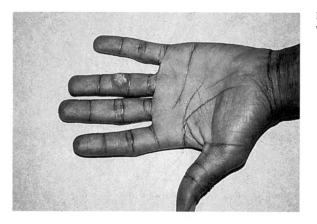

FIGURE 8–3
Viral wart. See Color Section 1.

causing hemorrhagic bullous lesions. These are best treated with doxycycline and ceftazidime.

## INFECTIONS IN PERSONS WITH DIABETES

Persons with diabetes are at risk for complications of hand infections, although foot infections are more typical. The tendency toward polymicrobial infection may require intravenous antibiotics and may demand surgical debridement.

## ANIMAL BITE

Animal bites and scratches, especially cat bites, are often contaminated by *Pasteurella multocida*. These infections have a rapid onset of cellulitis with serosanguineous drainage. Penicillin is the drug of choice, though antibiotics such as amoxicillin/clavulenate are also good choices to cover *Pasteurella* and other more common skin organisms. Infected animal bites can lead to septic tenosynovitis (see below). If there is a consideration of rabies (unprovoked bite, inability to observe animal for signs of rabies, or animal with a high endemic risk), rabies prophylaxis should be given. When in doubt, consult infectious disease specialists or local public health experts.

## HUMAN BITE

A wound inflicted by human bite commonly inoculates the hand with anaerobic streptococcus (Fig. 8–4). Wounds on the knuckles from a fistfight may enter the joint space, causing septic arthritis. Stiffness and destruction of the joint can be the consequence of neglect. Fresh wounds should be irrigated and explored to determine the extent of the wound. If there is no evidence of joint involvement or sign of infection, treat with elevation and antibiotics such as amoxicillin/clavulenate. Radiographs should be taken in all these injuries and may be repeated in follow-up to diagnose bone destruction. If there is bone destruction, consult a hand surgeon.

*Wounds on the knuckles from a fistfight may cause septic arthritis and eventual stiffness and destruction of the joint.*

FIGURE 8–4
Human bite. See Color Section 1.

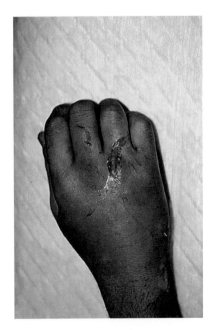

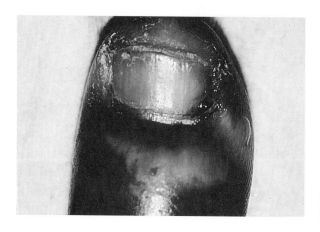

**FIGURE 8–5**
Paronychia. See Color Section 1.

## PARONYCHIA

*Paronychia* usually occurs from trauma to the cuticle and periungual tissues (nail-biting, manicures, and dishwashing) (Fig. 8–5). It is most serious in those with diabetes or circulatory abnormalities. An attempt should be made to abort the early infection by warm soaks, elevation, immobilization, and antibiotics such as clindamycin or erythromycin. Antimicrobial therapy is indicated, and it may be necessary to incise and drain with a #11 scalpel at the margin of the nail.

## PULP SPACE INFECTION

*For drainage of a felon, an aggressive longitudinal midline incision is preferred.*

Infection of the pulp space (felon) often results from minor trauma. The most common pathogenic organisms are staphylococcus and streptococcus. Most of these abscesses point to the center of the pad. An aggressive longitudinal midline incision over the felon is preferred for drainage, as fish-mouth and transverse incisions cause necrosis from ischemia and anesthesia of the tip. Untreated cases may develop osteomyelitis of the

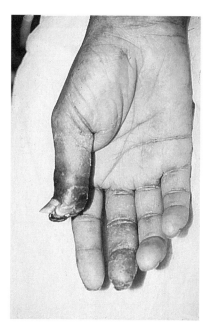

**FIGURE 8–6**
Untreated infection of a felon may lead to ischemia. See Color Section 1.

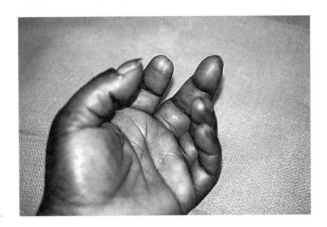

**FIGURE 8–7**
Septic tenosynovitis.

distal phalanx as well as ischemia from increased pressure in the closed space (Fig. 8–6).

## SEPTIC TENOSYNOVITIS

Flexor and extensor tendon sheaths are easily infected by puncture wounds, with *Staphylococcus* and *Streptococcus* the most common infecting organisms (Fig. 8–7). Unless promptly attended, secondary adhesions and stiffness produce serious disability. Tendon necrosis can also occur. The diagnosis is usually made by the presence of Kanavel's sign (uniform swelling of the digit, semiflexed position, tenderness over the entire sheath, and pain produced by passive extension of the finger). Patients with suspected suppurative tenosynovitis should be promptly referred to a hand surgeon for management, as decompression of the tendon sheath is required.

## DEEP FASCIAL SPACE INFECTION

The thenar and midpalmar spaces are potential planes of easy dissection, lying between the deep interosseous and adductor fascia and the fascia deep to the flexor and lumbrical compartments. Diagnosis of a deep fascial-space infection is based on swelling, palmar pain, and tenderness and loss of motion in fingers (Fig. 8–8). These infections require prompt surgical drainage.

**FIGURE 8–8**
Palmar abscess. See Color Section 1.

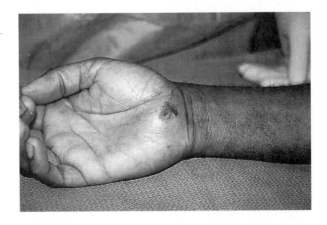

# Injuries

## TETANUS TOXOID

All patients with an open wound should be questioned about the status of tetanus prophylaxis. Patients who have been fully immunized within the past 10 years and who have a clean wound require no further prophylaxis. If the wound is tetanus-prone (contaminated, a puncture, or a wound containing devitalized tissue), a tetanus toxoid booster should be administered. If an immunization history is not available or is incomplete, tetanus toxoid should be given as a complete immunization course for clean wounds, and tetanus toxoid immunization, along with human tetanus immune globulin, should be given for tetanus-prone wounds.

## SUBUNGUAL HEMATOMA

*Subungual hematomas* usually follow crush injury to the tip of a finger (Fig. 8–9). This is a very painful condition, which is frequently associated with an underlying tuft fracture. If seen soon after development, the hematoma can be drained by making a small hole in the nail with a scalpel or drill or burning a small hole with a heated metal probe.

## FINGERTIP INJURIES

Fingertip injuries are very common in children. These wounds can be classified into simple lacerations and complex, crushed, or contaminated wounds (Fig. 8–10). It is important to note the level of injury, the amount of bone exposed, the obliquity of the injury, and the degree of involvement of the nail structures. The goal is to provide a stable, durable skin cover that protects the underlying bone and has pain-free sensation. Whenever possible, the nail bed should be repaired to avoid nail deformity. The examiner can close simple, clean wounds, but more complex or contaminated wounds may require specialized techniques to repair.

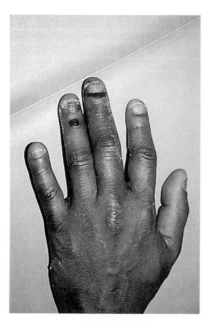

**FIGURE 8–9**
Subungual hematoma. See Color Section 1.

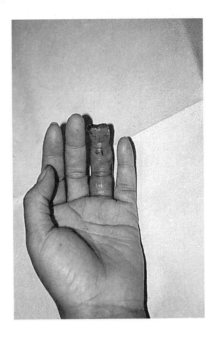

FIGURE 8–10
Fingertip injury.

## RING AVULSION INJURIES AND TRAUMATIC AMPUTATIONS

*Ring avulsion injuries* occur when a ring gets caught and pulled in a machine or door (Fig. 8–11) The injury can be severe enough to cause severance of the finger at the distal interphalangeal joint. Sometimes the avulsed skin or severed digits can be replanted. The severed part should be kept in a plastic bag and the bag immersed in ice prior to prompt transfer to a surgical center.

## CRUSH INJURIES OF HAND AND FOREARM

Crush injuries are usually caused by industrial accidents (Fig. 8–12). The surface wound may be deceptive with respect to the severity of the underlying injury, so radiographs

FIGURE 8–11
Ring avulsion injury. See Color Section 1.

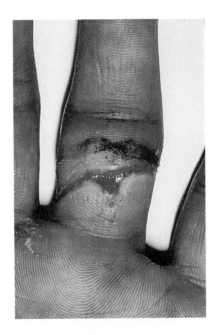

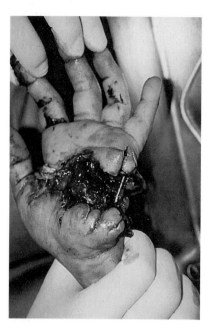

**FIGURE 8–12**
Crush injury. See Color Section 1.

should be obtained. Congestion and ischemia are common. When a compartment syndrome is suspected, immediate decompression is mandatory. These injuries should be referred to a hand surgeon.

## FOREIGN BODIES

Injuries involving foreign bodies are commonly neglected and present when cellulitis develops (Fig. 8–13). It is usually easy to detect and remove a foreign body that is protruding from the skin or is palpable under the skin. Fish hooks are an exception. They may be removed by cutting the hook and advancing it forward to prevent further damage by the wider barb. Deep foreign bodies may be difficult to remove, but they should be removed if symptomatic. When a foreign body is seen radiologically (Fig. 8–14), it can be located with a fluoroscope or guide needles and removed with very little damage to the surrounding structures. Deep foreign bodies that are not radiographically visible may require extensive exploration to remove, so they should be removed by someone with expertise in hand anatomy.

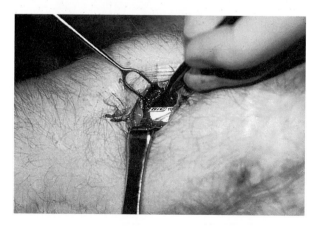

**FIGURE 8–13**
Foreign body. See Color Section 1.

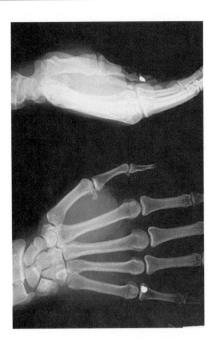

**FIGURE 8–14**
X-ray of hand showing foreign body.

## TENDON INJURIES

*Flexor tendon injuries* are classified according to topographic zones. Zone 2 injuries (from the distal palmar crease to the middle phalanx) are most unpredictable (Fig. 8–15). All flexor tendon injuries should be explored and repaired by a surgeon experienced in hand surgery in order to obtain optimum function. Each finger should be examined independently for flexor tendon function and associated nerve or vascular injuries.

*Extensor tendon injuries* are divided into five groups according to the anatomic location of the injury:

1. *Mallet finger*, when the injury (frequently an avulsion of the bony insertion of the tendon) is at the level of insertion into the distal phalanx. This may be corrected by splinting if less than one-third of the articular surface is involved.
2. *Boutonniere deformity*, where the injury is to the central slip of the extensor tendon, allowing the lateral bands to slip, causing flexion of the PIP joint. Although sometimes responsive to splinting, this may require surgical repair.
3. Extensor tendon injuries over the dorsum of a finger.

• ━━━
*All flexor tendon injuries should be explored and repaired by a surgeon experienced in hand surgery.*

**FIGURE 8–15**
Flexor tendon injury. Note the extended position of the index finger.

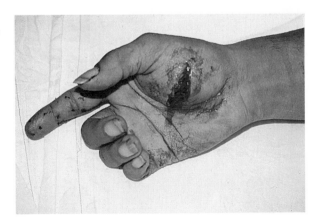

4. Injuries over the dorsum of the hand.
5. Tendon injuries over the wrist and forearm. All of these proximal tendon injuries require prompt surgical repair.

## NERVE INJURIES

Injuries to nerves of the hand can cause considerable functional disability. All lacerations of the hand and fingers should be assessed for nerve injuries prior to infiltration of local anesthetics. Consideration of the disability caused by the loss of nerve function should guide therapy and possibility of referral.

## BONE AND JOINT INJURIES

Bone and joint injuries are common after trauma. Signs and symptoms vary, and all these injuries should be assessed clinically and by radiographs. Undisplaced fractures of the second to fifth metacarpals or the phalanges can be treated with immobilization. Fractures that are compound, are open, are displaced, or involve the joint should be splinted and referred to a hand surgeon.

## LIGAMENTOUS INJURIES

Ligamentous injuries may cause acute or chronic subluxation of the joints. When involving the third and fourth digit, these injuries may respond well to immobilization. Subluxation at the border digits (thumb, second, or fifth digit) may reduce function, such as the ability to grasp and pinch. Some of these, such as "gamekeeper's thumb" (torn ulnar collateral ligament of the thumb), may require surgical repair.

## DISLOCATIONS OF DIGITS

Most dislocation of the fingers (Fig. 8–16) can be reduced under local anesthesia. An exception is the dislocation of metacarpophalangeal joints, which may require open reduction.

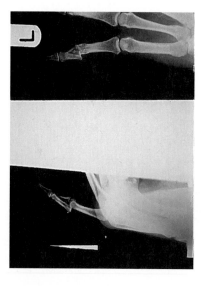

FIGURE 8–16
Dislocation of interphalangeal joint.

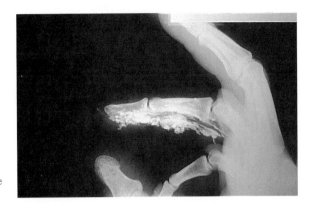

**FIGURE 8–17**
Paint gun injuries. Note the paint inside the tendon sheath.

## PAINT-GUN INJURIES

*Paint-gun injuries* are very serious injuries in which foreign material is injected into the tissue under considerable pressure (Fig. 8–17). These tend to spread through tissue planes. Radiologic examination of the extremities may show air in the soft-tissue planes and even evidence of radio-opaque material within the tissue planes. Extensive debridement is usually required; these injuries may even result in loss of parts.

*Paint-gun injuries are very serious injuries in which foreign material is injected into the tissue under considerable pressure.*

## FROSTBITE

Cold injuries occur when water crystallizes in the skin and subcutaneous tissue (Fig. 8–18). These generally occur as a result of exposure to extremely cold temperatures. Lack of adequate protection and the wind chill factor play a role in the development of frostbite. The usual symptoms are numbness followed by pain. The severity of the frostbite may not be clear until several days after thawing. As rewarming occurs, tingling and aching may increase. Management of frostbite is by rapid rewarming at 38°

**FIGURE 8–18**
Frostbite. See Color Section 1.

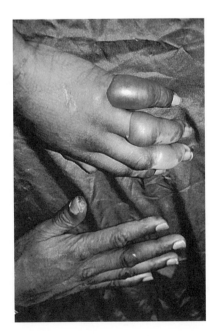

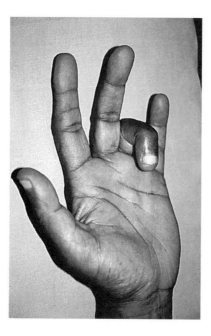

**FIGURE 8–19**
Trigger finger. Note the locked position of the finger.

to 40°C. Rewarming should be continued until all involved tissues are warm and hyperemic. Patients should cease smoking because it causes severe vasoconstriction and additional tissue damage. If deep injury is suspected, referral is appropriate.

## DEGENERATIVE DISORDERS

Degenerative disorders of the hand are due to wear and tear, especially of the interphalangeal joints. Patients usually present with swelling and pain. Crepitus may be elicited on examination. Radiographs usually reveal destruction of the joint surface to varying degrees. Nonsteroidal analgesics and physical therapy usually improve symptoms. Joint replacement is reserved for severe and intractable cases.

## STENOSING TENOSYNOVITIS

Tendons are covered with sheaths lined by synovium. When the tendons swell and thus cannot glide properly, it is painful and function is limited. Common examples of stenosing tenosynovitis are trigger finger and DeQuervain's disease. *Trigger finger* (Fig. 8–19) usually occurs at the level of the metacarpal head (A1 pulley), and *DeQuervain's disease* occurs at the radial side of the wrist. These can be treated with local injection of steroids and splinting. Recurrent cases may require surgical release.

## NEURAL ENTRAPMENT

*Nerve compression syndromes like carpal tunnel syndrome should be documented with nerve conduction studies.*

Carpal tunnel syndrome and compression of the ulnar nerve at the wrist (Guyon's canal) or elbow are common nerve-compression disorders. These injuries may be work related and should be documented with nerve-conduction studies. Advanced cases may present with contractures and muscle wasting, as in claw hand (Fig. 8–20). Splinting

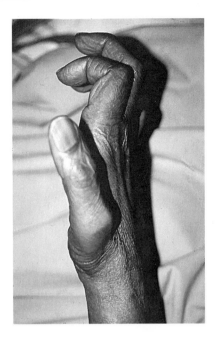

**FIGURE 8-20**
Ulnar claw hand. Note the wasting of intrinsic muscles of the hand and extension of the metacarpophalangeal joint.

and local steroids are useful in the early stage. When ineffective, the opinion of a hand surgeon should be obtained to consider decompression.

## DUPUYTREN'S DISEASE

*Dupuytren's disease*, also known as *Dupuytren's contracture*, is a nodular thickening of the palmar fascia that occurs most frequently in males, Northern Europeans, and individuals with alcoholic cirrhosis or vibrational trauma (Fig. 8-21). Early disease can be treated with physical therapy or local steroid injections, but most cases involve progressive contracture that causes limitation of function requiring fasciectomy.

**FIGURE 8-21**
Dupuytren's contracture.

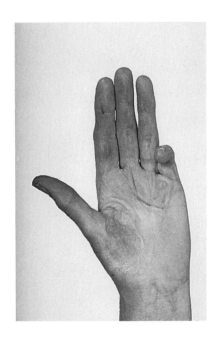

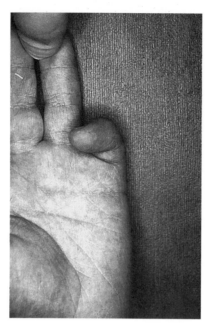

**FIGURE 8–22**
Clinodactyly.

## Congenital Anomalies

Congenital deformities are relatively common and present a diverse array and range of disorders. The common congenital disorders are *polyphalangism* (excess number of fingers), *syndactyly* (fusion of fingers), *clinodactyly* (curled fingers) (Fig. 8–22), *cleft hand* (Fig. 8–23), and *aplasia of the hand* (Fig. 8–24). Supernumerary digits may simply be removed at birth with ligature or excision, but other deformities are best treated by a hand surgeon.

**FIGURE 8–23**
Cleft hand.

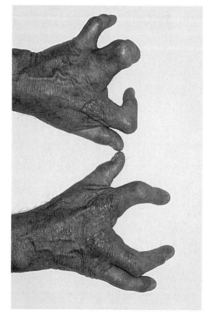

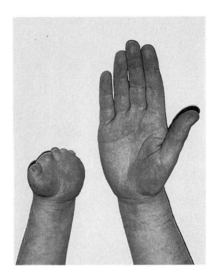

FIGURE 8–24
Aplasia of the hand.

# Tumors

## GANGLION CYSTS

*Ganglion cysts* are common tumors of the hand that originate from the connective tissue near the joints. They are usually located over the dorsum of the wrist (Fig. 8–25), over the radial aspect of the wrist, or at the base of the fingers. Treatment is by aspiration (frequently associated with recurrence), injection of steroid preparations, or excision by a skilled surgeon.

## INCLUSION CYSTS

There are no sebaceous glands in the palmar skin, but they do occur in the dorsal skin. Traumatic puncture wounds may drive small pieces of skin into the subdermal tissues.

FIGURE 8–25
Ganglion of the wrist.

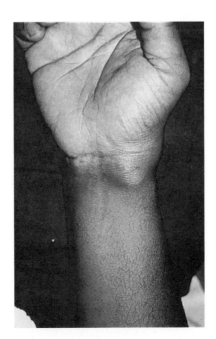

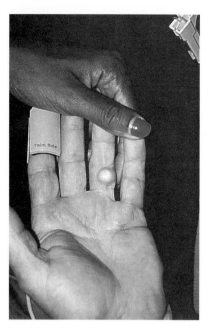

**FIGURE 8–26**
Inclusion cyst.

These cause inclusion cysts (Fig. 8–26), which are round, rubbery, and freely mobile. Treatment of choice is excision.

## LIPOMA

*Lipomas* are connective-tissue tumors that present with symptoms caused by nerve compression. These soft masses are present in the subcutaneous tissue (Fig. 8–27). They may enlarge slowly and become painful. Asymptomatic lipomas require no treatment.

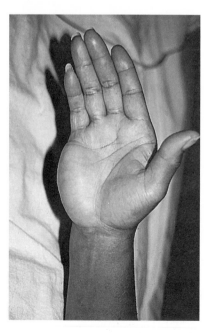

**FIGURE 8–27**
Lipoma of the palm.

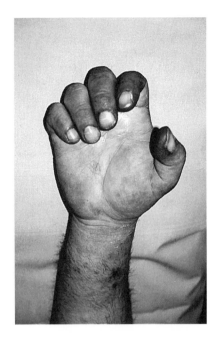

**FIGURE 8–28**
Ischemia of the hand from intra-arterial injection. See Color Section 1.

## ISCHEMIA OF THE HAND

*Ischemia of the hand* (Fig. 8–28) can occur from injection of various narcotic drugs into the soft tissue and vessels by drug addicts. These agents cause vascular sclerosis and subcutaneous fibrosis. This usually results in chronic ulceration, abscess, and pararthrosis.

## MALIGNANT TUMORS

Bowen's disease, squamous cell carcinoma, basal cell carcinoma, and malignant melanoma can occur in the hand. When suspected, these lesions should be biopsied. A subungual hematoma may be mistaken for a malignant melanoma.

## Conclusion

Primary care providers easily manage many hand injuries. Some, such as flexor tendon repair or surgical drainage of tenosynovitis, always require aggressive intervention by a hand surgeon. Although primary care providers may be capable of caring for injuries requiring simple surgical intervention (drainage of a felon or relocation and splinting of a mallet finger), attention to ultimate function requires skills that call for referral.

### When to Call the Surgeon about Hand Problems

• Infections of the hand that do not settle with antibiotics
• Suspicion of septic arthritis or tenosynovitis
• Any vascular compromise to hand or fingers
• Fingertip injuries with exposure of bone or loss of pulp
• Tendon injuries

- Fractures that are compound, open, displaced, or involve a joint
- Congenital anomaly of the hand

## RECOMMENDED READING

Clinics in Plastic Surgery. Hand Surgery Update 1. July 1996.

Green, DP: Operative Hand Surgery. Churchill Livingstone, 1993.

Kilgore, ES, and Graham, WP: The Hand: Surgical and Nonsurgical Management. Lea & Febiger.

Wilson, RF, and Walt, A: Management of Trauma: Pitfalls and Practice, ed 2. Williams and Wilkins, Baltimore, 1996.

# Involuntary Weight Loss

## GERALD GOODENOUGH, MD, and MAX M. COHEN, MD

## *Causes of Weight Loss*

Weight loss that is involuntary is always a problem and may be a marker for underlying conditions that must be addressed. Patient records kept by primary care providers should record weight over the entire time of the patient care.

Weight in adult humans is remarkably stable. The average American adult maintains his or her weight within 1 to 2 pounds (not withstanding a slow decline over time in old age). Generally accepted definitions of worrisome unintentional weight loss in adults are 5% loss of body weight over 6 months or 10% loss over 1 year. Either of these events should trigger a workup to determine the cause.

In general terms, weight loss is a result of one of the following mechanisms:

- poor intake
- loss of nutrients
- catabolic states
- hypermetabolic states
- dehydration

### POOR INTAKE

Poor intake is an inadequate intake of calories and nutrients causing weight loss. Underlying conditions (Table 9–1) may contribute to an inability to swallow properly, a lack of desire to eat, or an inability to procure food.

Several of these conditions or diseases contribute to satiety or early satiety. Some peptides and hormones that have been implicated in early satiety include norepineph-

*Weight loss that is involuntary is always a problem and may be a marker for underlying conditions that must be addressed.*

**TABLE 9–1**

## Causes of Failure to Eat or Drink Adequately

*Dysphagia*
Neuromuscular
  Stroke
  Myasthenia gravis
  Spasm
  Zenker's diverticulum
  Achalasia
Benign stricture of the esophagus
Neoplasm of the esophagus

*Anorexia*
Organic Disease
  Cancer, especially gastric and pancreatic
  Chronic infection
  Degenerative diseases
Drug Effects
  Alcohol
  Amphetamines
  Digoxin
  Opioids
  Thiazides
  Other drugs
Depression
  Anxiety-depression state
  Endogenous depression
  Exogenous depression
  Medication-induced depression
Altered Metabolism
  Cancer
  Fever
  Hypothermia
  Liver disease
  Metabolic disease

*Inability to Procure Food*
Lack of ambulation (bedfast persons)
Functional problems
Poverty

rine and corticotropin-releasing factor in depression, cytokines such as tumor necrosis factor, adepsin, IL 1 and IL 6 in cancer, AIDS, and other infections.

Tumor necrosis factor (previously known as cachectin), a product of activated blood monocytes and other reactive blood cells, has been shown to cause anorexia in laboratory animals. Cancer victims may also be affected by humoral substances such as bombesin and somatostatin.

### *When to Call the Surgeon about Poor Intake*

- When cancer is suspected and a search is necessary
- When parenteral access lines are necessary
- When enteral access is necessary
- When dysphagia is present
- When abdominal masses are discovered
- When there is a suspected gastrointestinal (GI) obstruction at any level

**TABLE 9–2**

### Causes of Nutrient Loss

*GI Tract*
Chronic Vomiting
    Bulimia
    Gastroparesis
    Gastric outlet obstruction
    Psychogenic
    Medication induced
Chronic Diarrhea
    Infection
    Malabsorption
    Secretory disorders
    Crohn's disease
    Ulcerative colitis
    Psychogenic diarrhea

*Urinary Tract*
Diabetes mellitus
Nephrotic syndrome
Nephritis

*Other*
Fistula (spontaneous or iatrogenic)
Phlebotomy
Dialysis
Paracentesis

## LOSSES FROM THE BODY

Losses of fluid and nutrients may contribute to weight loss. This includes losses from the GI tract, either by malabsorption or excess secretion into the lumen; losses from vomiting; and losses through the urine, as in diabetes mellitus. Table 9–2 shows categories of losses and their underlying causes.

*When to Call the Surgeon about Loss of Nutrients*

• For gastric outlet obstruction
• For other mechanical gut problems
• For severe or complicated cases of ulcerative colitis or Crohn's disease

## CATABOLIC STATES

Infectious diseases and malignancy are the two causes of catabolic states leading to weight loss (Table 9–3). In some cases, a failure of down-regulation in energy expenditure in the face of poor caloric intake has caused weight loss. This contributes to wasting. Interleukin-1 and tumor necrosis factor, both of which may be produced by cancers, are capable of increasing resting energy expenditure and can promote skeletal wasting.

    Humoral agents can contribute to catabolic wasting in infectious processes. Patients with AIDS have been shown to have higher resting energy consumption than normal people. Similar mechanisms can be seen in patients with chronic abscesses. Occult malignancy and hidden infections such as tuberculosis, fungal disease, ab-

*Occult malignancy and hidden infections such as HIV, tuberculosis, fungal disease, abscesses, and subacute bacterial endocarditis should be sought in patients with obscure weight loss.*

**TABLE 9–3**

| Causes of Catabolic Wasting |
| --- |

*Malignancy*
Leukemia and lymphoma
Cancer at any site
GI malignancy

*Infections*
Chronic bacterial infection
Chronic viral infection
Fungal infections
AIDS
Parasitic infestation

scesses, and subacute bacterial endocarditis should be sought in patients with obscure weight loss.

Congestive heart failure also may increase metabolic demands and lead to weight loss.

*When to Call the Surgeon about Catabolic Wasting*

• • • • • • • • • • • • • • • • • • • • • • • • • • • • • • • • • • • • • • • • • • • • • • • • • • • • • •

- For drainage of abscesses
- For any suspected solid- or hollow-organ malignancy

## HYPERMETABOLIC STATES

States causing excessively rapid metabolism and excessive energy expenditures can lead to weight loss (Table 9–4). Underlying causes can include hyperthyroidism, hyperparathyroidism, hyperadrenalism, pheochromocytoma, and the paraneoplastic syndromes. All of these increase the consumption of nutrients in the tissues beyond physiologic need. Enzymes are produced that convert muscle and fat into energy sources. Occasionally there is an increase in appetite, but usually the appetite diminishes, causing further weight depletion.

**TABLE 9–4**

| Hypermetabolic States |
| --- |

*Benign*
Hyperthyroidism
Hyperparathyroidism
Pheochromocytoma
Hyperadrenalism

*Malignant*
Lung cancer
Pancreatic cancer
Renal cancer
GI cancer
Paraneoplastic syndromes

*Iatrogenic/Self-Induced*
Thyroid pills
Diet pills
Street drugs

Hyperthyroidism, with its circulating thyroid hormones, increases consumption of energy at the expense of stored tissue sources. The patient may feel extra energy (especially in younger patients) or apathy and loss of appetite (common in older people). In hyperthyroidism, both increased metabolism and anorexia may cause loss of weight.

Hyperadrenalism and pheochromocytoma can produce beta-adrenergic agents that increase cardiac output and promote gluconeogenesis and energy consumption. Increased muscular use of energy results in a restless feeling as the hypermetabolic state is maintained.

In paraneoplastic syndromes, aberrant malignant cells produce abnormal peptides or hormones. Common sources for such tumors are the lungs, pancreas, kidneys, and GI tract. The primary tumor may be very small and difficult to find. These abnormal peptides and hormones can mimic those physiologically produced and can increase metabolism by mimicking the action of thyroid or adrenergic hormones.

Drugs such as thyroid pills can produce a hypermetabolic state. Consumption of diet pills, "energy" pills, or other substances also can produce hypermetabolic states. Cocaine increases metabolism and produces an energy "rush" along with suppression of the appetite. "Designer drugs" can produce similar states of increased metabolism.

### *When to Call the Surgeon about Hypermetabolic States*

- For hyperthyroidism (in patients who will not or should not take radioactive iodine)
- For hyperparathyroidism
- For search for suspected malignancy
- For pheochromocytoma

## DEHYDRATION STATES

Weight loss from dehydration may be acute or chronic but of course is rarely chronic and progressive. Physiologic deficiencies do not allow for very prolonged, chronic progressive dehydration. Patients with signs and symptoms of dehydration will rarely focus on the associated mild weight loss.

A specific history should be sought if dehydration is suspected. The history should include an account of fluid intake, fluid losses, weight record, history of illnesses, and triggering events. Laboratory data may be deceptive. For example, in a nitrogen-deficient patient, the blood urea nitrogen may not rise as expected with significant dehydration.

### *When to Call the Surgeon about Dehydration*

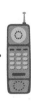

- Dehydration per se is never treated surgically

## *Approach to the Patient with Weight Loss*

The underlying cause must be sought in all cases of significant weight loss. The relative prevalence of various underlying causes varies by age. Cancer is the most common underlying medical problem found in middle-aged patients. In the elderly, however, physical and physiologic changes associated with aging and age-related disease that interfere with intake are the most common underlying problems. Malabsorption and hypermetabolic status are rare causes of weight loss in the elderly. In children, metabolic causes and psychosocial causes predominate.

*Cancer is the most common underlying medical problem found in middle-aged patients.*

An initial history, physical examination, functional assessment (including mental status), and selective laboratory evaluation should be done on all patients with unintentional weight loss of over 10% within the past year, or 5% within the past 6 months.

## HISTORY

Details in the history are important in patients with involuntary weight loss. The onset and duration of weight loss should be noted, as should changes in appetite and food intake. Changes in the home may alter patterns of food shopping and food preparation. Changes in medication may affect mood and appetite. Symptoms of depression also should be noted. Psychosocial stress and substance abuse can contribute to changes in appetite and eating patterns. Fear of food due to abdominal pain in a patient with atherosclerosis suggests "intestinal angina."

## PHYSICAL EXAMINATION

The physical examination should include general appearance and vital signs. Changes in skin color (e.g., jaundice) may suggest the cause of weight loss. A careful examination of the mouth, throat, and dentition may reveal lesions interfering with food intake. All lymph node basins should be examined for evidence of lymphadenopathy. A careful neurologic examination may show signs of chronic neurologic disease. Chest, abdominal, rectal, and pelvic exams are important, especially for detection of malignancy.

## FUNCTIONAL ASSESSMENT

Functional problems to be considered include:

- *Home environment.* Visit the patient's home and inspect the refrigerator to gather information about eating habits.
- *Physical functional abilities.* Assess walking ability, gait, and eating ability (handling utensils, cutting food, swallowing abilities).
- *Social considerations.* Look at the person's finances and the availability of caregivers, if appropriate.

## LABORATORY STUDIES

Laboratory studies should be used to screen for potential causes of weight loss, to pursue suspected diagnoses, and to monitor therapy. The following initial screening studies may be indicated depending on the clinical context; complete blood count (CBC), electrolytes, blood urea nitrogen (BUN), creatinine, serum hepatic enzymes, plasma glucose, serum protein and albumin, total iron binding capacity, $T_4$, $T_3$ uptake, thyroid-stimulating hormone (TSH), sedimentation rate, urinalysis, and stools for occult blood, ova, parasites, proteolytic enzyme, reducing substance, and fat. An HIV test and a TB skin test should be performed on at-risk individuals.

The possibility of occult malignancy should be examined. A chest x-ray, flexible sigmoidoscopy, Pap smear, mammography, and prostate-specific antigen (PSA) should be obtained in appropriate patients in whom no diagnosis is evident early in the workup. If malignancy is still suspect after all tests return negative, a bone scan may be helpful.

The subjective global assessment (SGA) divides patients into three categories based on the subjective analysis of the following:

- Degree and pattern of weight loss
- Change in oral intake
- Presence of GI symptoms
- Functional level
- Loss of subcutaneous tissue
- Muscle wasting
- Presence of edema or ascites

If the SGA indicates adequate intake of nutrients or that a poor food intake is unexplained or associated with apparent disease states, further studies are indicated.

## TREATMENT/MANAGEMENT

### Weight Loss Due to Poor Intake

Ensuring adequate intake may involve changing medications, ensuring the availability of food and help in eating, closely monitoring the amount eaten, and fixing dentures or repairing teeth. Emotional disease or a demented patient's refusal to eat involves ethical decisions along with medical ones. Other underlying disease (such as congestive heart failure, thyroid disease, or liver failure) should be immediately treated to the extent possible. The evaluation and management of weight loss should not ignore protein-calorie malnutrition as a problem itself. In the absence of a specific cause for the poor intake, increasing the food intake becomes the focus of the therapy. Enteral hyperalimentation or parenteral nutrition may be required in some patients. The enteral route is always preferred if available.

### Weight Loss Due to Malabsorption

If malabsorption is to blame for weight loss, the exact cause should be determined. The gut wall, the length of the gut, the transit time, and infections may all lead to malabsorption. Pancreatic failure also may lead to malabsorption. Treatment varies depending on the cause. Intravenous hyperalimentation may be required until the primary problem is resolved.

### Weight Loss Due to a Catabolic Process

Older patients should be encouraged to engage in as much activity as feasible because activity may improve appetite and the overall outlook. Cancer should be managed according to the primary site. Management may be aggressive or nonaggressive depending on the wishes of the patient and family. Infection is treated as appropriate for the organism and site of infection.

### Weight Loss Due to Hypermetabolic States

The underlying problem (usually hyperthyroidism) is specifically treated after the diagnosis is made.

### Weight Loss Due to Dehydration

In an elderly person with recent weight loss, dehydration must be suspected until disproven. If the history, examination, and laboratory data support the diagnosis, an adequate maintenance supply of fluids must be maintained. Replacement fluid should be given carefully while monitoring closely for signs of overhydration.

## RECOMMENDED READING

Koch, KL, and Stern, RM: Functional disorders of the stomach. Sem Gastrointest Dis 7:185–195, 1996.

Mathias, JR, and Clench, MH: Neuromuscular disorders of the gastrointestinal tract. Specific disorder that often gets a nonspecific diagnosis. Postgrad Med 97:95–108, 1995.

Plata-Soloman, CR: Anorexia during acute and chronic disease. Nutrition 12:69–78, 1996.

Reife, CM: Involuntary weight loss. Medical Clinics of North America 79:299–313, 1995.

Wise, GR, and Craig, D: Evaluation of involuntary weight loss. Where do you start? Postgrad Med 95:143–150, 1994.

# Problems with Feeding Tubes

## DAVID BOUWMAN, MD

Nutrition is an important therapeutic modality. The ability of the health care community to maintain patients through parenteral nutrition has improved over the last several decades, but enteral nutrition remains preferable. The advantages of using the gastrointestinal (GI) tract for nutrition include better gut integrity, lower cost, lower rate of septicemia, less chance of volume or electrolyte abnormalities, and broader range of caregivers who can manage the administration of the nutrition. The technology of feeding tube placement involves access at various levels of the GI tract. Feedings via tube are replete with difficulties. This chapter differs from most of the others in this book in that it does not cover an organ system, but it does cover an aspect of patient care that frequently requires surgical consultation: the use of feeding tubes and common associated problems (Table 10–1).

## When to Use a Feeding Tube

The primary care provider is frequently faced with patients requiring nutritional supplements. If the patient is willing and able to eat the problem is easy to solve. If not, the practitioner is faced with a problem. Identifying the patient who would benefit from placement of a feeding tube and enteral nutrition is best approached by answering the following three basic questions (Table 10–2).

### IS MALNUTRITION PRESENT OR IMPENDING?

If there is no pre-existing deficit, nutritional equilibrium can be maintained by providing 20 kcal/kg per day if the patient is expending energy at a resting state. These requirements may increase to 30 or even 40 kcal/kg per day if the patient becomes more physically active or if hypermetabolic states such as sepsis occur. To assess the patient's initial nutritional status, the body mass index (BMI), using height and weight, is an easy

TABLE 10-1

| **Decision Points Concerning Feeding Tubes** |
| --- |
| Deciding when to use a feeding tube |
| Selecting the appropriate feeding tube |
| Managing tube feedings |
| Avoiding common feeding problems |
| Managing difficulties seen with tubes |
| Deciding when to terminate the feeding tube |

approximation. Obese patients also benefit from nutrition when acutely starved. Knowing the clinical details of the diagnosis that interrupted the patient's oral intake aids in prediction of the need for nutrition. For example, a patient with a head and neck carcinoma may face an extended course of radiation, chemotherapy, and surgery, which may be predicted to extend over months. Early institution of caloric repletion results in overall lower morbidity for such patients.

## IS THE GI TRACT USABLE FOR FEEDING?

Mechanical patency, absence of distal fistulae, and adequate gut motility are necessary for food to be processed by the GI tract. Usually these qualities are easy to ascertain, but in certain situations only trial feedings through a temporary access route, such as a transnasal feeding tube, can help determine whether the GI tract is usable.

## IS THERE A CLEAR TREATMENT GOAL?

Medical ethicists agree that both hydration and enteral nutrition are therapeutic modalities requiring a deliberate decision for implementation. The institution of tube feedings is clearly undesirable in comatose or preterminal patients in whom prior directives or present directives of the family specify the prolongation of life to be an unacceptable goal. The same standards of appropriateness should be applied to the use of enteral nutrition as to any other intervening therapeutic modality in terminally ill patients. Decisions for patients with personal or family ambivalence may be arduous and time-consuming but should be squarely faced.

When the answer to all three questions is "yes," tube feedings are indicated. That is, when there is an inability to maintain oral nutrition in a patient with an intact GI tract and a reasonable treatment goal, tube feedings should be instituted.

## *Selection of the Appropriate Feeding Tube*

Three factors must be considered in deciding the methodology for tube feeding in an individual patient: the appropriate level of the GI tract at which to introduce feedings,

TABLE 10-2

| **Questions to Ask When Considering Tube Feeding** |
| --- |
| Is malnutrition already present or expected to develop? |
| Is the small bowel capable of absorption of enteral feedings? |
| Does nutrition serve an identifiable treatment goal? |

TABLE 10–3

**Factors Determining Appropriate Feeding Tube Selection**

Correct GI site for feeding
Expected duration of feeding
Level of acceptable operative risk

the duration for which the tube will be needed, and the patient's complication risk for tube placement (Table 10–3). All three factors are influenced by the etiology of the patient's problem, which is always functional or mechanical disruption of the oropharynx or upper digestive tract.

Causes of functional disruptions are usually neurologic but occasionally psychiatric. If the stomach is available and the esophagus is patent, a transnasal tube or a percutaneous endoscopic gastrostomy (PEG) tube is the first choice for establishing a feeding route. Occasionally, patients with gastroparesis secondary to diabetic neuropathy may require jejunostomy. Inability to protect the upper airway may dictate more distal introduction of tube feedings because reflux of feedings into the oropharynx may cause massive aspiration. X-ray contrast studies overestimate the incidence of esophageal reflux and should not be used. Use of a transnasal feeding tube for trial feedings with food coloring as a marker allows monitoring of tracheal aspiration. If colored secretions are found on nasotracheal suctioning, then the stomach is an unacceptable level of the GI tract for feeding. Indwelling feeding tubes that cross the esophagogastric junction may increase the likelihood of reflux and aspiration.

*X-ray contrast studies overestimate the incidence of esophageal reflux and should not be used.*

Mechanical obstructions of the oropharynx or esophagus are usually due to neoplasms, trauma, caustic burns, or surgical interventions. Except in cases of gastric outlet obstruction, the stomach is usable, and if there is no aspiration, feeding at the stomach level is an excellent choice. When the esophagus is passable, PEG tubes are ideal. If the esophagus is blocked, access is obtained by a direct transabdominal approach using radiologic guidance, minilaparotomy, or laparoscopy. The choice of the exact feeding tube to be installed will depend on the availability of expertise with the various placement techniques.

The ideal choice of tube is based in part on the expected duration of use. When the problem lies in the very proximal GI tract and is accompanied by a patent esophagus and no aspiration, transnasal feeding tubes are an excellent short-term solution. Such tubes are placed and managed by many primary care providers. PEG tubes are an excellent solution for intermediate- or long-term problems, and gastrostomies are excellent choices for very long-term access. PEG tubes require a surgeon, a gastroenterologist, or an interventional radiologist for placement. Long-term access to the jejunum may be obtained by open or laparoscopic jejunostomy. Open gastrostomy or jejunostomy requires a surgeon's expertise.

The examiner must assess the patient's risk for invasive placement procedures that require anesthesia. Although placement of an open jejunostomy may be the best technical choice, if the patient cannot tolerate anesthesia or a minilaparotomy, a jejunostomy is not the right choice.

## How to Manage Tube Feedings

The examiner must choose the content of the feeding and administration techniques and must also arrange for surveillance of both the apparatus and the patient.

Many commercial tube feedings are available. The parameters differentiating these feedings from one another include fiber content, osmolality, and level of predigestion of the foodstuff (ranging from an elemental diet through a partially digested diet to a more crude liquid-nutrient puree). Preparations will deliver in the range of 1 to 1.5 kcal/

mL. Disease-specific preparations are also available: limited glucose for glucose intolerance, limited acid ash for renal failure, limited aromatic amino acids for hepatic failure, and a lactose-free preparation for lactase deficiency. Disease-specific preparations are relatively expensive.

*Feeding at the gastric level provides the advantage of bolus feedings with some variation in osmolality.*

Feeding at the gastric level allows the advantage of bolus feedings with some variation in osmolality. All gastric bolus feedings should begin with measurement of residual gastric volume by aspiration of gastric contents through a catheter-tip syringe. If the residual volume is below 100 to 150 mL, gastric emptying is adequate and a bolus feeding can be instilled. The feeding tube should be rinsed before capping, and 2 to 3 hours should be allowed for gastric emptying before instituting the next feeding. A volume of up to 4 mL/kg at each feeding is well tolerated by the average patient. This allows boluses of 200, 300, or even 400 mL to be placed into the stomach. It may be possible to feed the patient adequately during daylight hours, allowing a respite for uninterrupted sleep at night. A nonrecumbent position after instillation of feedings is an additional precaution against reflux. If high-viscosity feedings containing fiber are being instilled, a pump may be needed. Continuous feeding into the stomach is discouraged because the advantage of checking residual volumes is lost.

*In both gastrostomy and jejunostomy patients, disuse atrophy of gut mucosa may require several days of reduced feedings before the patient can reach targeted caloric and volume intake.*

Feedings into the duodenum or jejunum with access by transnasal tube or jejunostomy must be by continuous infusion because the stomach's osmolal buffering capacity and controlled emptying are bypassed. To control rates accurately, pumps should be used rather than gravity systems. Rates of infusion should start at 10 to 20 mL/hr and work up to 70 or even 80 as tolerated. The nursing staff must monitor the patient for diarrhea or abdominal distress. Symptoms of dumping, with diaphoresis, abdominal cramping, and distention, may occur. In both gastrostomy and jejunostomy patients, disuse atrophy of gut mucosa may require several days of reduced feedings before the patient can reach targeted caloric and volume intake. Continuous infusion of tube feedings should not last for more than 4 to 6 hours before replacement of the feeding solution. The entire infusion set should be replaced periodically. Only fresh, sterile suspensions should be used. Bacterial overgrowth is a recognized problem of hanging large volumes in reservoirs at the bedside and is the most common cause of diarrhea.

*Bacterial overgrowth is a recognized problem with hanging large volumes in reservoirs at the bedside and is the most common cause of diarrhea.*

Medications can be instilled through feeding tubes. For stomach-level feeding, liquid preparations of any oral medication may be used in the customary dosage and schedule. Jejunal administration of medications is more difficult. Uptake by direct infusion into the jejunum is not ensured and should be checked with a pharmacist. Direct infusion of nonsteroidal anti-inflammatory drugs into the jejunum has been associated with ulceration and bleeding.

Urinary output and specific gravity are good baselines for ascertaining whether the volume and basic electrolyte content being provided are adequate for the individual patient. To avoid overhydration, calculation of tube-feeding regimens should take into account the additional volume of free water used to rinse the tubes. Conversely, water may need to be added to maintain some patients in a volume range where their renal function allows their kidneys to adequately maintain homeostasis of fluid and electrolytes. The ability of patients capable of taking sips to drink water as they desire it may allow the patient's intrinsic thirst mechanism to help titrate volume requirements. The clinician's expertise in maintaining NPO (nothing by mouth) patients in an adequate hydration status by the use of IVs alone can be transferred directly to the calculation of tube feedings.

## How to Avoid Problems Common with Tube Feedings

The four common problems associated with tube feedings occur in pairs: ileus (or obstruction), aspiration, electrolyte disorders and diarrhea.

## ILEUS AND ASPIRATION

We have already discussed assessment of aspiration risk and its occurrence. Health care professionals who order tube feedings assume responsibility to prevent the subsequent development of aspiration. Pneumonia or respiratory distress in tube-feeding patients should lead to an in-depth reevaluation of the possibility of aspiration. Gastroparesis or reduced bowel motility is usually the inciting factor. Urinary tract infections or other non–GI-related foci of sepsis often induce paralytic ileus, with gut distention, regurgitation, and aspiration. Tube feedings must be discontinued until the problem is resolved. Mechanical bowel obstruction may also occur. Feeding tubes with inflated balloons have repeatedly been the cause of new obstructive symptoms, frequently discovered only after aspiration.

## ELECTROLYTE DISORDERS AND DIARRHEA

Since most tube-fed patients do not control their enteral intakes, health care providers assume responsibility for checking the adequacy of hydration. Intake-output volumes, urine-specific gravity, and periodic serum electrolytes are the most useful parameters. Diuretics and abnormal fluid losses (such as volume losses from diarrhea) compound the difficulties and require close surveillance.

The most common and recognized problem with tube feedings is diarrhea. Contamination of feedings, with direct introduction of pathogenic bacteria into the GI tract, is a major cause of diarrhea. Careful preparation and storage of bacteria-free nutrients administered through clean and periodically replaced administration sets are required. The availability of sterile canned preparations has somewhat reduced this problem. Fastidious rinsing of the tubes after feeding is important. The actual osmolal load of the feeding is seldom the source of diarrhea in patients past the initial institution of feedings. Adequate caregiver training in the identification of the type of feeding being administered to a patient is crucial. Unwitting administration of bolus feedings via jejunostomy tubes invariably causes diarrhea. This quickly depletes both volume and electrolytes in malnourished patients who already have reduced potassium stores and reduced fluid space. Cessation of tube feeding and IV replacement of electrolytes are required until diarrhea resolves. Specific antibiotics may be needed if the gut has been colonized.

*Contamination of tube feedings, with direct introduction of pathogenic bacteria into the GI tract, is a major cause of diarrhea.*

# Difficulties Common to Feeding Tubes

Clinicians responsible for tube feedings must recognize which tube is being used and be able to identify abnormalities (Table 10–4).

## MISIDENTIFICATION OF TUBES

An iatrogenic problem with feeding tubes is their misidentification: Tube feedings have been instilled into the balloons of feeding tubes, causing intestinal obstructions requir-

---

**TABLE 10–4**

### Problems with Feeding Tubes

Misuse of lumens
Accidental removal or partial dislodgment
Obstruction of tubes
Painful tube sites
Changing feeding tubes

ing laparotomy; tube feedings have been administered into tracheostomy cuff balloons, causing fatal respiratory arrests; IV medications have been administered into feeding tubes; and tube feedings have been given intravenously. All members of the nursing team and care-giving family members must recognize the lumens of all tubes and understand which lumen is appropriate for administering tube feedings and medications.

## ACCIDENTAL REMOVAL OR DISPLACEMENT

Accidental removal of the tube is not uncommon. When this occurs soon (1–7 days) after placement of the tube, peritonitis is a potential danger because the hole in the stomach or the jejunum may function as a free perforation. This is a surgical emergency. To avoid the catastrophe of instillation of tube feedings into the peritoneal cavity, tubes should be reinserted very cautiously, with soluble-contrast radiographs to confirm replacement. If immediate replacement is impossible, nasogastric suction and antibiotics should be instituted. Serial abdominal examination for progressive peritoneal signs is required. If peritonitis develops, the area must be surgically repaired.

Accidental removal of tubes from mature gastrostomies or jejunostomies is not likely to result in peritonitis. In these cases, expeditious reintubation with an appropriately sized catheter is usually possible and re-establishes a feeding route. A radiograph with contrast is advisable to ensure proper positioning of the tube.

A related phenomenon is tube displacement. In some cases, a tube may advance further into the gut via peristalsis. Tubes with small external hubs have been lost entirely into the GI tract. If a Foley catheter is used as a gastrostomy tube, it may advance and be functioning as a jejunostomy. This is an occasional cause of new-onset diarrhea. Such a tube may be pulled back into the stomach after the balloon has been deflated. It is possible to tear the pylorus by failing to deflate the balloon before pulling the tube back.

Tubes may also be displaced outward, with the balloon or retaining dome migrating into the abdominal wall. This may be subtle while feedings are still tolerated. Any previously asymptomatic tube that is now locally painful and has an apparently normal external site needs to be examined for outward dislodgment. This may be checked by carefully backing off the external retaining bar. Push the tube down through the bar, rather than pulling up on the bar, to avoid further outward displacement. An appropriately positioned tube will slide easily into the stomach with inward pressure on the tube and then return to its seated position with gentle traction. If the tube appears to be fixed in position and cannot be pushed in, the retaining balloon or dome may have eroded through the stomach into the abdominal wall. Feedings should be discontinued until correct placement can be ascertained by endoscopy.

*Repeated fixation stitches are not suitable for tubes intended for long-term use; site infections and abscesses are inevitable.*

Long-term gastrostomies or jejunostomies with mucosal stomas are designed for simple reintubation. Thus, the problem of displacement does not exist because of the direct permanent access to the GI tract. Balloons should be left routinely deflated in these stomas. Accidental removal and displacement of any tube can be avoided by fastening the tube to the skin with tethering tape. Repeated fixation stitches are not suitable for tubes intended for long-term use; site infections and abscesses are inevitable.

## TUBE OBSTRUCTION

Another common problem with feeding tubes is tube obstruction. The rate of obstruction is directly related to the diameter of the tube; the small, weighted transnasal tubes are very prone to obstruction. The rate of obstruction is also related to the type of feeding, with dietary preparations containing fiber being major offenders. Medications also may cause obstruction by precipitation, especially if pills are crushed and infused.

Care must be taken to rinse tubes thoroughly after every use. Carbonated beverage or hydrogen peroxide can percolate sediments out of the tube. Mucolytic solutions can open tubes with proteinaceous concretions. At no time should tubes be capped with residual medication or food substances within the tube. If a tube becomes obstructed, judicious use of a guidewire through the tube may unplug it, but vigorous efforts can cause guidewires to leave the lumen of the tube and perforate a viscus. Obstructed tubes that cannot be cleared must be replaced. Repeated obstruction of tubes indicates the need for careful review of tube care for a given patient.

## PAINFUL TUBE SITES

A common problem with feeding tubes in conscious patients is complaints of tube-site irritation. Visual inspection of the site is important. If retaining sutures are in place, there will frequently be cellulitis and dermal abscesses at the stitch sites. Remove all stitches and depend on secure taping to keep the tube in place. Tube infections occur acutely if tubes have been inserted through small skin incisions that tightly seal around the tube and create a closed subcutaneous tube tract. This situation may lead to an abscess, which will require incision and drainage. The first feedings given after opening these abscesses must contain food coloring as a marker to see whether there is leakage around the tube. Leakage around tubes requires cessation of enteral feedings until the tract has scarred down. If the tube is a gastrostomy, pharmaceutical blockade of acid production speeds the resolution of the leak.

Granulation tissue around the tube can be a source of secretions and irritation to the patient. Aggressive cauterization with silver nitrate is effective. Care must be taken not to enlarge the tube-opening site to the point of leakage, which is particularly common in cachectic patients. One cause of granulation is excessive tube motion at the skin level, which can be addressed by more careful taping and dressing of the tube site. These problems happen most frequently in very obese or very thin patients.

Occasionally a patient's continued complaints of disability arising from tube-site pain are an indication that the patient's overall adaptation to the disease process is deteriorating. In a system of denial, the patient focuses on the tube as the source of all troubles. Conversely, some patients may become agitated at the prospect of having tube feedings discontinued.

## CHANGING THE TUBE

Occasionally tubes must be changed because of obstruction or because the tube itself has physically deteriorated. Understanding the type of tube involved is important. A transnasal tube can simply be extracted and replaced by a nurse or other health care professional. In matured gastrostomies with balloon feeding tubes, simple deflation of the balloon, extraction of the tube, and replacement with an identical tube is possible. Replacement with a Foley catheter of the appropriate French scale works well when PEG tubes are changed. Most PEG tubes are designed for traction extraction in the office. Replacement procedures must be within the repertoire of clinicians caring for feeding tubes because gastrostomy tracts close within hours if tubes are not replaced. Individual practitioners should be aware of the types of tubes being used in each of their patients so that a visiting nurse on the evening shift can call and obtain accurate instructions for tube replacement. If a gastrostomy or jejunostomy cannot be replaced and the tract closes, a surgeon will be needed for tube placement. If a specialized device such as a gastrostomy button becomes dislodged, it may be replaced with the original, provided the introduction obturator is available.

*Replacement procedures must be a part of the repertoire of clinicians caring for feeding tubes because gastrostomy tracts close within hours if tubes are not replaced.*

## When and How to Terminate Feeding Tubes

A mistake to be avoided in terminating feeding tubes is the premature removal of an invasively placed tube that cannot be replaced without submitting the patient to an additional procedure. Familiarity with the patient's ability to maintain oral intake, the specific diagnosis, and additional proposed therapy are important. It may be an error to remove a PEG tube from a patient who is eating after head and neck surgery but is facing radiation therapy in the next 2 weeks. Edema from the radiation may return the patient to a dysphagic situation. Conversely, discontinuation of easily placed tubes such as transnasal gastric feeding tubes may be indicated to give the patient a short rest.

Tube identification is important so patients with Foley catheters as feeding tubes can have them removed in the examiner's office without referral for further procedures. PEG tubes can also routinely be removed as an office procedure if the particular tube is recognized.

## Conclusion

Primary care practitioners should be familiar with the indications for use of a feeding tube and should know the most appropriate access routes for the types of patients commonly seen in their practices. The basic repertoire should include use of a standard transnasal feeding tube, use of a standard gastrostomy tube, and overall management of a jejunal feeding tube. It is not possible to recognize every tube on the market, but the primary care provider should be familiar with the tubes used in his or her particular practice. The choice of tubes used should be influenced by care-provider familiarity, level of home care available, and whether adequate specialty consultation exists for placement.

Placement of a feeding tube and institution of a feeding regimen may be relegated to a specialist, but subsequent care frequently is provided by the primary care provider. Feeding tubes are an overall integrated part of ongoing patient management. With attention to both details and broad principles, the appropriate use of feeding tubes will benefit patients, health care providers, and family.

### *When to Call the Surgeon about Feeding Tube Issues*

- For placement of gastrostomy or jejunostomy
- For replacement of a displaced or blocked tube (if a chronic tract is not present)
- For intraperitoneal complications of feeding tubes

### RECOMMENDED READING

Drickamer, MA, Cooney, LM, Jr: A geriatrician's guide to enteral feeding. J Amer Geriatrics Soc 41:672–679, 1993.

Kirby, DF, et al: American Gastroenterological Association technical review on tube feeding for enteral nutrition. Gastroenterology 108:1282–1301, 1995.

Minard, G: Enteral access. Nutrition in Clinical Practice 9(5):172–182, 1994.

Rodman, DP, Gaskins, SE: Optimizing enteral nutrition. American Family Physician 53:2535–2542, 1996.

# Jaundice

## FRANK CELESTINO, MD, and CHRISTOPHER STEFFES, MD

*Jaundice* is the yellow discoloration of sclerae, mucous membranes, and skin caused by accumulation of bilirubin. It becomes noticeable in adults when the serum bilirubin (normally 0.2–1.2 mg/dL) ranges approximately between 2.5 and 3.0 mg/dL, whereas in newborns the threshold for visible jaundice is between 5 and 6 mg/dL.

Although recognizing jaundice is usually quite simple, finding the underlying cause can be challenging. Jaundice due to extrahepatic obstruction usually requires surgical attention. Unfortunately, the clinical and biochemical presentation of biliary obstruction may be nonspecific and indistinguishable from hepatocellular disorders. This chapter reviews the pathophysiology, differential diagnosis, and diagnostic evaluation of jaundice, with emphasis on the rapid detection of extrahepatic biliary obstruction using laboratory tests and imaging studies.

*Jaundice due to extrahepatic obstruction usually requires surgical attention.*

## Pathophysiology and Differential Diagnosis

Bilirubin is a breakdown product of hemoglobin. Total plasma bilirubin concentration varies directly with bilirubin production and inversely with hepatic bilirubin clearance. Mechanisms responsible for jaundice include excess bilirubin production, decreased hepatic uptake, impaired conjugation, intrahepatic cholestasis, hepatocellular injury, and extrahepatic obstruction (Table 11–1). Excess production, decreased uptake, and impaired conjugation lead to a predominance of unconjugated bilirubin, whereas conjugated hyperbilirubinemia is the result of intrahepatic cholestasis, hepatocellular injury, or extrahepatic obstruction. It is important to realize, however, that more than one pathophysiologic process may be present in a single patient or disorder. For example, cirrhotic patients may have both hepatocellular dysfunction and hemolysis.

TABLE 11–1

### Differential Diagnosis of Jaundice by Pathophysiologic Mechanisms

***Unconjugated hyperbilirubinemias***
*Excessive production:* hemolysis, ineffective erythropoiesis, reabsorption of hematomas
*Decreased hepatic uptake or impaired conjugation:* Gilbert syndrome, Crigler-Najjar syndrome, physiologic jaundice of the newborn, congenital hypothyroidism, breast-milk jaundice

***Conjugated hyperbilirubinemias***
*Intrahepatic cholestasis:* hepatitis, drug-induced cholestasis, primary biliary cirrhosis, graft-versus-host disease, diffuse infiltrative disorders or malignancies, Dubin-Johnson or Rotor syndromes, hepatocellular carcinoma, pyogenic or parasitic abscesses
*Hepatocellular injury:* hepatitis, drug- or toxin-induced injury, congestive heart failure, pregnancy, pre-eclampsia, sepsis, ischemia, Wilson's disease, hemochromatoses, X-antitrypsin deficiency, cirrhosis, galactosemia
*Extrahepatic obstruction:* choledocholithiasis, strictures, pancreatic cancer, primary sclerosing cholangitis, chronic pancreatitis, AIDS cholangiopathy, cholangiocarcinoma, metastatic lesions to porta hepatis

## *Evaluation*

### HISTORY

The history of jaundiced patients' present illness and their past medical histories are important. Pertinent findings could include a history of recent travel to countries where parasitic or infectious diseases are common or a social habit such as intravenous drug abuse, which may increase the patient's risk of hepatitis.

Clues from the history that suggest extrahepatic obstruction in the jaundiced patient include abdominal pain, fever and rigors, prior biliary surgery, old age, prior history of gallstones, and absence of exposure to hepatotoxins or hepatitis. A history of recurrent episodes of rigors suggests a stricture or multiple small stones. It is important to remember that the absence of abdominal pain does not rule out obstruction. Weight loss may suggest the presence of an underlying malignancy.

*Clues from the history that suggest extrahepatic obstruction in the jaundiced patient include abdominal pain, fever and rigors, prior biliary surgery, old age, prior history of gallstones, and absence of exposure to hepatotoxins or hepatitis.*

### PHYSICAL EXAMINATION

Extrahepatic obstruction is suggested on physical examination by fever, abdominal tenderness, multiple abdominal scars, abdominal mass, or a palpable nontender gallbladder (Courvoisier's sign). The presence of Charcot's triad (fever, abdominal pain, and jaundice) suggests ascending cholangitis, which is caused by obstructing gallstones 90% of the time. Adding hypotension and altered mental status to this picture (i.e., Reynold's pentad) is said to be pathognomonic of severe suppurative cholangitis. Massive hepatic enlargement (more than 6 cm below the costal margins) occurs in some instances of extrahepatic obstruction but also occurs in severe passive hepatic congestion, advanced infiltration, and severe metastases. A small liver, signs of portal hypertension, asterixis, peripheral edema, spider angioma, gynecomastia, or palmar erythema suggests cirrhosis.

### LABORATORY STUDIES

*Disproportionate elevations of alkaline phosphatase compared to the transaminases suggest either extrahepatic obstruction or intrahepatic cholestasis.*

Initial laboratory tests in the jaundiced patient should include a total serum bilirubin with fractionation, complete blood count, reticulocyte count, urinalysis, peripheral blood smear, serum transaminases, alkaline phosphatase, gamma glutamyl transpeptidase, albumin, and prothrombin time. Disproportionate elevations of alkaline phosphatase (greater than three to four times normal) compared to the transaminases (less than two to three times normal), combined with conjugated hyperbilirubinemia, suggests either extrahepatic obstruction or intrahepatic cholestasis. Very low levels of alkaline phosphatase (less than half of normal) or very high transaminase levels (more than 10 times normal) argue against extrahepatic obstruction. Normalization of a prolonged prothrombin time following vitamin K administration strongly implies an obstructive etiology. An elevated serum amylase also may point to an extrahepatic problem.

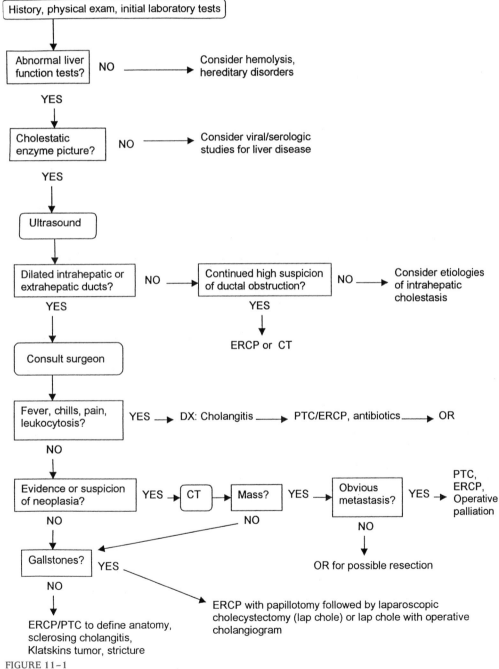

FIGURE 11-1

A rational algorithm for the evaluation of the jaundiced patient. CT = computed tomography, ERCP = endoscopic retrograde cholangiopancreatography, PTC = percutaneous transhepatic cholangiography, OR = operating room.

## IMAGING STUDIES

In many cases, hepatocellular disease can be distinguished from intrahepatic cholestasis and extrahepatic obstruction on the basis of the clinical data and laboratory results just mentioned, but cholestasis and obstruction may be indistinguishable without further testing. The distinction is critical to subsequent management because mechanical obstruction will require direct surgical, endoscopic, or radiologic intervention to restore bile flow. The presumptive clinical impression of obstruction must be confirmed by imaging techniques because studies have revealed that 25% of patients suspected of having obstruction turn out to have hepatocellular cholestasis on more definitive testing.

Ultrasonography, computed tomography (CT), percutaneous transhepatic cholangiography (PTC), and recently developed three-dimensional magnetic resonance cholangiography (MRC) can all achieve visualization of the biliary tree. Ultrasound has emerged as the initial imaging modality of choice due to its lesser expense, lack of radiation, noninvasiveness, portability, and widespread availability. It is over 90% specific and, if jaundice has been present for at least a week, 80% to 90% sensitive in detecting obstruction. Ultrasound also has a sensitivity of over 90% for the detection of stones. Nonetheless, factors such as obesity or excess abdominal gas can cause an ultrasound study to be ineffective. CT scanning offers excellent imaging of the liver, biliary tree, and pancreas. As a noninvasive alternative to ultrasound, CT is more expensive and less sensitive to the presence of stones. Conversely, CT is preferable for cases of malignant obstruction.

Should a very strong clinical suspicion of extrahepatic obstruction remain despite a normal ultrasound, an endoscopic retrograde cholangiopancreatography (ERCP) is preferred over PTC in most centers because of the versatile endoscopic treatment options available to treat the cause of the obstruction (endoscopic sphincterotomy, stone extraction, stricture dilation, or placement of a stent). PTC can be used if ERCP fails. It should be noted that some authorities suggest proceeding directly to ERCP (or PTC) and skipping the noninvasive study when there is very strong clinical suspicion of obstruction. This approach, although more invasive, offers significant cost savings. Other studies such as hepatobiliary scintigraphy, intravenous cholangiography, oral cholecystography, plain abdominal films, and upper gastrointestinal series offer little valuable information in the setting of biliary obstruction and are best avoided. Liver biopsy is usually contraindicated in the setting of obstructive ("surgical") jaundice because it may lead to a biliary-peritoneal fistula, but biopsy is sometimes useful in the differential diagnoses of confusing cases of intrahepatic cholestasis. Figure 11–1 depicts a rational algorithm for the evaluation of the jaundiced patient given these principles.

## *Management*

Therapy for hyperbilirubinemia, of course, depends on the underlying cause. Two-thirds of patients over age 60 have extrahepatic obstruction as the etiology. Once a ductal abnormality has been demonstrated by ultrasound or CT scan, consultation with a surgeon experienced in further management of extrahepatic obstruction is warranted. Therapeutic endoscopic and radiologic procedures are important adjuncts in the management of these patients and in some cases have supplanted surgical techniques. An experienced surgeon should assist in coordinating the employment of these various techniques, as operative intervention is probable in most cases. Avoiding unnecessary procedures before definitive operation is medically and economically advantageous.

PTC and ERCP can be used to directly assess the biliary tree. Drains may be placed to externally decompress the biliary tree, or stents may be placed through obstructing

*An experienced surgeon should assist in coordinating therapeutic endoscopic and radiologic procedures, as operative intervention is probable in most cases.*

lesions. Endoscopic papillotomy (sphincterotomy) permits placement of catheters and baskets for clearing the common bile duct of gallstones in a retrograde fashion. These are important techniques for patients who are not candidates for surgery and for patients with disseminated malignant disease in whom palliative drainage is needed. Also, percutaneous and endoscopic techniques may complement the laparoscopic technology that is often employed in biliary surgery.

Once the examiner makes the diagnosis of extrahepatic biliary obstruction, management of common conditions should commence, as discussed in the following paragraphs.

## ACUTE CHOLANGITIS

*Acute cholangitis* (suppurative infection of the biliary tree) is an acute, life-threatening situation in which timely decompression of the biliary tree and the use of broad-spectrum antibiotics is necessary. Often patients need to be admitted to an intensive care unit for hemodynamic monitoring because they are septic and unstable. Broad-spectrum combination antibiotic therapy should be used to deter common biliary pathogens. Urgent decompression is necessary, either surgically or by endoscopic or invasive radiologic techniques, if there is not a prompt response to antibiotic therapy. Depending on the etiology of the obstruction, PTC or ERCP may be the initially preferred approach to decompressing the biliary tree, but if these fail to resolve the sepsis, emergent operation is indicated.

*Acute cholangitis (suppurative infection of the biliary tree) is an acute, life-threatening situation in which timely decompression of the biliary tree and the use of broad-spectrum antibiotics are necessary.*

## CHOLEDOCHOLITHIASIS

The trend in care for patients with common duct stones has moved away from open surgery. An ERCP is performed initially to clear the duct of stones by retrograde techniques after an ampullary papillotomy. If the duct is successfully cleared this way, a laparoscopic cholecystectomy is the next step. If the common duct is not cleared preoperatively, a common bile duct exploration should be performed at operation. This involves opening the common bile duct, with intraoperative placement of a t-tube to drain externally. The t-tube should be left in place for at least 3 weeks, allowing for postoperative cholangiography. Retained (missed) stones can be removed via the t-tube tract or via ERCP.

## BENIGN BILE DUCT STRICTURES

Bile duct strictures are usually posttraumatic, following diagnostic instrumentation (ERCP or PTC) or surgery. The incidence of bile duct stricture is higher after laparoscopic cholecystectomy than after open cholecystectomy. A preoperative workup should be coordinated by the surgeon to help plan the operation. Placement of stents or drains preoperatively is necessary only if the patient has cholangitis.

## MALIGNANCY

In the workup of pancreatic, ampullary, or common bile duct malignancy, much effort and expense are often wasted on repeated or redundant preoperative imaging studies after a diagnosis has been made. Since resection can be performed with low morbidity and mortality for not only cure but also palliation, most patients should be considered candidates for exploration.

Preoperative placement of stents in many cases wastes resources because the patient will be operated on soon after. Stents have also been shown to increase operative complications because they allow greater access of bacteria to the biliary tree. Furthermore, preoperative biliary drainage employed to reduce serum bilirubin does not minimize postoperative complications.

A CT scan is necessary to assess for ductal dilatation, obvious metastases, and the location and extent of the mass. ERCP is occasionally helpful in defining the anatomy but usually is not needed. The findings of jaundice and a mass in the distal duct are enough to commit the surgeon in most cases to a pancreaticoduodenectomy unless there are obvious metastases or unless the portal vein, superior mesenteric artery, or other vital structure is involved. Biopsies of pancreatic masses are notoriously inaccurate and unnecessarily delay operation.

## ACUTE CHOLECYSTITIS

Most cases of acute cholecystitis are not accompanied by clinically evident jaundice. Quite often the inflammation surrounding a severe case of acute cholecystitis leads to mild elevations of the serum bilirubin or an increased alkaline phosphatase. The findings of acute cholecystitis are usually shown by ultrasonography or a radionuclide biliary scan using technetium-labeled N-substituted iminodiacetic acids (HIDA or DISIDA). After treatment with antibiotics and cholecystectomy, the jaundice usually resolves. As in any case of jaundice or increased alkaline phosphatase, an operative cholangiogram will be performed at the time of cholecystectomy to rule out lesions in the common bile duct.

## SCLEROSING CHOLANGITIS

*Sclerosing cholangitis* is an uncommon disorder characterized by multiple and diffuse biliary ductal strictures. The etiology is unknown. The diagnosis is suggested by ultrasonography and ERCP. Management of this disorder is complex and usually requires transfer of the patient to a center experienced in its management.

### *When to Call the Surgeon about a Jaundiced Patient*

- Dilated intrahepatic ducts
- Fever, chills, leukocytosis
- Severe abdominal pain, especially right upper quadrant
- Dilated common bile duct
- Pancreatitis
- Recent right upper quadrant surgery
- Pancreatic mass on imaging study
- Gallstones on imaging study

### RECOMMENDED READING

Banerjee, B: Extrahepatic biliary tract obstruction—modern methods of management. Postgraduate Medicine 93(4):113, 1993.

Barloon, TJ, et al: Diagnostic imaging to identify the cause of jaundice. Amer Fam Phys 54(2):556, 1996.

Frank, BV: Clinical evaluation of jaundice. JAMA 262:3031, 1989.

Johnston, DE, Kaplan MM: Pathogenesis and treatment of gallstones. N Engl J Med 328(6):412, 1993.

Lai, ECS, et al: Endoscopic biliary drainage for severe acute cholangitis. N Engl J Med 326:1582, 1992.

Richter, JM, et al: Suspected obstructive jaundice—a decision analysis of diagnostic strategies. Ann Intern Med 99:46, 1983.

Sampliner, RE: Jaundice. In Greene, HL, et al (eds): Decision Making in Medicine. Mosby-Year Book, St. Louis, 1993, p 150.

Scharschmidt, BF: Bilirubin metabolism, hyperbilirubinemia, and approach to the jaundiced patient. In Bennett, JC, Plum, F (eds): Cecil Textbook of Medicine. WB Saunders, Philadelphia, 1996, p 755.

# Gastrointestinal Bleeding

STEVEN TENNENBERG, MD,
DAVID JACKSON, MD,
and ROBERT A. KOZOL, MD

Bleeding of the gastrointestinal (GI) tract is a frequent symptom that prompts patients to seek medical evaluation. Most, if not all, of these patients will require invasive diagnostic testing. Some will require inpatient hospitalization, often with elective or emergent surgical consultation. This chapter discusses the different ways in which GI bleeding is manifest and suggests rational and cost-effective plans for its evaluation and management.

## Occult GI Bleeding (Guaiac-Positive Stool)

### FECAL OCCULT BLOOD TESTING

Fecal occult blood testing is done in the context of screening for asymptomatic disease or for evaluation of complaints referable to the GI system, such as abdominal pain, change in bowel habits, or history of possible blood loss from the bowel. It should be part of the workup of any patient who is discovered to have iron-deficient (microcytic) anemia. It is very sensitive and will detect as little as 10 to 15 mL of blood loss in the GI tract.

Multiple factors may contribute to lack of validity for this type of testing. Foods such as red meat (including processed meats) and raw fruits and vegetables (especially melons, radishes, turnips, horseradish, broccoli, and cauliflower) can produce positive results. Vitamin C in excess of 250 mg per day may also lead to false-positive results. Use of aspirin and other nonsteroidal anti-inflammatory drugs (NSAIDs) may cause small amounts of blood loss that can be detected on the cards. Although this can be due to gastric mucosal irritation from the drug, it could also be due to a significant lesion. At-home sampling is not accurate in patients with known bleeding from hemorrhoids or blood in the urine or for women around the time of a menstrual period, owing to possible contamination from these sources. Strictly following package instructions for obtaining a stool sample may be unappealing to some patients and may lead to no testing or inappropriate sampling techniques.

## HISTORY AND PHYSICAL EXAMINATION

When evaluating a patient with guaiac-positive stool, the examiner should obtain a detailed history and review of the upper respiratory system to exclude a history of epistaxis, poor oral or dental hygiene, or hemoptysis, all of which could lead to swallowed blood. Symptoms of gastroesophageal reflux disease, peptic ulcer disease, abdominal pain, bloating, change in bowel habits, and history of hemorrhoids should also be elicited. The examiner also should request a dietary history for the several days preceding obtaining the stool samples. Any history of previous GI problems, such as peptic ulcer disease or diverticular disease, may direct the questioning of the patient. One goal of the history should be to determine whether pathology is in the upper or lower GI tract. This should guide the initial diagnostic workup.

A general physical exam should determine any vital-sign instability, check for skin pallor, and carefully examine the nasal and oropharyngeal regions. The examiner also should perform or request a complete abdominal exam, perianal evaluation, and digital rectal exam. Stool on the examining finger should undergo an occult blood test. The sporadic nature of blood loss for any of a number of pathological processes may lead to a positive or negative result.

## LABORATORY EVALUATION

Laboratory evaluations should include a hemoglobin or hematocrit and a platelet count estimate. If the history or physical findings suggest a coagulopathy or possible liver dysfunction, a prothrombin time (PT) and a partial thromboplastin time (PTT) should also be obtained.

## DIAGNOSTIC EVALUATION

The patient's symptoms or history should direct the initial evaluation. Upper abdominal, epigastric, and midsternal chest pain suggests an esophageal, gastric, or duodenal etiology. Upper endoscopy (esophagogastroduodenoscopy or EGD) is the method of choice to evaluate these areas. Advantages of EGD compared to upper GI contrast studies include its greater sensitivity in detecting lesions that cannot be seen on contrast studies (e.g., gastritis) and the ability to biopsy any potentially malignant lesions.

For the same reasons, colonoscopy is preferable to barium enema for evaluating the colon. If a complete and satisfactory colonoscopy is not possible, usually due to bowel tortuosity, an air-contrast barium enema may be performed to evaluate the more proximal colon. Mass lesions seen with a barium enema would then require surgical evaluation for diagnosis and therapy.

Obviously, if the initial endoscopic procedure of either the upper or lower tract is negative, the complementary procedure should be performed. If both prove to be negative, the examiner should consider obtaining a small-bowel follow-through x-ray study.

*The advantages of EGD compared to upper GI contrast studies include greater sensitivity in detecting lesions that cannot be seen on contrast studies (e.g., gastritis) and the ability to biopsy any potentially malignant lesions.*

## DIFFERENTIAL DIAGNOSIS AND TREATMENT

The differential diagnosis of occult blood in the stool includes any source of bleeding along the GI tract. Oronasopharyngeal sources such as chronic nosebleeds, poor dental hygiene with loss of blood caused by brushing or flossing, and pharyngeal neoplasia may be found. Esophageal pathology including reflux esophagitis, esophageal cancer, and slowly bleeding esophageal varices could lead to a positive occult blood test. Gastritis, gastric erosions, and peptic ulcer disease account for most upper GI bleeding. The possibility of gastric malignancy should also be considered.

Colonic sources include angiodysplasia in 40% to 60% of cases in individuals over 60 years of age, diverticulosis in those over 50 years of age, colon polyps, and colorectal malignancies. Anal fissures and hemorrhoids usually present with bright red blood in the stool or on toilet tissue. Although hemorrhoids may produce positivity on fecal occult blood testing, the examiner should never initially attribute guaiac-positive stool to them; a full GI workup is required to rule out other concomitant sources, particularly colorectal cancers in older patients.

Treatment of most conditions causing occult bleeding is medical, such as H2 blockers for peptic ulcer disease, gastritis, and esophagitis. Many colonic causes of guaiac-positive stools can be treated at the time of diagnosis through the colonoscope. Polyps can be removed and large-bowel angiodysplastic lesions cauterized. Diverticular bleeding, which in the elderly population is a significantly more likely cause, usually stops with conservative therapy. Hemorrhoids, anal fissures, and other local anal pathology can often be treated conservatively or with minor office procedures.

The examiner should seek surgical consultation for any source of bleeding that persists despite medical therapy, such as a nonhealing gastric or duodenal ulcer. Biopsy-proven malignancy of the upper or lower GI tract also requires surgical evaluation for further therapy.

## Upper GI Bleeding

*Upper gastrointestinal (UGI) bleeding* is defined as bleeding that originates in the UGI tract from the esophagus to the ligament of Treitz (the junction between the fourth portion of the duodenum and the jejunum). It is more common in males than in females and can be a life-threatening disorder. The mortality associated with UGI bleeding is higher in older patients. Bleeding lesions of the UGI tract most commonly present as *hematemesis* (vomiting bright red blood or material resembling coffee grounds) or, in the absence of vomiting, as *melena* (dark tarry stools). Rapid UGI bleeding may also present as bright red blood per rectum (BRBPR) because blood is a cathartic and can pass through the bowel quickly. This is why all patients with apparent lower GI bleeding (discussed later) should have a nasogastric tube placed to rule out UGI bleeding. If the lesion bleeds small volumes intermittently, the patient may present simply with anemia with or without fecal occult blood. Patients with significant upper GI bleeding present with hematemesis or melena.

Hematemesis and melena are frightening symptoms, which will lead most patients straight to the nearest emergency department. These patients will often be volume depleted. Mild volume depletion may present with tachycardia only. Severe volume depletion will present with hypotension (shock) and possibly varying levels of mental status changes. All of these patients will require rapid evaluation and resuscitation.

### INITIAL EVALUATION AND RESUSCITATION

When a patient presents with a history of significant recent or ongoing GI bleeding (hematemesis, melena, or *hematochezia* [the passage of BRBPR or maroon blood per rectum]), the examiner must make an initial assessment of hemodynamic stability. Routine vital signs (heart rate and blood pressure) should be checked and orthostatic measurements obtained if possible. Normal vital signs with significant orthostatic changes may indicate up to a 20% blood-volume loss. The presence of baseline tachycardia (heart rate [HR] >100), hypotension (systolic blood pressure [BP] <90), or both is the hallmark of a hemodynamically unstable patient and indicates a blood-volume loss of up to 30% to 40%.

Patients who present with unstable vital signs require aggressive fluid resuscitation including the following:

- placing two large-bore IVs
- an initial fluid bolus of 1 to 2 liters of isotonic crystalloid solution (lactated Ringer's solution or normal saline) over 30 to 60 minutes
- continued IV fluid infusion at a rate of $\geq$150 mL/hr.

Transfusion of packed red blood cells can usually wait until a hemoglobin of less than 10 mg/dL is documented and cross-matched blood is available. Continued IV fluid therapy should be gauged clinically by monitoring hourly urine output (requiring a Foley catheter) and the need for transfusion by following serial complete blood counts (CBCs). We advocate maintaining a urine output of $\geq$0.5 mL/kg body weight per hour, and a hemoglobin of 10 mg/dL in all actively bleeding patients.

## HISTORY & PHYSICAL EXAMINATION

The history of a patient with upper GI bleeding should focus on three subjects. First, as with any case of GI bleeding, a systems review should determine whether the patient may have a disorder of coagulation. Thus, excessive menstrual periods, prolonged bleeding from minor cuts and scrapes, or prolonged bleeding after a tooth extraction would be suggestive. Second, the patient should be asked about acute and chronic ethanol intake and use of NSAIDs. Alcohol and NSAIDs can contribute to upper GI bleeding and are further discussed later in this chapter. Third, any history of prior GI bleeding should be elicited. Many diseases discussed in this chapter are recurrent or chronic problems (peptic ulcer, esophageal varices).

Physical examination begins with the vital signs. Tachycardia and orthostatic drops in blood pressure are indicative of hypovolemia. The skin should be examined for signs of coagulopathy, such as petechia and ecchymoses. The patient should be examined for signs of cirrhosis such as ascites, palmar erythema, Dupuytren's contracture, caput medusae, and "spider" angiomas. There are no specific physical findings with peptic ulcer, gastritis, or Mallory-Weiss tear.

## LABORATORY EVALUATION

The laboratory evaluation of a patient with upper GI bleeding includes a CBC and a platelet count. In cases of NSAID use, a bleeding time to evaluate platelet function should be obtained. In cases of suspected alcohol abuse or cirrhosis, a prothrombin time and a liver function panel including a serum albumin will help establish the magnitude of the disease.

## DIAGNOSTIC EVALUATION

Patients with hematemesis require upper endoscopy. Most cases of UGI bleeding stop spontaneously. If the patient is stable and has stopped bleeding, the upper endoscopic examination may be performed in the same fashion as other elective endoscopy. If the initial endoscopic examination reveals a stomach full of clotted blood, the endoscopic may decide to stop at this point. A large-caliber tube (Ewald type) is passed via the mouth, and the stomach is lavaged and suctioned to remove the clots. Endoscopic examination can then proceed.

If the patient continues to vomit blood, there is great risk of aspiration of blood

*Patients with hematemesis require upper endoscopy.*

- *The four most common causes of hematemesis are erosive gastritis, peptic ulcer disease, esophageal varices, and Mallory-Weiss tear.*

- *Obtain an early surgical consultation on all cases of major upper gastrointestinal bleeding.*

into the bronchial tree during endoscopy. Under these conditions, the safest course is to intubate the patient to help protect the airway during the endoscopic examination.

Very few cases will require surgical therapy. The four most common causes of hematemesis are erosive gastritis, peptic ulcer disease, esophageal varices, and Mallory-Weiss tear. Gastritis and bleeding peptic ulcer generally respond well to medical therapy. Most cases of Mallory-Weiss tear resolve without any specific therapy. Patients with bleeding esophageal varices are usually treated via endoscopic therapy (injection sclerotherapy or endoscopic rubber banding). It is wise to obtain an early surgical consultation on all cases of major UGI bleeding. This consultation allows the surgeon and patient to establish a relationship with an understanding of surgical care should it become necessary. This is far preferable to having the patient meet the surgeon during a rapid trip to the operating room.

*Melena* consists of voluminous black, tarry stools. It occurs when blood remains in the GI tract for at least 8 to 12 hours, while bacteria degrade the hemoglobin into hematin and other dark pigments. Melena can occur with as little as 50 mL of blood loss but usually involves more. Patients with melena and intravascular volume depletion are resuscitated the same way as a patient with hematemesis. Patients with melena require upper endoscopy with the same differential diagnosis as listed earlier (peptic ulcer, gastritis, esophageal varices, and Mallory-Weiss tear). If a patient has melena and a negative upper endoscopic examination (including no blood in the stomach or duodenum), he or she may have a right-sided colonic lesion, which can be sought with colonoscopy, or a primary small-bowel lesion (tumor or arteriovenous malformation). The differential diagnosis would also include a Meckel's diverticulum with heterotopic gastric mucosa. This can be diagnosed with a Meckel's radionuclide scan.

## DIFFERENTIAL DIAGNOSIS AND TREATMENT

- *About 80% of all gastrointestinal bleeding stops spontaneously.*

- *In cases of massive GI bleeding, the clinician cannot be timid with resuscitation.*

About 80% of all gastrointestinal bleeding stops spontaneously. Therefore, time is on the side of the patient. Resuscitation and supportive care are paramount. Adequate volume restoration is critical in the establishment and maintenance of adequate urine output and the stabilization of vital signs. In cases of massive GI bleeding, the clinician cannot be timid with resuscitation. The situation calls for large-bore IV lines and boluses of 500 to 1000 mL of crystalloid as rapidly as possible. Blood should be type- and cross-matched with the initial blood draw. The first (baseline) hemoglobin (Hgb) and hematocrit (Hct) will be falsely high due to acute volume depletion. After 30 to 60 minutes of resuscitation, a more accurate Hgb/Hct will reflect the magnitude of the bleed. Blood transfusions should be given to maintain a Hgb/Hct level of 10/30 during an acute bleeding episode. Specific or directed therapy is not possible unless the bleeding lesion

TABLE 12–1

## Causes of UGI Bleeding

*Esophagus*
Reflux esophagitis
Esophageal varices
Esophageal cancer

*Stomach*
Gastritis
Mallory-Weiss tear
Gastric ulcer
Gastric cancer
Gastric varices

*Duodenum*
Peptic ulcer disease (duodenal ulcer)
Aortoenteric fistula

has been identified—usually by endoscopy. Table 12–1 lists the common causes of UGI bleeding that can present as hematemesis or melena. Most cases are managed nonsurgically.

## GASTRITIS

Bleeding from gastritis usually appears in the form of a diffuse ooze from erosions in the body and fundus of the stomach. Erosive gastritis occurs with stress such as major medical or surgical illness, burns, and trauma. Gastritis may also occur following NSAID use, aspirin use, or alcohol abuse. With resuscitation and anti-acid (H2 blockers or antacid) therapy, most cases resolve within 24 hours of presentation. It is indeed rare to require surgical therapy for hemorrhage from gastritis.

## PEPTIC ULCER DISEASE

Most peptic ulcers are related to *Helicobacter pylori* infection or to NSAID use. Significant bleeding is more common from duodenal ulcers than from gastric ulcers. If the bleeding stops, more than 90% of ulcers will heal with appropriate medical management, which includes H2 blockers or proton pump inhibitors and anti-*Helicobacter pylori* treatment if such infection is documented. Persistent bleeding from an ulcer may be managed endoscopically with a heater probe, cautery, laser, or injection therapy. Cases with visible vessels in the ulcer bed or pulsatile arterial flow visible on EGD exam often require surgery.

*Most peptic ulcers are related to* Helicobacter pylori *infection or to NSAID use.*

## MALLORY-WEISS TEAR

Mallory-Weiss tears usually present as hematemesis after a patient has experienced retching or vomiting from another cause. The increased pressure generated in the proximal stomach just below the gastroesophageal (GE) junction causes the mucosa in this area to tear and bleed. Although most occur in the proximal stomach, some do occur at the distal esophagus or GE junction. Most such tears stop bleeding spontaneously. If active bleeding is noted at the time of upper endoscopy, the area may be heater probed, coagulated, or injected with epinephrine. Only if these measures fail is surgical intervention necessary.

## ESOPHAGEAL VARICES

Patients with esophageal varices have portal hypertension. In the United States, most cases in adults are due to cirrhosis of the liver from alcohol abuse. Patients therefore have varying degrees of hepatic dysfunction and are often malnourished. The bleeding may be potentiated by coagulopathy due to inadequate production of clotting factors. Patients in shock from massive bleeding may be managed with insertion of a Sengstaken-Blakemore (S-B) tube or a Minnesota tube. This stops bleeding from varices by pressure tamponade and buys the clinician time (usually 24–48 hours) for planning. Insertion of an S-B tube is a complicated procedure and should be undertaken only by personnel familiar with its insertion and care. After 24 hours, the balloons may be deflated as the endoscopist is poised for immediate repeat endoscopy with injection sclerotherapy or rubber banding of the varices.

If an S-B tube is unavailable or fails to arrest bleeding, the patient may be started on a vasopressin drip (0.2–0.46 units/min IV). This treatment slows mesenteric and portal blood flow. A potential side effect is cardiac ischemia secondary to coronary vasoconstriction, so many authorities recommend concomitant nitrates (IV or transdermal) for prophylaxis.

Ideal therapy for bleeding esophageal varices is variceal ablation via sclerotherapy or rubber banding. Surgical portal-systemic shunting has fallen into disfavor because of high morbidity and mortality rates. The TIPS procedure (transvenous intrahepatic portal systemic shunt) can be used in recalcitrant cases.

## REFLUX ESOPHAGITIS

Patients with reflux esophagitis often present with a history of dyspepsia or heartburn. Bleeding from reflux esophagitis almost always stops spontaneously with institution of appropriate medical therapy. This includes H2 blocker or proton pump inhibitor therapy and measures to prevent gastric content reflux, such as elevating the head of the bed and avoiding eating close to bedtime.

# Mild Lower GI Bleeding (Hematochezia)

As previously mentioned, the passage of BRBPR or of maroon blood per rectum, either alone or mixed with stools, is termed *hematochezia*. This section focuses on hematochezia resulting from mild lower (LGI) bleeding that is not hemodynamically significant and usually does not require transfusion. This type of LGI bleeding has also been referred to as *outlet-type bleeding*. Moderate to severe LGI bleeding is discussed later.

## HISTORY AND PHYSICAL EXAMINATION

The examiner should consider a number of important factors in the patient's history. Previous episodes might suggest a more chronic problem. Details such as the presence of pain and the character of stools are helpful. Pain is usually present when bleeding results from an anal fissure or inflammatory bowel disease but is generally absent in other common causes such as hemorrhoids, neoplasm, or radiation proctitis. It is important to determine whether the stool is coated or streaked with blood versus bloody. Does blood drip from the anus after defecation? Has there been a change in bowel habits or weight loss along with the bleeding?

Depending on the amount of blood loss the patient reports, the examiner should clinically assess the patient's volume status to rule out more significant acute blood loss. (See next section.)

A thorough rectal exam is mandatory. Inspection of the external anus should note the presence of external skin tags or prolapsing hemorrhoids signaling internal hemorrhoidal disease. Perianal fistulous openings are visible with Crohn's disease. Digital exam may detect a palpable cancer.

*All patients with mild LGI bleeding should have a thorough rectal exam.*

## LABORATORY EVALUATION

The chronicity and severity of rectal bleeding can be determined with a CBC looking for anemia with microcytic indices. A coagulation profile is indicated if the review of systems suggests a coagulation disorder, but bleeding in a patient with a coagulopathy (such as one receiving chronic anticoagulation) should not be attributed to the coagulopathy alone. A full workup for a mucosal lesion should be undertaken.

## DIAGNOSTIC EVALUATION

*Radiologic studies are of limited value in the initial evaluation of hematochezia.*

Radiologic studies are of limited value in the initial evaluation of hematochezia. A barium enema may be useful to rule out other lesions after identification of a bleeding source, such as one in the anorectal area, has been found. The examiner must never initially attribute rectal bleeding to hemorrhoids alone; a full examination of the colon (either with colonoscopy or barium enema) is necessary to rule out other causes.

Examination for mild hematochezia requires a thorough evaluation of the entire colon and rectum. If the history or digital rectal exam suggests anal pathology, evaluation can usually begin with anoscopy. This can be done in a clinic setting if properly equipped, in an outpatient endoscopy suite, or in the operating room. If anal pathology is highly suspected or evident on initial evaluation, many examiners favor formal evaluation under anesthesia (usually caudal or spinal block) with anoscopy in the operating room. This allows for definitive diagnosis as well as interventional therapy if indicated, such as banding or sclerotherapy of hemorrhoids or lateral sphincterotomy for anal fissure.

If the initial evaluation does not necessarily point toward anal canal pathology, many practitioners would proceed with flexible sigmoidoscopy or colonoscopy. Although flexible sigmoidoscopy can be performed with less patient preparation and usually without intravenous sedation, it cannot evaluate the entire colon. Conversely, colonoscopy requires more patient preparation and IV sedation but does allow for the entire colon to be evaluated. For the evaluation of a patient with rectal bleeding, we recommend colonoscopy so that the entire colon can be evaluated. Obviously, if a flexible sigmoidoscopy is performed and no pathology to account for the bleeding is found, a colonoscopy is indicated.

## DIFFERENTIAL DIAGNOSIS AND TREATMENT

Table 12–2 lists many of the causes of mild rectal bleeding. Bleeding internal hemorrhoids should initially be treated conservatively with a regimen of aggressive management of constipation (ducosate sodium, psyllium, increased dietary fiber). Perianal symptomatology can be managed with sitz baths or over-the-counter remedies. We do not recommend steroid-based creams. If conservative therapy fails, or if the hemorrhoids are large or very symptomatic on presentation, intervention with either banding, injection sclerotherapy, or infrared coagulation is recommended. Surgical excision is reserved for large, symptomatic hemorrhoids or for when conservative or lesser therapies fail. Anal fissures can often be managed conservatively but occasionally require surgical intervention (lateral internal sphincterotomy).

**TABLE 12–2**

### Causes of Mild Rectal Bleeding

*Anorectum*
Internal hemorrhoids
Anal fissure
Cancer
Radiation proctitis

*Colon*
Colonic polyps
Cancer
Inflammatory bowel disease
Angiodysplasia
Diverticulosis
Infectious colitis

*Small Intestine*
Meckel's diverticulum
Jejunal diverticulum
Small bowel neoplasm

Colonic polyps can usually be managed colonoscopically and only require surgical excision if they are too large to be removed endoscopically. Colorectal cancers obviously require surgical evaluation. More detailed discussion on anorectal disorders appears in Chapter 17.

## Massive Lower GI Bleeding

*The patient with massive LGI bleeding represents a true medical emergency.*

The patient who presents with massive LGI tract bleeding represents a true medical emergency. This patient must be treated with a very high level of urgency.

### INITIAL EVALUATION AND RESUSCITATION

*LGI bleeding* originates at or distal to the level of the ligament of Treitz (the junction of the fourth portion of the duodenum and the jejunum). The designation of "massive" is arbitrary but for our purposes will be defined as any degree of rectal bleeding associated with evidence of intravascular volume depletion, as assessed by vital signs (tachycardia, hypotension) or the passage of large quantities of gross blood or clots from the rectum (hematochezia, even in the presence of stable vital signs). Usually, these patients will require blood transfusions early in their hospital stay. In general, massive LGI bleeding occurs less frequently than UGI bleeding, but its exact incidence is not known. Initial evaluation and resuscitation is the same as discussed for UGI bleeding.

Nearly all LGI bleeding originates in the colon; only sporadic cases (about 5%) originate in the small bowel. In about 10% of cases, the source of rectal blood is the UGI tract. Because a significant or rapid UGI bleed can present as LGI bleeding, a nasogastric (NG) tube should be placed early in the patient's evaluation to rule out the possibility of a UGI source. A positive NG aspirate or lavage (with the presence of blood or "coffee grounds") will obviously diagnose an UGI source. A negative aspirate or lavage, particularly if bile is present, is highly predictive (although not 100% conclusive) of the absence of an UGI source, and the tube may be removed.

### HISTORY AND PHYSICAL EXAMINATION

A detailed history or physical should not be allowed to delay initial evaluation or resuscitation when a patient has major LGI bleeding, but some valuable points can be gleaned from a limited history. The patient's age is important because angiodysplasia and diverticular bleeding are common in elderly patients and inflammatory bowel disease is more common in younger patients. Knowledge of previous episodes of bleeding or known diagnoses of diverticulosis, angiodysplasia, or inflammatory bowel disease is important. To establish a sense of the severity of the bleeding, its duration and nature should be sought. Lightheadedness, dizziness, or fainting are indicative of significant volume depletion. Most cases of LGI bleeding are painless. A history of pain or weight loss might alert the examiner to the possibility of colon cancer. The abdominal exam is usually benign, but the presence of a mass is important to note. Finally, a digital rectal exam is mandatory to confirm the presence of blood and define its exact character (i.e., gross blood vs. melena). In addition, large rectal cancers can often be felt.

### LABORATORY EVALUATION

Along with the placement of IV lines, laboratory tests should obviously be performed early in the patient's evaluation and must include a CBC with platelet count, as well as coagulation studies (PT, PTT), if indicated. A type and cross (usually for 4 to 8 units) should also be sent, in the event that blood transfusions are necessary.

## DIAGNOSTIC EVALUATION

Conventional radiologic studies such as barium enema have no role in the evaluation of severe LGI bleeding. In fact, a barium enema may only delay and obscure subsequent studies such as endoscopy or angiography.

Although somewhat controversial, we recommend an initial attempt at colonoscopy if the bleeding has stopped and the NG aspirate is negative. As often happens, if the bleeding is episodic and stops and the patient is stabilized, colonoscopy can follow a formal prep. If bleeding is ongoing or a full prep cannot be performed, colonoscopy may still be helpful but is decidedly more difficult and less diagnostic. Overall diagnostic accuracy ranges from 70% to 90%. Occasionally, colonoscopy may offer an opportunity for therapeutic intervention in the form of endoscopic removal of a polyp or management of angiodysplasia.

Although obtaining a specific diagnosis is important, surgical consultation relies on two advanced modalities that can provide information to localize bleeding to a specific region of the colon. This is important to the surgeon, who is often faced with a difficult decision about the need for limited versus near- or sub-total colectomy to manage life-threatening LGI bleeding. These modalities are radionuclide scanning with 99m-technetium–labeled red blood cells ($^{99}$mTc-RBC) and angiography.

$^{99}$mTc-RBC scans have the advantage of detecting active bleeding at a rate as low as 0.1 cc/min, and the scanning procedure can be repeated for up to 24 hours, which may be helpful in cases of intermittent bleeding. Their disadvantage is that they sometimes lack precise localization, so some practitioners regard them as unreliable. On the other hand, the test is sometimes specific enough to localize bleeding to the small bowel or to a major segment of the colon (i.e., right-sided versus left-sided), and this information can be very useful to the surgeon in planning an operation or in deciding about performing an arteriogram as well.

Angiography has the advantage of precise localization when positive but requires active bleeding at a rate of 0.5 to 1.0 cc/min. In addition, infusional therapy (i.e., vasopressin) or embolization is an option, particularly for patients who refuse surgery or are prohibitively high surgical risks. Its disadvantages sometimes include its more invasive nature, the need for contrast use, the amount of time it consumes, and limited availability.

*Angiography has the advantage of precise localization when positive.*

Other modalities occasionally required include enteroclysis (small-bowel follow-through, particularly when upper and lower endoscopy is negative and a small-bowel source is suspected), Meckel's radionuclide scanning, and small-bowel endoscopy.

## DIFFERENTIAL DIAGNOSIS AND TREATMENT

In general, the clinician should contact a surgeon early in the management of any patient with significant LGI bleeding. Even though up to 80% of cases will stop spontaneously, avoiding a delay in surgical consultation can be life-saving for those patients who require surgery. Most surgeons will recommend emergency surgery if the patient requires 4 to 6 units of transfused blood, the bleeding has not stopped, and nonoperative modalities such as therapeutic colonoscopy or angiography have failed. If the bleeding has stopped or is recurrent, a decision regarding elective surgery to prevent recurrent bleeding should be tailored around the specific diagnosis and the patient's overall clinical situation.

The most common causes of massive LGI bleeding are diverticulosis and angiodysplasia (Table 12–3). Significant diverticular bleeding is thought to occur in no more

TABLE 12-3

## Causes of Major LGI Bleeding

**Upper GI tract** (10% of diagnosed cases)
**Small intestine** (5% of diagnosed cases)
    Angiodysplasia
    Meckel's diverticulum
    Aortoenteric fistula
    Neoplasm
    Crohn's disease
**Large intestine** (85% of diagnosed cases)
    Angiodysplasia
    Diverticulosis
    Neoplasms
    Inflammatory bowel disease
    Ischemia
    Colitis (radiation/infectious)
    Hemorrhoids
**Undiagnosed** (10%)

than 3% to 5% of patients with diverticulosis. Bleeding is usually attributed to right-sided diverticuli and stops spontaneously in 80% to 90% of cases. Of patients who develop diverticular bleeding, only 10% to 25% of cases will become recurrent. In the emergency setting, surgery usually involves a subtotal colectomy or segmental resection (e.g., a right hemicolectomy) if the bleeding can be accurately localized. Only limited data support vasopressin infusion or embolization via arteriography; these procedures are usually recommended only for high-risk patients.

Angiodysplastic lesions are found incidentally in about 3% to 6% of patients undergoing colonoscopy. Most are present in the cecum and right colon. Fewer than 10% of patients with angiodysplasia develop bleeding. Again, bleeding stops spontaneously in 80% of patients, but the rebleed rate is as high as 25% to 50%. Most cases of significant bleeding can be diagnosed and managed colonoscopically (using electrocautery or laser). Surgical resection (usually right hemicolectomy) is required if bleeding cannot be controlled endoscopically.

### *When to Call the Surgeon about GI Bleeding*

- Any bleeding that persists despite medical therapy
- Early consultation in all cases of major upper or lower GI bleeding
- Bleeding peptic ulcer with a "visible vessel"
- Bleeding from GI tract malignancies

## RECOMMENDED READING

DeMarkles, MP, Murphy, JR: Acute lower gastrointestinal bleeding. Med Clin N Amer 77:1085–1100, 1993.

Friedman, LS (ed): Gastrointestinal Bleeding I and II. Gastroenterology Clinics of N America, Dec 1993 (vol 22) and March 1994 (vol 23).

McDermott, JP, Caushaj, PF: Lower gastrointestinal hemorrhage. In Cameron, JL (ed): Current Surgical Therapy, ed 5. Mosby, St. Louis, 1989, pp. 254–257.

Peterson, WL, Laine, L: Gastrointestinal bleeding. In Sleisenger MH, Fortran, JS (eds): Gastrointestinal Disease. WB Saunders, Philadelphia, 1993, pp. 162–192.

Sleisenger, MH, Fordtran, JS (eds): Gastrointestinal Diseases, ed 5. WB Saunders, Philadelphia, pp. 162–192.

# Chapter 13

# Abdominal Pain

ALAN M. ALELMAN, MD,
and DAVID FROMM, MD

Abdominal pain is a common complaint that the primary care examiner encounters. The most frequent diagnoses are nonspecific abdominal pain, acute gastroenteritis, pelvic inflammatory disease, and urinary tract infection (Table 13–1). These four diagnoses account for 60% to 70% of all diagnoses. There is a similar pattern among individuals who are evaluated in the emergency department for nontraumatic abdominal pain. Most individuals with abdominal pain can be easily managed in the office and will not need to be evaluated by a surgeon, but about 10% need to be referred to a specialist. Half of these patients are seen by general surgeons and another third by gynecologists. Less than 10% of patients presenting with abdominal pain are admitted to the hospital for evaluation and treatment. Although most individuals can be managed without the aid of a surgeon, the primary care provider needs to know when to call a surgeon. The main task for the practitioner is to differentiate a surgical problem that requires prompt attention from a self-limited, benign process.

Our purpose in this chapter is neither to list all of the conditions causing abdominal pain nor to spell out how to make the diagnosis. Rather, we will provide a general approach to dealing with abdominal pain, offer reminders of the most frequently omitted physical diagnostic maneuvers, and then discuss when to call a surgeon. We will also focus on the acute abdomen, since the question of whether or not to consult a surgeon occurs most frequently with this problem.

## History

The patient's history is the most important aspect for diagnosis. Whether or not the pain is acute in onset or chronic; located in a specific area, generalized, or radiating; solitary or associated with other symptoms sets off a diagnostic algorithm that lends focus to specific parts of the physical examination and diagnostic studies. Without a

TABLE 13-1

| **Final Diagnoses for the Presenting Symptom of Abdominal Pain in the Family Practice and Emergency Department Settings** | | |
|---|---|---|
| Diagnosis | Family Practice (%)* | Emergency Department (%)† |
| Abdominal pain, nonspecific | 50.4 | 41.3 |
| Acute gastroenteritis | 9.2 | 6.9 |
| Urinary tract infection | 6.7 | 5.2 |
| Irritable bowel syndrome | 5.8 | |
| Pelvic inflammatory disease | 3.8 | 6.7 |
| Hiatal hernia or reflux | 2.3 | |
| Diverticulosis | 2.2 | |
| Diarrhea, cause undetermined | 1.6 | |
| Cholelithiasis | 1.6 | 3.7 |
| Tumor, benign | 1.4 | |
| Duodenal ulcer | 1.4 | 2.0 |
| Urolithiasis | 1.3 | 4.3 |
| Appendicitis | 1.1 | 4.3 |
| Ulcerative colitis | 0.9 | |
| Muscular strain | 0.9 | |
| Other | 9.5 | |

*Data from Adelman, A: Abdominal pain in the primary care setting. J Fam Prac 25:27–32, 1987.

†Data from Brewer, RJ, et al: Abdominal pain: An analysis of 1000 consecutive cases in a university hospital emergency room. Am J Surg 131:219, 1976.

thorough and detailed history, the clinician runs the risk of setting off on the wrong track for making a diagnosis.

Diagnosis in most patients is relatively straightforward. The most difficult cases often occur among elderly and severely immunocompromised patients. Such individuals can have a catastrophic intra-abdominal event with a meager history and few or no physical findings. There are few absolutes in diagnosing abdominal pain. Diagnosis is made by assembling clues into a reasonable list of possibilities. The next step is to determine whether surgical attention is required to minimize morbidity and mortality.

Single symptoms, such as pain, anorexia, or vomiting, may not be indicators of serious pathology, but the clinician must not summarily dismiss these symptoms as indications of a self-limited problem. Most clinicians look for symptom complexes rather than placing too much emphasis on a single symptom to help them differentiate the cause for the abdominal pain.

It is helpful to have an organized approach in the evaluation of abdominal pain. This is particularly important when the diagnosis is not initially clear because an orderly, consistent review of the course of the patient's situation very often suggests the diagnosis.

*• ▬▬*

*Elderly and severely immunocompromised patients can have a catastrophic intra-abdominal event with a meager history and few or no physical findings.*

## ONSET OF PAIN

Pain of sudden onset (i.e., within seconds or minutes) is generally caused by perforation or rupture of an organ, blood vessel (e.g., aneurysm or rectus sheath hematoma), or tumor. Aortic dissection, torsion of the testicle or ovary and mesenteric vascular occulsion also can present with sudden pain. Pain of more gradual onset, developing over hours or days, generally indicates an inflammatory process (e.g., appendicitis, diverticulitis, cholecystitis, pancreatitis, abscess), obstruction, or impending rupture (e.g., ectopic pregnancy, tumor, aneurysm, peptic ulcer). Pain that develops slowly over days or weeks is generally more characteristic of neoplasm or chronic inflammation.

## ANTECEDENT EVENTS

A recent or even remote history of trauma always alerts one to a missed organ injury. Abdominal pain following a recent invasive diagnostic procedure, such as endoscopy, may indicate an organ injury due to the procedure. Left lower-quadrant pain occurring shortly after a bowel movement is more indicative of acute diverticulitis, whereas pain relieved by a bowel movement is more consistent with irritable bowel disease. Pain that wakes a patient is more common with organic than functional disease, although the difference is not statistically significant. Strenuous physical activity associated with acute-onset abdominal pain might well be due to muscle sprain, which can be difficult to distinguish from peritoneal irritation on examination.

- *A recent or even remote history of trauma should always alert one to a missed organ injury.*

## PAST HISTORY

A history of a previous condition as well as past surgical procedures may afford important clues. A misconception is that a history of significant weight loss makes the actual diagnosis of the abdominal pain less urgent. Although the weight loss may be associated with an intra-abdominal malignancy, acute (and even curable) complications of the malignancy can occur. Furthermore, weight loss associated with a benign condition does not exclude an acute complication of the underlying illness. Severely immunocompromised patients (e.g., a chemotherapy patient with a white blood cell count of <1000/mm$^3$, an AIDS patient with a CD4$^+$ count <200/mm$^3$, or a transplant recipient) can present with unusual problems related to opportunistic infections, neutropenic enterocolitis, graft-versus-host disease, or tumors (e.g., Kaposi's sarcoma, lymphomas), or with protean manifestations of more common problems.

Medications may complicate the evaluation of abdominal pain. Patients taking corticosteroids may have significant masking of serious abdominal conditions. Anticoagulants (even if coagulation parameters are within therapeutic range) or drugs known to cause pancreatitis also warrant diagnostic consideration.

- *A misconception is that a history of significant weight loss makes the actual diagnosis of the abdominal pain less urgent.*
- *Severely immunocompromised patients can present with unusual problems or with protean manifestations of common problems.*
- *Patients taking corticosteroids may have significant masking of serious abdominal conditions.*

## LOCATION

When coupled with other signs and symptoms, location of pain can be helpful, but location alone may not be a reliable indicator of the anatomic sites involved. For example, patients with irritable bowel syndrome (IBS) may present with pain anywhere in the abdomen. Abdominal pain that the patient can localize to a limited area is generally indicative of parietal peritoneal irritation. More diffuse pain or pain in the midline is generally characteristic of distention of an organ, ischemia, or smooth muscle contraction.

The site of radiation is often important. Shoulder pain that is not aggravated by arm motion suggests irritation of the peritoneal surface of the diaphragm (e.g., pancreatitis, perforated ulcer). Right subscapular pain suggests biliary colic. Pain in the region of the 12th rib may be renal or pancreatic in origin. Low sacral pain may be a manifestation of genital tract or rectal pathology. Radiation of pain to the inguinal or genital area may be due to a kidney stone, appendicitis, or groin hernia. Periumbilical pain suggests a small-bowel origin, but pain from the same source may also occur in the epigastrium.

It is helpful to distinguish between radiation and migration of pain. *Radiation* generally implies that the pain occurs in association with another site. In contrast, *migration* implies that the location of the pain has shifted to a different, albeit contiguous, site. Migration is more typical of appendicitis or a perforation that gradually spreads its contents to other areas of the peritoneal cavity. Thus, a perforated duodenal ulcer may begin with epigastric pain, but the pain may migrate to the right lower abdominal quadrant as duodenal contents migrate along the right pericolic gutter.

## CHARACTER

*Renal colic typically increases, reaches a short peak, then decreases. In contrast, biliary colic typically increases, reaches a plateau, and later decreases.*

Knowing the character of the pain (e.g., steady, progressive, radiating, or colicky) is often helpful. *Colic* is intermittent visceral pain and its origin is frequently suggested by its location. Most often, right renal colic can be distinguished from biliary colic. Renal colic typically increases, reaches a short peak, then decreases. In contrast, biliary colic typically increases, reaches a plateau, and later decreases. If the plateau of supposed biliary colic lasts more than 5 hours, a different diagnosis should be considered even though it may still involve the biliary tract (e.g., acute cholecystitis). The constant nature of the peak biliary pain is due to passage or lodgment of a stone causing proximal distention; the muscle of the gall bladder and especially of the bile ducts is sparse and does not undergo strong intermittent contraction. Small-bowel colic generally is periumbilical in nature.

Vague, central abdominal pain always poses difficulty in diagnosis, especially in the elderly, because this may be the first sign of acute mesenteric vascular ischemia.

## PROGRESSION

*Cramping pain that changes to a constant pain generally indicates a situation requiring operation, but pain that appears to improve does not necessarily preclude it.*

Progressive worsening of the pain may indicate that a significant disease process is occurring. Cramping pain that changes to a constant pain generally indicates a situation requiring operation. But pain that appears to improve does not necessarily indicate the absence of significant disease requiring operation. For example, a perforated ulcer may initially seal and reperforate; a bowel obstruction may temporarily relieve itself only to recur and strangulate in a short period.

## VOMITING

*Vomiting that follows the onset of pain strongly suggests a surgical abdomen.*

The character of the vomitus can be an important clue in diagnosis. Persistent vomiting of clear fluid suggests gastric outlet obstruction, but the subsequent appearance of small-bowel contents suggests intestinal obstruction. An important feature is the odor of the vomitus. *Feculent* vomitus refers not to a stool-like appearance but rather to the odor. Feculent odor is the result of bacterial overgrowth occurring with small intestinal obstruction of more than several hours' duration. Blood in the vomitus may indicate a stress ulcer or erosive gastritis. These are usually secondary to some other condition—most often sepsis.

Timing may also be important. Vomiting that follows the onset of pain strongly suggests a surgical abdomen.

## OTHER SYMPTOMS

*A patient lying still with pain suggests peritonitis, while moving about in a writhing manner suggests colic. Leaning forward, rocking backward and forward, or lying in the fetal position suggests pancreatitis. Psoas irritation causes the patient to lie with the leg flexed at the hip and knee.*

Pain associated with syncope or fainting may be due to hypovolemia secondary to dehydration or blood loss. Pain worsened by breathing or change in body position may be associated with peritoneal irritation.

## *Physical Examination*

Just observing the facial expression and the extent or ease of the patient's movements gives a clue as to the acuteness of the situation. For example, a patient lying still with pain suggests peritonitis; a patient moving about in a writhing manner suggests colic. Leaning forward, rocking backward and forward, or lying in the fetal position suggests pancreatitis. Psoas irritation causes the patient to lie with the legs flexed at the hip and knee. When patients keep their eyes closed during abdominal palpation, a psychological cause for the pain is possible; patients with organic disease usually keep their eyes open. The predictive power of a positive "closed-eye test" is 79% and the predictive power of a negative test is 65%.

An often-overlooked determination is whether the abdomen is scaphoid, flat, or distended. A normal patient who has had no oral intake for about 8 hours will have a scaphoid abdomen. A flat abdomen in this circumstance or its progression from scaphoid to flat may be a significant clue to a progressive condition, the nature of which may not be initially apparent. The distinction between scaphoid, flat, and distended lies along an imaginary line running from xiphoid to symphysis pubis. If the abdominal wall lies at the line, the abdomen is flat. Change of the abdominal wall during a period of observation is an important clue.

Many texts are replete with discussion about the significance of bowel sounds, but few objective data support their diagnostic import.

The presence of peritonitis can at times be extremely difficult to determine. The least sensitive means for detection of peritonitis is the determination of rebound done by initial deep palpation. If peritonitis is present, voluntary guarding develops in response to subsequent examinations. Furthermore, deep palpation with sudden release of abdominal pressure can result in a whiplash effect on the mesentery, which causes pain in an otherwise normal abdomen. Abdominal pain on coughing and detectable guarding on percussion are more reliable signs of peritonitis. The significance of "tenderness" in the absence of other peritoneal signs is difficult to determine. Detection of such tenderness often varies among examiners. Extra-abdominal conditions such as pneumonia or pleurisy can cause abdominal pain that mimics focal peritonitis. A clue to the presence of such a condition is when compression of an adjacent area of the abdomen does not increase the pain. With peritonitis, the pain increases.

*Abdominal pain on coughing and detectable guarding on percussion are more reliable signs of peritonitis than deep palpation with rebound.*

In the appropriate clinical setting, a tip-off to the presence of free air is the loss of hepatic dullness to percussion over the right lower anterior thorax. This finding does not distinguish between pneumoperitoneum and emphysema, however.

It is often helpful to determine whether the patient's pain is out of proportion to physical findings. If so, it is dangerous to assume that the pain is psychological, however. Pain out of proportion to physical findings also suggests acute pancreatitis, mesenteric ischemia (including strangulating obstruction), biliary colic, and renal colic.

*Pain out of proportion to physical findings may indicate acute pancreatitis, mesenteric ischemia (including strangulating obstruction), biliary colic, or renal colic.*

Examiners often omit important elements of physical diagnosis. Determination of a psoas sign (lying the patient on the side opposite the pain and passively hyperextending the thigh posteriorly) is one such element. Aggravation of the pain by this maneuver generally indicates the presence of retroperitoneal inflammation in the vicinity of the psoas muscle. A positive obturator test (pain on flexing and passively internally rotating the thigh) may be an indication of a pelvic appendicitis or irritation of the pelvic peritoneum. Peritonitis limited to the pelvis does not cause abdominal wall rigidity but is suggested by pelvic examination. In addition to determining whether a gynecologic problem is the cause of pain, the clinician can detect metastatic nodules or even feel fluid in the pouch of Douglas on simultaneous examination of the vagina and rectum.

Murphy's sign (tenderness and short cessation of breathing during mid inspiration as moderate pressure is applied to the right subcostal area) is considered by some to be classic for acute cholecystitis, but the sign may also be positive in the presence of acute hepatitis and right heart failure, causing distention of the hepatic capsule.

Right-sided pelvic pain occurring during right lateral distention of the rectum by the examining finger can be a sign of an inflamed appendix lying deep within the pelvis. However, the sign is frequently misinterpreted and is often said to be positive when in fact the patient has uncomplicated appendicitis outside of the pelvis.

The presence of a pulsatile mass is always of concern, but it is not only a sign of an aneurysm; it can be a pulse transmitted to a mass overlying the aorta or iliac vessels. As a general rule, a transmitted pulse is perpendicular to the abdominal wall, whereas an aneurysmal pulse is routed at a 45° angle from the abdominal wall. Evaluation of femoral pulses is often overlooked but may be a tip-off to a dissection if pulses are absent or asymmetric.

## Laboratory and Radiologic Studies

In general, too much emphasis is placed on laboratory and radiologic studies in the evaluation of abdominal pain. Such studies can confirm suspicions, but they rarely provide information that is not already suspected. There is no "routine" set of studies that should be ordered. Instead, testing should be based on the history and physical examination.

### LABORATORY STUDIES

Blood leukocyte count (WBC) is often ordered in the evaluation of acute abdominal pain. Although an elevated WBC ($>$12,000/mL) may suggest inflammation or infection, its absence does not rule out either. The trend of serial WBCs is important when observing a patient. Elderly patients are less likely to have an elevated leukocyte count with a surgical abdomen.

### RADIOLOGIC STUDIES

An abdominal series or flat plate of the abdomen is often not helpful in the workup for acute abdominal pain. In a study of patients being evaluated for abdominal pain with an abdominal series, the x-ray gave a specific diagnosis, such as free air or obstructive pattern, in less than 15% of patients. In most cases the x-ray did not change the clinical diagnosis. Chest radiographs give a specific abdominal diagnosis, such as free intra-abdominal air, in only 3% of examinations. In the case of appendicitis, abdominal radiographs are often not helpful. Even if positive, the findings are nonspecific. Barium enema, abdominal computed tomography (CT) scanning, and ultrasonography may be appropriate in certain individuals, but their use should not be routine.

## What If the Diagnosis Is Not Apparent?

*Withholding pain medication from someone who is writhing with abdominal pain and thus cannot give a coherent history is an archaic practice. Assuming the patient is not in shock, a single intravenous dose of an opioid can be exceedingly helpful.*

If the diagnosis of acute-onset abdominal pain is not apparent, the safest approach is to observe the patient. It is also an opportune time to consult a surgeon. Observation entails more than periodic measurement of vital signs or repeated tests. Repetitive examination (preferably by the original examiner) is key.

The archaic practice of withholding pain medication from someone who is writhing with abdominal pain results in the patient's inability to give a coherent history. Assuming the patient is not in shock, a single intravenous dose of an opioid (which generally lasts for no more than 1 hour) can be exceedingly helpful. This approach will only blunt, not mask, peritoneal signs. However, many surgeons prefer to see the patient before medication is administered in order to get a better appreciation of the patient's baseline condition.

## When Should a Surgeon Be Consulted?

There is no argument that a surgeon should be called about an acute situation requiring surgery. However, it also is important to involve a surgeon early in the course of a

TABLE 13-2

## Nonsurgical Causes for Significant Abdominal Pain

Acute hepatitis
Congestive heart failure
Lower-lobe pneumonia
Pulmonary embolism
Pancreatitis
Sickle-cell anemia
Crohn's disease
Urinary retention
Urosepsis
Diabetic acidosis
Myocardial infarction
Porphyria
Gastroenteritis

disease process that has the potential for requiring operation. In addition, in the case of an acute abdomen, it may be less expensive to obtain early surgical consultation rather than order expensive tests such as ultrasound that may not alter the patient's evaluation or management. It is important to determine the necessity for operation before catastrophic or irretrievable events occur. Treating acute cholecystitis or diverticulitis with antibiotics before the surgeon evaluates the patient can significantly mask a complication that is better treated by early operation.

Very often, a collaborative effort is effective in making a determination about the urgency of the situation, which may be perceived differently based on one's medical background. In difficult cases, at the very least, a surgeon may indicate that the patient's situation does not require immediate surgical attention or that further acute observation might be beneficial.

A surgeon should certainly be consulted when a patient appears with abdominal pain that follows a recent surgical procedure, because this may be a manifestation of an important complication. Even vague pain may be significant. For example, vague abdominal pain following a laparoscopic procedure may be a manifestation of a sterile biliary fistula.

Consulting a surgeon does not mean that operation is necessarily indicated. Few conditions are made worse by exploratory laparotomy or, in appropriate circumstances, laparoscopy. Medical conditions that mimic a surgical problem but may be worsened by anesthesia or operation are listed in Table 13-2. Note that most of these conditions can be excluded with an appropriate history. If a patient has an acute abdomen, hours should not be wasted in testing for obscure diagnoses. In contrast to the list of nonsurgical causes of abdominal pain, Table 13-3 lists common surgical causes

*Treating acute cholecystitis or diverticulitis with antibiotics before the surgeon evaluates the patient can significantly mask a complication that is better treated by early operation.*

*If a patient has an acute abdomen, hours should not be wasted in testing for obscure diagnoses.*

TABLE 13-3

## Common Surgical Causes of Abdominal Pain

Acute cholecystitis
Acute appendicitis
Mesenteric ischemia
Leaking aneurysm
Bowel obstruction
Perforated peptic ulcer
Perforated diverticulitis

for acute abdominal pain. Finally, the old aphorism "When in doubt, consult" holds true for primary care providers as well as for surgeons.

### *When to Call the Surgeon about Abdominal Pain*

- Acute abdominal pain
- Unexplained abdominal pain following a recent surgical procedure
- Peritoneal signs on physical exam
- Pain out of proportion to physical exam
- Pain worsening under observation
- Diagnosis is doubtful

## RECOMMENDED READING

Adelman, A: Abdominal pain in the primary care setting. J Fam Prac 25:27–32, 1987.

Adelman, A, and Koch, H: New visits for abdominal pain—The NAMCS experience. Fam Med 23:122–6, 1991.

Brazaitis, MP, and Dachman, AH: The radiologic evaluation of acute abdominal pain of intestinal origin: A clinical approach. Med Clin North Am 77:939–61, 1993.

Brewer, RJ, et al: Abdominal pain: An analysis of 1000 consecutive cases in a university hospital emergency room. Am J Surg 131:219, 1976.

Lewis, FR, et al: Appendicitis: A critical review of diagnosis and treatment in 1000 cases. Arch Surg 110:677–84, 1975.

Silen, W: Cope's Early Diagnosis of the Acute Abdomen. Oxford University Press Inc, 1987.

# Urologic Problems

MARKO R. GUDZIAK, MD
and JOSEPH C. KONEN, MD

Patients often present to their primary care providers with various urinary complaints including dysuria, frequency, hematuria, incontinence, nocturia, slow stream, urgency, or inability to void. Urinary symptoms may be classified as *irritative* or *obstructive*, but in reality symptoms often have mixed etiology. Obstructive symptoms include weak stream, straining, feeling of incomplete emptying, postvoid dribbling, intermittency, and hesitancy. Irritative symptoms include nocturia, frequency, urgency, urge incontinence, and dysuria; these have been thought to be due to an overactive bladder. Such complaints may be caused by reasonably benign conditions such as a simple cystitis or the introduction of a new medication. On the other hand, these same symptoms may be associated with other disease processes such as delirium or may be harbingers of serious or malignant diseases such as bladder or renal cancers. In short, urinary complaints cannot be ignored.

## Recurrent Urinary Tract Infections

For the most part, neither simple cystitis nor pyelonephritis present a diagnostic dilemma. Patients commonly present with typical irritative voiding symptoms such as dysuria, frequency, urgency, urge incontinence, or suprapubic pain. Urinalysis most often reveals pyuria and bacteriuria. Hematuria, malaise, fever, and flank pain indicate a severe cystitis or involvement of the upper urinary tract (ureters and kidneys). In men, perineal pain suggests prostatitis, and scrotal pain suggests epididymo-orchitis. When urinary tract infections or irritative symptoms are recurrent, a more thorough workup is needed since the etiology is often obscure. Women in whom simple cystitis occurs fewer than 3 or 4 times per year and responds readily to oral antibiotics need not be worked up further. If urinary tract infections are associated with fevers, occur more frequently than 3 or 4 times per year, or are difficult to treat, further evaluation is indicated. In men, all urinary tract infections deserve further workup unless a clear

**141**

source such as prostatitis, orchitis, or epididymitis is identified and easily treated. Immunodeficiency, particularly due to HIV, should be considered in the appropriate clinical setting.

The typical complaints of patients with recurrent urinary tract infections are the irritative symptoms mentioned earlier, although none of these symptoms is specific for infections. The patient may relate that the symptoms improve or abate with antibiotics and often for several days or weeks after completing a course of antibiotic therapy. The symptoms then recur. Sometimes the symptoms do not improve at all with antibiotics.

The first goal in a patient with recurring symptoms is to document that the patient does in fact have recurrent urinary tract infections. Simple urinary dipsticks showing nitrite- and leukocyte esterase-positive urine and even microscopic examination showing bacteria or leukocytes or both may not be sufficient to establish that an infection exists. Recurrent urinary tract infection should be documented by urine cultures. Women who cannot provide a good, clean-catch midstream specimen need to be catheterized to obtain the urine for urinalysis and culture to avoid vaginal contamination. Mixed flora or lactobacillus on a culture is usually a sign of contamination. Patients are often treated empirically for presumed urinary tract infections, and when the symptoms do not improve, subsequent cultures frequently reveal that the urine is sterile. Similarly, in the absence of positive urine cultures, one cannot assume that the symptoms were caused by an infection just because the patient states that he or she felt better after courses of antibiotics. Irritative voiding symptoms due to other causes (Table 14–1) can wax and wane, so presumed responses to antibiotic treatment may actually be coincidental improvement. Careful questioning may reveal that symptoms did abate at times following administration of antibiotics but at other times the symptoms were unchanged or may have worsened with antibiotics. These findings are clues that the patient's symptoms may be unrelated to infection. Finally, it is important to show in the face of multiple recurrence of symptoms whether the urine cultures always yield the same organism, different organisms with each occurrence, or multiple organisms.

Once there is bacteriologic evidence for recurrent urinary tract infections, a careful history should again be acquired. It may become apparent that a woman is having recurrent bouts of cystitis only after intercourse. So called "honeymoon cystitis" may clear simply by instructing the patient to void after intercourse or by prescribing a single oral dose of prophylactic antibiotics to be taken before or soon after intercourse. Recurrent infections with the same organism may indicate inadequate treatment of a urinary tract infection, with actual persistence of the infection and not a recurrence. This can occur with infected stones or foreign bodies such as catheters or internal stents, which, once infected, cannot be sterilized by antibiotics and should be removed. Recurrence with a different organism each time is more consistent with reinfection.

*Recurrent urinary tract infection should be documented by urine cultures.*

*Recurrent infections with the same organism may indicate persistence of the infection and not a recurrence.*

TABLE 14–1

**Causes of Irritative Symptoms Other Than Infection**

Bladder cancer
Bladder carcinoma in situ (CIS)
Bladder stones/foreign bodies
Distal ureteral stone
Interstitial cystitis
Urethral stricture
Benign prostatic hyperplasia
Bladder neck dysfunction
Detrusor instability
Neurogenic vesical dysfunction

Recurrent urinary tract infections with multiple organisms often suggest an enterovesical fistula, particularly when associated with pneumaturia.

In general, the workup for recurrent urinary tract infections involves searching for an anatomic or structural deficit (Table 14–2). Recurrent urinary tract infections that started in childhood suggest congenital abnormalities. On the other hand, an elderly man or a patient with long-standing bladder outlet obstruction or a poorly contractile bladder may have incomplete emptying and urinary stasis, which predisposes one to urinary tract infection. The differential diagnosis needs be tailored to the patient and his or her presentation. Indwelling Foley or suprapubic catheters are a prime cause of recurrent urinary tract infections. Whenever possible, intermittent catheterization should be substituted for an indwelling catheter. Intermittent catheterization is associated with fewer complications, especially urinary tract infections. One should elicit a history of stones, previous genitourinary or pelvic surgery, sexually transmitted diseases, and neurologic disease. Patients with neurogenic vesical dysfunction should be referred to a urologist.

*Patients with neurogenic vesical dysfunction should be referred to a urologist.*

On directed physical examination, the clinician should check for flank tenderness, flank masses, abdominal masses, suprapubic fullness, a palpable bladder with dullness to percussion, and signs of neurologic disease. In women, the examiner should check for anterior vaginal wall masses or tenderness suggestive of a urethral diverticulum. In men, examination of scrotal contents, including the epididymis and testes, and digital rectal examination to assess the prostate are mandatory. If incomplete bladder emptying or urinary retention is suspected, a postvoid residual (PVR) should be measured. A PVR exceeding 100 mL is abnormal.

Radiographic evaluation is obligatory when the physical examination is unrevealing; most anatomic abnormalities cannot be found on physical examination. In a woman with a low suspicion of upper tract involvement (i.e., no suggestive signs or symptoms such as fever, flank pain, or history of stones) a renal ultrasound (RUS), if absolutely normal, is enough to screen for upper tract abnormalities. A voiding cystourethrogram (VCUG) is necessary to assess for ureteral reflux and for urethral and bladder diverticula. If there is a strong suspicion of an upper tract abnormality, or if the renal ultrasound is abnormal, the examiner should order an intravenous pyelogram (IVP), which provides much more anatomic detail.

Men are less prone to urinary tract infections than women. In men, if urinary retention is ruled out by a low postvoid residual and there are no signs of prostatitis or epididymo-orchitis to explain the urinary tract infection, an IVP is the preferred test to visualize the anatomy. In this setting, the likelihood of finding an upper tract abnormality and the yield of the IVP are higher (e.g., showing a ureteral stone or ureteral pelvic junction (UPJ) obstruction).

If a patient is allergic to intravenous contrast, retrograde pyelograms in combination with a renal ultrasound can provide equivalent anatomic information but do not provide information on function. If an enterourinary fistula is suspected, prescribing

**TABLE 14–2**

### Anatomic and Structural Abnormalities Associated with Recurrent Urinary Tract Infections

Vesicoureteral reflux
Ureteropelvic junction obstruction
Urethral diverticulum
Bladder diverticulum
Ureteral obstruction (stones, adynamic segment, stricture, extrinsic mass)
Incomplete bladder emptying (BPH, urethral stricture, iatrogenic injury, neurogenic causes)
Foreign body (catheters)
Infected stone
Fistulas (enterourinary, vesicovaginal)

oral charcoal and checking for charcoal in urinary sediment is a good screening test. Cystourethroscopy is, however, the most specific and accurate method not only for identifying fistulas but also for assessing the urethra and subtle bladder abnormalities. Cystograms, computed tomography (CT) scans, and barium studies of the bowel (which may show vesicovaginal fisculae (VVF) or enteroureteral fistulae) may also help identify fistulae.

Treatment of recurrent urinary tract infections is first aimed at correcting any underlying structural or functional problems. From the primary care standpoint, the examiner should first employ urine cultures to determine if the patient does indeed have recurrent urinary tract infections. Women who have infrequent cystitis without signs of invasive or upper tract involvement can be treated expectantly and encouraged to drink moderate amounts of fluids in order to decrease the frequency of infections. Most other scenarios involving recurrent urinary tract infections should be referred to a urologic surgeon because treatment often involves surgical correction of an anatomic, structural, or functional abnormality of the urinary tract. For example, urethral dilation may improve symptoms of recurrent UTI's in women even when repeated attempts to document infection have failed.

### *When to Call the Surgeon about Urinary Tract Infections*

- After documenting recurrent urinary tract infections
- When symptoms persist but the examiner cannot identify the etiology
- When urinary tract infections are frequent (>3–4/yr) or severe in women
- When any urinary tract infection in men is not easily explained or treated
- When a child has any (even just one) urinary tract infection
- When any anatomic, structural or functional abnormality is identified

## *Urinary Incontinence*

Urinary incontinence affects an estimated 12 million individuals in the United States and is most prevalent in the elderly. Approximately 38% of women and 19% of men over 60 years of age experience urinary incontinence. Over half of institutionalized elderly people are incontinent. Urinary incontinence, however, affects patients of all ages and of both sexes.

Even though urinary incontinence is very bothersome, alters lifestyles, can affect health, and can be expensive owing to the cost of pads or diapers, many patients do not complain of urinary incontinence to their primary care provider. Embarrassment or the assumption that urinary incontinence is just a normal part of aging or that nothing can be done about it leads to patient underreporting. Similarly, health care providers who are unfamiliar with the treatment of urinary incontinence or who mistakenly consider it unimportant may downplay or ignore the complaint. Thus, the most important step in the diagnosis of urinary incontinence is eliciting a history of the incontinence so that the issue can be addressed. Urinary incontinence may be due to significant pathology and should not be ignored, particularly when associated with irritative voiding symptoms, urgency, urge urinary incontinence, dysuria, or frequency.

In general, urinary incontinence has two main causes: (1) bladder dysfunction, that is, a bladder that does not hold, store, or empty urine appropriately; or (2) urethral dysfunction, that is, weakened or incompetent urinary sphincters (Fig. 14–1). Some patients have a combination of both bladder and urethral dysfunction. Factors outside the urinary tract, many of them reversible, can also cause incontinence (Table 14–3). These factors are more common in the elderly. In addition, normal age-related changes in the lower urinary tract can cause or predispose to urinary incontinence. These include uninhibited detrusor contractions, increased nocturnal diuresis, decreased blad-

*Urinary incontinence may be due to significant pathology and should not be ignored, particularly when associated with irritative voiding symptoms, urgency, urge urinary incontinence, dysuria, or frequency.*

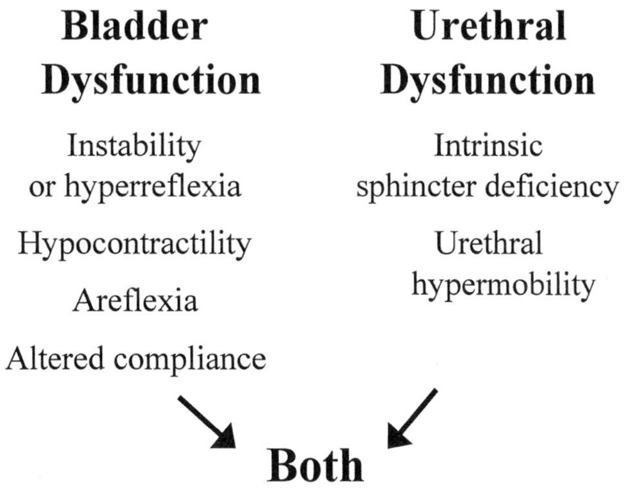

**Bladder
Dysfunction**

Instability
or hyperreflexia

Hypocontractility

Areflexia

Altered compliance

**Urethral
Dysfunction**

Intrinsic
sphincter deficiency

Urethral
hypermobility

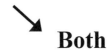

**Both**

FIGURE 14–1
Etiology of urinary incontinence.

der contractility and capacity, urethral shortening, and sphincteric weakening in women and prostatic enlargement in men.

Reversible causes of urinary incontinence, those usually outside the urinary tract, should be ruled out first, particularly in an elderly patient. A thorough history and physical exam is very helpful. The examiner may address relevant factors by using items listed in the mnemonic DIAPPERS (see Table 14–3). Altered mental status with decreased awareness of fullness and disinhibition can lead to urinary incontinence. All patients should be assessed for urinary tract infection, a very easily treated cause. Postmenopausal atrophy of estrogen-sensitive vaginal and urethral tissue can lead to poor coaptation of the urethral walls and relative sphincteric incompetence. This can be diagnosed by observing atrophy of the vaginal walls with petechiae and friability. Oral or topical estrogens can alleviate the problem, if there are no contraindications to estrogen administration. Another overlooked but reversible cause of urinary incontinence is altered psychological states—particularly severe depression.

Many medications also can lead to urinary incontinence (Table 14–4). Diuretics can cause a high urine output, which overwhelms a tenuously compensated lower urinary tract. Sedatives can alter mental status. Drugs with anticholinergic effects can diminish bladder contractility and lead to urinary retention and overflow incontinence. Such drugs include antipsychotics, antidepressants, opioids, antihistamines, and antispasmodics, among others. Sympatholytics and sympathomimetics can affect the bladder neck and the proximal and prostatic urethra. Over-the-counter nasal decongestants and combination cough preparations frequently bring about acute urinary retention in late middle-aged and older men. Thus, the examiner should inventory all medications, including over-the-counter drugs, in a patient with urinary incontinence.

Endocrine disorders such as hypercalcemia and hyperglycemia can cause signifi-

*Postmenopausal atrophy of estrogen-sensitive vaginal and urethral tissue can lead to relative sphincteric incompetence.*

*Over-the-counter nasal decongestants and combination cough preparations may bring about acute urinary retention in older men.*

TABLE 14–3

| **Reversible Causes of Urinary Incontinence** |
|---|

**D** - Delirium/confusional states
**I** - Infection
**A** - Atrophic vaginitis
**P** - Psychological/depression
**P** - Pharmaceuticals
**E** - Endocrine (hypercalcemia, hyperglycemia)
**R** - Restricted mobility
**S** - Stool impaction

**TABLE 14-4**

**Medications Associated with Urinary Incontinence**

Sedatives/hypnotics
Diuretics
Anticholinergics
Sympatholytics
Sympathomimetics

cant diuresis, mental status changes, or both. Patients with restricted mobility due to arthritis, deconditioning, severe congestive heart failure, coronary artery or pulmonary disease, physical restraints, or just a fear of falling may not be able to get to a bathroom in time. Finally, for reasons that are yet unclear, stool impaction can cause urinary retention and then overflow urinary incontinence.

These potentially reversible causes of urinary incontinence should always be investigated first, because correcting the underlying problem often resolves the incontinence or at least diminishes it. Many patients, however, will also need more thorough evaluation of established causes for incontinence.

## URINARY INCONTINENCE IN MEN

### Urethral Dysfunction

Men should be referred to a urologist once reversible causes have been ruled out. Urinary incontinence is very unusual in men and indicates a pathologic process that deserves specialized urologic evaluation. Incontinence due to de novo sphincteric weakness is rare in men. Iatrogenic injury during surgery, pelvic radiation therapy, trauma, certain spinal cord injuries, or neurologic disease can cause sphincteric deficiency (Table 14-5). Treatment of intrinsic sphincter deficiency in men is difficult. Urodynamic evaluation and surgical therapy is usually required.

### Bladder Dysfunction

Uninhibited or hyperreflexic detrusor contractions, areflexia, or altered bladder compliance (the loss of elasticity of the bladder wall, leading to high urinary storage pres-

**TABLE 14-5**

**Causes of Intrinsic Sphincter Deficiency (ISD)**

| | |
|---|---|
| Men: | Radical prostatectomy |
| | Prostatectomy for benign disease |
| | Prostatic cryosurgery |
| Women: | Previous anti-incontinence surgery |
| | Estrogen insufficiency |
| | De novo (idiopathic) |
| Both: | Myelodysplasia |
| | $T_{12}$ spinal cord injury |
| | Pelvic and urethral trauma |
| | Extirpative pelvic surgery |
| | Pelvic radiation therapy |
| | Indwelling urethral catheters |

sure) can all lead to significant complications, including infections, stones, hydronephrosis, and even renal failure. Non-neurogenic causes of bladder dysfunction in men include bladder outlet obstruction, direct trauma, and radiation therapy. Neurogenic causes of bladder dysfunction, such as spinal cord injury, multiple sclerosis, iatrogenic injury to pelvic nerves during rectal surgery, and diabetic cystopathy, can lead to upper urinary tract deterioration if not appropriately treated. All patients with neurogenic bladders need urodynamic evaluation of their bladders and should be referred to a urologist because the incidence and severity of complications are high. Even for an elderly man with urge incontinence following a stroke, empiric treatment with anticholinergics such as oxybutynin can be dangerous. In men, the incidence of bladder outlet obstruction rises with increasing age, and anticholinergics can induce urinary retention. As a rule of thumb, every male presenting with urinary incontinence should have a postvoid residual measured by catheterization or ultrasound to rule out incomplete emptying or urinary retention as a cause of overflow incontinence.

*Every male presenting with urinary incontinence should have a postvoid residual measured by catheterization or by ultrasound.*

## URINARY INCONTINENCE IN WOMEN

### Urethral Dysfunction

Urinary incontinence is more common in women than in men. Women may develop idiopathic incompetence of the intrinsic or internal urinary sphincter, which does not occur in men. Nevertheless, intrinsic sphincter deficiency has multiple etiologies in both sexes (see Table 14–5). Weakening of pelvic musculature and fascia leads to various degrees of pelvic prolapse and loss of urethral support, also called urethral hypermobility. Prolapse or loss of support can render the urinary sphincteric mechanism ineffective. This phenomenon occurs only in women, in whom the vagina serves as a potential point of weakness in the pelvic floor. In a given female patient, both intrinsic sphincter deficiency and urethral hypermobility may contribute to sphincteric dysfunction.

Sphincteric incompetence, depending on its severity, causes varying degrees of stress urinary incontinence. If the sphincteric unit is still somewhat competent, stress urinary incontinence may occur only with vigorous activity, coughing, sneezing, or heavy lifting. As the sphincter becomes more incompetent, lesser degrees of activity will cause incontinence. If the sphincter is completely nonfunctional, incontinence may be total and occur even at rest. Incontinence caused by sphincteric weakness only, not accompanied by significant bladder dysfunction, will usually be worse during the day and with increased activity and be better at rest or while sleeping. Sphincteric incompetence due to intrinsic sphincter deficiency or urethral hypermobility is accompanied by urge incontinence and detrusor instability in 30% to 40% of patients. Patients with both stress urinary incontinence and urge incontinence are said to have "mixed" incontinence.

### Bladder Dysfunction

As in men, bladder dysfunction in women has multiple etiologies. Uninhibited detrusor contractions in the absence of any neurologic disorder are called *detrusor instability*. The usual symptom is urge incontinence. Detrusor instability can be idiopathic. Very rarely it is the result of prolonged bladder outlet obstruction in women. Obstruction rarely occurs in women who have not had urethral or bladder surgery or trauma.

*Detrusor hyperreflexia*, by definition, is the presence of uninhibited bladder contractions, which are due to neural injury or disease such as spinal cord injury or multiple sclerosis. Women as well as men with this disorder should be referred to a urologist. Patients with *detrusor areflexia*, a noncontracting bladder due to neurogenic causes, also should be referred. A bladder may be hypocontractile owing to myogenic injury

*Any patient with a postvoid residual of more than 100 mL or signs of renal insufficiency needs evaluation by a urologist.*

resulting from acute or chronic overdistention, overall patient debility, diabetic cystopathy, or simple aging. Hypocontractility leads to incomplete emptying and can be accompanied by instability, a condition known as detrusor hyperactivity with impaired contractility (DHIC). Measuring a postvoid residual will rule out poor emptying. Normally, a postvoid residual should be less than 20 mL, but one of less than 80 to 100 mL may be acceptable, particularly in the elderly, if the individual is reasonably asymptomatic and has normal renal function. Any patient with a postvoid residual of more than 100 mL or signs of renal insufficiency needs evaluation by a urologist.

Loss of normal bladder compliance can only be assessed by urodynamics. Patients at risk for altered compliance include those with previous pelvic radiation, pelvic surgery, spinal cord injury, spina bifida, or a long-term indwelling catheter. These patients should see a urologist.

### Evaluation of Urinary Incontinence

Evaluation of urinary incontinence should begin with a history to determine whether it is related to activity or straining (stress incontinence) and whether its pattern includes urgency, frequency, or diurnal variation. Does the patient report postvoid fullness or urge incontinence? Has the patient had previous pelvic or genitourinary surgery, neurologic disease, herniated disc, diabetes, trauma, or pelvic radiation? On physical examination, the examiner should palpate the abdomen to assess for a distended bladder, assess lumbosacral innervation, and perform a pelvic exam to assess for prolapse or any degree of anterior vaginal wall laxity. One should also look for signs of vaginal atrophy in postmenopausal women. A rectal examination can help exclude impaction and allow for assessment of sphincteric tone. Measuring a postvoid residual is imperative, as is a urinalysis to rule out infection. Hematuria requires a separate workup, as discussed later in this chapter. Ultimately, urodynamic studies are often needed to fully assess the causes of urinary incontinence and to guide therapy.

## TREATMENT OF URINARY INCONTINENCE

A woman with mild stress urinary incontinence and mild prolapse or urethral hypermobility may respond to conservative measures such as clock or timed voiding. The idea is to have the patient empty her bladder on a schedule and not wait until she has the desire to void, keeping the bladder from getting very full and thus making it easier for a weak sphincter to resist abdominal pressure (coughing, sneezing, straining) as an expulsive force of urine. Kegel exercises, which are highly touted, should be tried but are overrated and often do not make a significant difference. Low-dose sympathomimetics such as pseudoephedrine 15 mg PO (by mouth) bid (twice daily) can help. In theory they do so by stimulating the alpha adrenergic receptors in the proximal urethra and intrinsic sphincter, increasing its tone. Anticholinergic agents such as imipramine (10–25 mg PO bid) or others listed on Table 14–6 can also help to increase functional bladder capacity in women. They should not be used in men without prior evaluation for outlet obstruction. Women with severe stress urinary incontinence or moderate or

TABLE 14–6

### Commonly Used Anticholinergic Medication

Oxybutynin (Ditropan) 2.5 to 10 mg PO bid (twice per day) to qid (four times per day)
Imipramine (Tofranil) 10 to 25 mg PO bid to tid
Hyoscyamine (Levsin) 0.125 to 0.375 mg PO tid (three times per day) to qid
Propantheline (Pro-Banthine) 7.5 to 30 mg PO tid to qid

severe prolapse, and those unresponsive to conservative measures, should see a urologist.

Women with only urge incontinence and a low postvoid residual usually respond very well to timed or clock voiding; by the time they have the urge to void they will often develop an uninhibited detrusor contraction resulting in urge urinary incontinence. Various forms of "bladder training" are also helpful but require both a dedicated therapist and a compliant patient. Anticholinergic agents (see Table 14–6) are an adjunct to timed voiding; they rarely eliminate detrusor instability completely. If anticholinergics are used alone, without timed voiding, urge incontinence often will continue but be less frequent. Anticholinergics do not generally increase warning time. Once the patient feels full, urination will still be precipitous. Anticholinergics do allow the bladder to hold more before the patient develops the desire to void, which allows for a less frequent schedule of timed voiding while still maintaining continence.

*Women with only urge incontinence and a low postvoid residual usually respond very well to timed or clock voiding.*

### When to Call the Surgeon about Urinary Incontinence

- Incontinence in a male
- Neurologic disease
- Renal insufficiency
- Postvoid residual >100 mL
- No response to conservative measures
- Reversible causes excluded

## Hematuria

### URINALYSIS AND CAUSES OF HEMATURIA

Virtually all patients presenting with hematuria, whether gross or microscopic, need to be evaluated. First, however, the examiner should define what is significant hematuria. *Gross hematuria*, blood in the urine visible to the naked eye, is always significant and always deserves further workup. Urine may appear red for reasons other than blood, of course; many possible causes are listed in Table 14–7.

When microhematuria is found on urinalysis, one must consider what degree of microhematuria is regarded as abnormal and deserving of further workup. Several factors must be considered. "Normal" individuals may excrete red blood cells (RBCs)

TABLE 14–7

| **Causes of Red Urine** |
| --- |
| Hematuria |
| Myoglobinuria |
| Hemoglobinuria |
| Urobilinogenuria (hemolytic anemia) |
| Acute intermittent porphyria (turns red in sunlight) |
| Porphyria erythropoietica |
| Chronic heavy metal poisoning (lead, mercury) |
| Food pigments (beets, blackberries) |
| Rifampin |
| Phenolphthalein (Ex-Lax, alkaline pH only) |
| Phenothiazines |
| Diphenylhydantoin |
| Nitrofurantoin |

**TABLE 14-8**

### Common Urologic Causes of Hematuria

Urinary tract infection
Bladder tumor
Renal tumor
Ureteral tumor
Benign prostatic hypertrophy
Trauma
Sickle-cell disease or trait
Tuberculosis
Renal infarction
Renal vein thrombosis
Coagulation and platelet deficiencies
Exercise
Hypercalciuria
Vasculitis
Chemical or radiation cystitis

*Hematuria is often intermittent even with significant pathology.*

in their urine on a continuous basis, but a finding of only 3 to 5 RBCs per high-power field (hpf) on a fresh, properly collected and centrifuged urine specimen may be abnormal. Urine analysis is often repeated for such findings, but one needs to be cautious because hematuria is often intermittent even with significant pathology. One could miss significant disease by not acting on one urinalysis showing microhematuria. If one chooses not to act on a single urinalysis that showed 3 to 5 RBC/hpf, then patients should be re-evaluated with at least two or three repeat urinalyses on separate occasions. One episode of gross hematuria or high-grade microhematuria (more than 20 RBC/hpf) always requires further evaluation.

To detect blood in the urine, urinary dipsticks rely on a peroxidase reaction in the test strip, which is catalyzed by hemoglobin or myoglobin to cause a color change. Several factors can give false-positive results from both dipstick testing and microscopic urinalysis: contamination with blood from menstrual flow or preputial tears; high specific gravity with more concentrated urine following exercise or accompanying dehydration and ingestion of ascorbic acid, other vitamins, or foods with high levels of oxidants. False negatives with a dipstick are unusual. Dipsticks are about 90% sensitive for finding >3 RBC/hpf and may be used for screening, but they are not very specific and have a high degree of false positives. A dipstick positive for blood needs to be confirmed with a microscopic analysis of centrifuged urine. False-negative microscopic analysis in the presence of a positive urinary dipstick for blood may occur if RBC lysis occurs prior to examination. This is most likely to occur in hypotonic urine (specific gravity <1.007) that has not been examined immediately after being provided.

It is also important to know whether RBCs in the urinary sediment are glomerular or nonglomerular in origin. Bleeding from a glomerular source, usually indicating nephrologic disease and glomerulonephritis, is characterized by dysmorphic, irregularly shaped RBCs and red-cell casts and is almost always associated with proteinuria. With urologic hematuria one usually finds normal-appearing RBCs with a round or crenated border. Nephrologic hematuria will not be covered in this chapter. The etiology of urologic hematuria (Table 14-8) varies with the patient's sex and age.

*With urologic hematuria, one usually finds normal-appearing RBCs.*

## HEMATURIA EVALUATION

The diagnostic evaluation of hematuria starts with a history and physical examination. The patient should be asked about other symptoms that may help establish a differential diagnosis: dysuria, frequency, fever, flank pain, colic. One should ask about recent trauma, history of urinary tract infections, stones, renal disease, cancers, chemotherapy, or pelvic radiation therapy. Smoking and exposure to chemicals can be risk factors for urothelial malignancies. On physical exam, the clinician should check for flank tenderness and masses. The abdomen should be examined for tenderness, masses, and bladder distention. The prostate should be palpated for nodules and enlargement. In women, it is advisable to palpate the urethra for masses during the pelvic exam. The male urethra should be assessed for palpable nodules or strictures. Urinalysis should be performed as previously discussed and urine cultures should be performed especially if there are any irritative symptoms.

In the presence of hematuria, especially in asymptomatic individuals, radiographic examination of the upper urinary tract (kidneys and ureters) is essential. This is usually done with an intravenous pyelogram (IVP). Cystoscopy is mandatory and is used to evaluate the lower urinary tract (bladder and urethra). Urine cytology should be performed for all patients, and urine should be cultured as needed. If a patient has abnormal renal function or an allergy to intravenous contrast, then a renal ultrasound should be performed to evaluate the kidneys, and retrograde pyelography should be done at the time of cystoscopy to evaluate the ureters and collecting system. Ureteroscopy may be indicated. The primary care provider may initiate the workup, but urologic consultation is necessary in all cases of significant hematuria not related to infection and that fails to completely resolve with therapy, because cystoscopy is essential to complete the diagnostic workup.

One should never ignore hematuria in a patient receiving anticoagulant therapy or nonsteroidal anti-inflammatory agents. Anticoagulant therapy will often unmask genitourinary lesions at an earlier stage.

Microhematuria clearly associated with an acute cystitis, which is then documented to resolve on follow-up urinalyses, does not need to be referred.

### *When to Call the Surgeon about Hematuria*

- Any significant hematuria
- Hematuria occurring in a patient receiving anticoagulants
- Hematuria not associated with acute cystitis and not resolved with antimicrobial therapy

## Disorders of the Prostate

Discomfort resulting from disorders of the prostate may range from a vague, mild sensation of fullness to exquisite pain in the perineal or rectal area. Discomfort may be localized to a well-defined area, but more often is diffuse and may be perceived in the floor of the pelvis, throughout the pelvic area, the scrotum and testicles, the suprapubic area, groin, or beyond. The discomfort may also be referred to the lower lumbar and sacral areas of the back. In general, one should consider disorders of the prostate in any man who complains of discomfort in his ''bathing suit'' area.

The complex of symptoms commonly known as *prostatism* includes obstructive and irritative symptoms of the lower urinary tract. In fact, the term *lower urinary tract symptoms* (LUTS) is a more descriptive and preferred term because these symptoms are not specific for the prostate. One cannot assume that the cause of these symptoms is an enlarged prostate. Other diseases also should be included in the differential diagnosis (see Table 14–1). Irritative symptoms include dysuria, urinary frequency, and urgency. Obstructive symptoms include decrease in the caliber and force of the urinary stream, hesitancy in initial voiding, a sensation of incomplete emptying of the bladder, and postvoid dribbling. The International Prostate Symptom Score (I-PSS, Table 14–9) is a useful tool to measure the frequency of symptoms and how much they bother men. Scores range from mild (score of ≤7) to moderate (8–19) to severe (≥20).

TABLE 14–9

## International Prostate Symptom Score (I-PSS)

| | Not at all | Less than 1 time in 5 | Less than half the time | About half the time | More than half the time | Almost always | Your score |
|---|---|---|---|---|---|---|---|
| **1. Incomplete emptying** Over the past month, how often have you had a sensation of not emptying your bladder completely after you finished urinating? | 0 | 1 | 2 | 3 | 4 | 5 | |
| **2. Frequency** Over the past month, how often have you had to urinate again less than 2 hours after you finished urinating? | 0 | 1 | 2 | 3 | 4 | 5 | |
| **3. Intermittency** Over the past month, how often have you found you stopped and started again several times when you urinated? | 0 | 1 | 2 | 3 | 4 | 5 | |
| **4. Urgency** Over the past month, how often have you found it difficult to postpone urination? | 0 | 1 | 2 | 3 | 4 | 5 | |
| **5. Weak stream** Over the past month, how often have you had a weak urinary stream? | 0 | 1 | 2 | 3 | 4 | 5 | |
| **6. Strain** Over the past month, how often have you had to push or strain to begin urination? | 0 | 1 | 2 | 3 | 4 | 5 | |
| | None | 1 time | 2 times | 3 times | 4 times | 5 or more times | |
| **7. Nocturia** Over the past month, how many times did you most typically get up to urinate from the time you went to bed at night until the time you got up in the morning? | 0 | 1 | 2 | 3 | 4 | 5 | |
| **Total I-PSS Score =** | | | | | | | |

### Quality of Life Due to Urinary Symptoms

| | Delighted | Pleased | Mostly satisfied | Mixed—about equally satisfied and dissatisfied | Mostly dissatisfied | Unhappy | Terrible |
|---|---|---|---|---|---|---|---|
| If you were to spend the rest of your life with your urinary condition just the way it is now, how would you feel about that? | | | | | | | |

## PROSTATODYNIA

*Prostatodynia*, or discomfort in the region of the prostate gland, is a common condition, but one which men probably underreport. The condition is not well understood but is probably multifactorial in origin. Sitting in warm water, resuming usual sexual activity patterns, or frequently changing sitting positions may be helpful for relieving prostatodynia. Aspirin or other anti-inflammatory agents may also be effective. Cold showers or baths, especially after sexual excitement, can aggravate the condition, probably through additional contraction of periprostatic tissues.

## ACUTE PROSTATITIS

*Prostatitis* is the inflammation of the prostate gland. Symptoms of acute prostatitis include increased discomfort in the perineal area, perhaps radiating to the lower back; dysuria; malaise; and possibly fever and chills. Often signs of both irritative and obstructive voiding dysfunction are present. Infection is the most common cause; other possibilities include significant trauma or pelvic radiation.

Digital rectal examination (DRE) usually reveals a tender, warm, swollen, "boggy" prostate. Prostatic secretions obtained from prostatic massage are almost always abnormal, but massage should not be performed when acute prostatitis is suspected because the procedure is usually painful and may result in bacteremia. Examination of the urine may be normal or show pyuria. Bacteriuria often, but not always, accompanies acute prostatitis. Urine cultures may reveal the causative infectious agent. Both gram-positive aerobes (*Enterococcus* and *Staphylococcus* species) and gram-negative aerobes (*Escherichia*, *Proteus*, *Klebsiella*, *Enterobacter*, and *Pseudomonas* species) are common causative agents. Uncommon infectious causes include gonococcal, tuberculous, mycotic, and parasitic agents. Other suspected but unproven agents include viruses, ureplasmas and chlamydia.

Treatment should be directed toward the causative agent, and choice of therapy should be guided by culture results. Initial treatment with trimethoprim/sulfa combination or fluoroquinolones is usually effective.

Unrecognized or inadequately treated acute prostatitis may result in prostatic abscesses. Men with diabetes or chronic renal insufficiency or who are immunocompromised are at greater risk for developing a prostatic abscess, as are those who have had a recent urethral catheterization or instrumentation. Abscesses vary greatly in their presentation, but the diagnosis should be entertained in cases of acute febrile urinary retention with a tender prostate. Imaging studies using CT or transrectal ultrasound usually confirm the diagnosis. Surgical consultation should be sought for treatment because drainage and antibiotics are required.

*Men with diabetes or chronic renal insufficiency or who are immunocompromised are at greater risk for developing a prostatic abscess, as are those who have had a recent urethral catheterization or instrumentation.*

## CHRONIC PROSTATITIS

Most men with chronic prostatitis present with moderate symptoms of irritative voiding dysfunction and unilateral or bilateral discomfort in the "bathing suit" area. Other men complain of pain on ejaculation or hematospermia. Some men with chronic prostatitis have clear evidence of an antecedent episode of acute prostatitis, but for most the cause is unknown. Both infectious and irritative chemical reflux etiologies have been proposed.

Physical examination of the prostate may reveal a normal, tender, or "boggy" gland. Even though bacteriologic evidence for infection may not be found, many men with chronic prostatitis respond at least temporarily to courses of antibiotics, especially trimethoprim/sulfa, doxycycline, or fluoroquinolones. However, failure to improve or completely resolve is common. Short courses of anti-inflammatory agents, stool softeners, or both may help, as may warm to hot sitz baths. Irritative voiding symptoms may also be relieved with oxybutynin or hysocyamine or alpha blockers.

## BENIGN PROSTATIC HYPERTROPHY

*Benign prostatic hypertrophy* (BPH) is extremely common and is predominantly a quality-of-life problem. Almost every male living into his eighth decade will have histologic evidence of BPH. However, only half will develop palpable prostatic enlargement, and only half of these will develop sufficient symptoms to undergo surgical resection. Even so, transurethral prostatectomy (TURP) is the most common surgical procedure performed on men in the United States today.

The quality-of-life problem for men arises from the need to balance the annoyance of BPH symptoms and potential complications of untreated BPH with unintended side effects of surgical and pharmacologic treatments. In general, even without therapy, symptom progression is uncommon. Stabilization and even improvement of symptoms is the normal course of events. Progression to complications such as acute urinary obstruction, urinary tract infection, obstructive uropathy, or renal failure is rare. Because symptoms often wax and wane, and risk of serious complications is relatively low, an initial "wait-and-see" management approach is often in the man's best interest. However, urologic consultation should be sought for men with signs and symptoms of persistent obstruction.

*Urologic consultation should be sought for men with signs and symptoms of persistent obstruction.*

Detection of nodules, consistency, and tenderness may be important for other diagnostic considerations, but by itself DRE is a poor screening tool for either BPH or prostate cancer. Because the examiner cannot feel the entire prostate gland in three dimensions, DRE is a poor estimator of gland size.

Measurement of prostate-specific antigen (PSA) should also not be considered a screening tool for BPH. PSAs are not specific for prostate cancer; they are often elevated, sometimes markedly, in BPH. Hence the absolute value of PSA cannot be used with any certainty to differentiate between BPH and prostatic carcinoma.

The differential diagnosis for BPH depends on the nature of the symptoms. Purely irritative symptomatology may accompany urinary tract infections, prostatitis, bladder cancer, bladder calculi, interstitial or radiation-induced cystitis, and uninhibited bladder contractions that may result from cerebrovascular accidents. Pure obstructive symptoms may be due to urethral stricture, prominent urethral valves, prostate cancer, bladder neck contracture, or a poorly contracting bladder in response to paraplegia. Mixed obstructive and irritative symptoms may result from neurologic insults such as spinal cord injury, multiple sclerosis, or Parkinson's disease. Usually an adequate history and a few laboratory tests will make the diagnosis clear.

Evaluation for BPH should begin with a careful history supplemented by use of the International Prostate Symptom Score (see Table 14-9) to semiquantitate urinary symptomatology. The examiner should evaluate the prostate by a DRE, realizing that significant BPH may exist even if the DRE seems normal. In most cases of BPH the gland will be enlarged, symmetrical, elastic, and firm. The abdomen should also be palpated and percussed for signs of bladder distention.

Laboratory evaluation should include a urine analysis with at least a qualitative measurement for blood and leukocyte esterase activity, if not microscopic examination. If the urinalysis is abnormal, the urine should be cultured. If cultures are negative and hematuria is detected, a workup to rule out carcinoma and stones should continue. Serum creatinine should also be measured at the initial evaluation and repeated along with periodic urine analysis in symptomatic men, especially those undergoing "watchful waiting" protocols. Obstructive uropathy is uncommon but can occur in 10% of men who have asymptomatic or "silent" prostatism.

If the urine analysis and serum creatinine are normal, other studies are not likely to contribute significantly to management decisions. Unless complications are suspected, an intravenous pyelogram, renal ultrasonography, cystometrics, or cystoscopy has no clear value. Measurements of postresidual volume and urine flow rates have poor reproducibility and usually add little to the diagnosis. Pressure flow studies may be useful in differentiating neurogenic and decompensated bladder conditions from BPH. Transrectal ultrasound may help in measuring large glands, especially when surgery is considered, because open prostatectomy may be preferred over transurethral resection for glands weighing more than 60 grams.

Management strategies should keep the interests of the patient clearly in mind and must balance the risk of complications from disease progression, side effects from therapy, lost time from work or avocations, and both short- and long-term treatment costs. Comparing serially performed I-PSS is useful in evaluating response to therapy.

In general, watchful waiting should be the treatment of choice for men who are not moderately to severely dissatisfied by their symptoms. This is an especially appropriate strategy for men whose total I-PSS score is less than or equal to 7, but it should also be considered as an option for men with higher scores. The risk is low that significant complications will develop during a period of noninterventional observation. Men should be instructed to report increases in severity or frequency of symptoms between evaluations. Even if symptoms are not progressing, men with BPH should be re-evaluated at least yearly with the I-PSS, DRE, urinalysis, serum creatinine and PSA.

Alteration of lifestyle should be recommended to all men with significant BPH symptoms, regardless of other treatment options they might select. In particular they should avoid alpha-adrenergic stimulants such as decongestants and cough syrups, which can increase prostatic muscular tone. Avoiding anticholinergic and antihistaminic medications may also be helpful. Reducing late-evening fluids and caffeine after dinner may be effective in lessening the frequency of nocturia. Cold, immobility, and excessive alcohol ingestion may also precipitate acute urinary retention in men with significant BPH and should be avoided.

Pharmaceutical approaches should be considered as the second line of intervention after watchful waiting. Presently these include the use of alpha-adrenergic blockers and 5$\alpha$-reductase inhibitors. However, 5$\alpha$-reductase inhibitors may work best when the prostate gland is especially large (>60 grams). Because finasteride effectively reduces the size of the prostate gland, PSA levels may fall about 50%. Clinicians following PSA levels should remember to draw new baseline levels after men have been taking finasteride for 4 to 6 months.

Invasive or surgical treatments should be considered when other strategies have failed, when the prostate gland is estimated to be markedly enlarged (>60 grams), or when the patient has expressed a preference for a urologic opinion. Referral to a urologist is also appropriate for refractory urinary retention after a trial of catheterization or for men who experience recurrent urinary tract infections, hematuria, or signs of renal insufficiency, all of which suggest significant obstruction caused by something other than BPH.

Surgical options for symptoms and bladder outlet obstruction secondary to BPH include simple prostatectomy (suprapubic, retropubic), transurethral prostatectomy (TURP), laser prostatectomy (TULIP, VLAP), transurethral incision of the prostate (TUIP), microwave ablation of the prostate, transurethral vaporization of the prostate (TUVP), and many other new, emerging technologies.

Urologic consultation is mandated for patients with prostatism accompanied by any of the conditions listed on the following "When to Call the Surgeon" table.

## PROSTATE CANCER

Adenocarcinoma of the prostate is the most commonly occurring solid tumor in Americans today. Although as many as one-third of men over the age of 50 may be harboring a silent type of the cancer, very few will ever become clinically apparent. Only a quarter of the men who develop prostate cancer will die from it. In general, prostate cancers are slow growing. Men who develop prostate cancer in their seventies are more likely to die from other causes—especially cardiovascular diseases. Although the attention paid to screening activities for prostate cancer has increased, using either DRE or PSA, there is no long term evidence that early detection and treatment have any significant favorable effect on survival.

Nearly all prostate carcinomas arise in the peripheral zones of the gland, not near the prostatic urethra. Hence the early stages of prostate cancer usually have no symptoms. When symptoms do develop, they are usually obstructive and may be identical to those caused by BPH. Late symptoms are usually due to distant metastasis—most commonly to bone. These symptoms include bone pain (especially in the back), weight loss, anemia, dyspnea, lymphedema, azotemia, ureteral obstruction, and neurologic symptoms.

Surgical consultation should be sought if prostatic masses or nodules are detected or if there is an elevated PSA, so that core-needle biopsies can be performed transrectally under ultrasound guidance or transperineally. Urologic recommendations should also be sought about the complex array of potential therapies. Depending on the stage of the tumor and the patient's age and health status, these may range from observation to hormonal and other pharmacologic interventions aimed at palliation to aggressive treatments aimed at cure.

### *When to Call the Surgeon about Prostate Disorders*

- Prostatic abscess
- Prostatic hyperplasia with signs of persistent obstruction such as:
  —refractory urinary retention after a trial of catheterization
  —recurrent urinary tract infections, hematuria, or signs of renal insufficiency
- "Prostatism" accompanied by:
  —hematuria
  —elevated prostate-specific antigen
  —renal insufficiency
  —previous genitourinary surgery
  —history of genitourinary malignancy
  —neurologic disease (e.g., Parkinson's disease, multiple sclerosis, stroke, long-standing diabetes with signs of neuropathy)
  —elevated postvoid residual (>100 mL)
  —urinary retention
  —bladder stones
  —no response to medical management
  —symptoms in patient <45 years old
- Prostatic masses or nodules
- Elevated PSA

### RECOMMENDED READING

Benign Prostatic Hyperplasia (BPH) Guidelines Panel: Diagnosis and treatment. AHCPR Pub No. 94-0582, February 1994.

Cooner, WH, and Roberts, GR: Prostate Disease: An American Family Physician Monograph. American Academy of Family Physicians. Kansas City, MO, 1992, pp 1–24.

Gudziak, MR, and Rudy, DC: Urinary incontinence. In Rahel, R (ed): Conn's Current Therapy. WB Saunders, Philadelphia, 1995.

Lepor, H, et al: The efficacy of terazosin, finasteride, or both in benign prostatic hyperplasia. N Engl J Med 335:533, 1996.

Mariani, AJ: The evaluation of adult hematuria. AUA Update Series 1989, Vol VIII, Lesson 23.

Urinary Incontinence Guideline Panel: Urinary incontinence in adults: Clinical practice guidelines. AHCPR Pub. No. 92-0038, Rockville, MD, AHCPR, Public Health Service, US Dept. of Health and Human Services, March 1992.

Urinary Tract Infections. Urol Cl NA, Vol 13, No. 4, Nov 1986.

# Chapter 15

# Pelvic Pain and Genital Tract Infections

S. GENE MCNEELEY, Jr, MD,
and HOWARD B. MCNEELEY, MD

## *Pelvic Pain*

Pelvic pain is a nonspecific symptom arising from the urogenital tract, gastrointestinal tract, or musculoskeletal system and is a common presenting complaint for women seeing their primary care providers. Although surgical intervention is unnecessary in most women with acute or chronic pelvic pain, an unnecessary delay in the diagnosis of ectopic pregnancy or adnexal torsion, for example, not only affects her immediate well-being, but also can have long lasting effects on her reproductive potential.

### CLINICAL EVALUATION OF PELVIC PAIN

When evaluating a woman with pelvic pain, a thorough history, including a complete obstetric and gynecologic history, is of paramount importance (Table 15–1). The onset of pain may coincide with menses (dysmenorrhea) or worsen with menses or at other times during the menstrual cycle, such as with ovulation. Assess menstrual regularity and irregular or otherwise abnormal bleeding. Inquire about factors that may exacerbate or alleviate her symptoms. Ask women of childbearing age about symptoms of pregnancy (amenorrhea, nausea, vomiting, and breast soreness or engorgement). Obtain a sexual history, consisting of sexual orientation, number of partners, new partners, contraceptive methods, and sexual satisfaction. Question the woman thoroughly as to gastrointestinal, urologic, and musculoskeletal symptoms and pre-existing or concurrent conditions.

Physical examination includes a general assessment of wellness or distress, including vital signs. The abdomen should be inspected and auscultated. Palpation should determine the area of maximum tenderness and whether rebound tenderness exists. A complete pelvic exam should include inspection of the external genitalia, visualization of the cervix with a bivalve speculum, and an endocervical culture or probe test for

**TABLE 15-1**

| **Obstetric and Gynecologic History** |
|---|
| Gravidity and parity |
| Chief complaint |
| Menstrual history |
|    Last normal menstrual period |
|    Menarche |
|    Duration and interval |
|    Menstrual flow |
|    Abnormal bleeding |
|    Pain |
| Obstetric history including complications |
| Gynecologic history |
|    Prior disorders and surgery |
|    Sexually transmitted diseases |
|    Contraception, present and past |
| Sexual health |
|    Activity, orientation, satisfaction, problems |
| Specific review of gastrointestinal and genitourinary symptoms |

*Neisseria gonorrhoeae* and *Chlamydia trachomatis*. After removing the speculum, perform a bimanual examination to determine the position and size of the uterus, the presence of uterine tenderness, pain with cervical movement, and the presence of adnexal tenderness or adnexal mass. Additional laboratory tests that may be helpful include a sensitive pregnancy test, complete blood count, and urinalysis. Pelvic ultrasound, preferably transvaginal, is the most helpful radiologic exam to evaluate pelvic pain.

## DYSMENORRHEA

*Dysmenorrhea* is defined as painful menstruation and may be further classified as primary or secondary. *Primary dysmenorrhea* is due to prostaglandin-mediated uterine contractions and occurs in 30% to 75% of women. The onset of dysmenorrhea is usually within 1 year of establishing ovulatory cycles. In 15% to 30% of women, dysmenorrhea is severe and interferes with the completion of daily tasks. During menstruation, excessive prostaglandin F2$\alpha$ is produced in the endometrium, causing intense uterine contractions. Other symptoms caused by this prostaglandin include nausea, vomiting, and diarrhea. Prostaglandin E2 is also released in the uterus. It may account for heavy menstrual flow as it produces vasodilatation and inhibits platelet aggregation. The pelvic examination will be normal in most circumstances. Primary dysmenorrhea should not be confused with dysmenorrhea due to imperforate hymen. In such circumstances, the pain is due to accumulation of blood in the vagina and uterine cavity (hematocolpos and hematometra) and peritoneal endometrial implants. Nonsteroidal anti-inflammatory drugs inhibit prostaglandin synthesis and are mainstays of the treatment of primary dysmenorrhea. Combination oral contraceptives are also effective.

*Secondary dysmenorrhea* is defined as acquired painful menstruation due to identifiable anatomic or clinical causes (Table 15-2). Peritoneal and adnexal disorders such as infection or endometriosis may produce an inflammatory response or may stretch or distort the peritoneum and pelvic structures by scarring. Uterine abnormalities such as leiomyomas and adenomyosis produce symptoms by stretching the peritoneum or impinging on neighboring structures. Physical examination may reveal evidence of uterine or adnexal enlargement or tenderness. Pelvic ultrasound is an important aid in this clinical setting. More expensive imaging studies (computed tomography [CT] scan and magnetic resonance imaging [MRI]) are not recommended in the initial workup of secondary dysmenorrhea, but they may be very helpful as confirmatory tests (e.g., MRI

*More expensive imaging studies (CT scan and MRI) are not recommended in the initial workup of secondary dysmenorrhea, but they may be very helpful as confirmatory tests.*

**TABLE 15-2**

| Causes of Secondary Dysmenorrhea |
|---|
| Endometriosis |
| Uterine fibroids |
| Uterine polyps |
| Adenomyosis |
| Cervical stenosis |
| Congenital genital-tract malformations |
| Pelvic adhesions |

is very specific for adenomyosis). Conditions causing secondary dysmenorrhea usually do not require surgical consultation in an urgent or emergency setting. Medical or surgical treatment is specific to the diagnosed condition and is beyond the realm of this chapter.

If the patient's pain continues throughout the menstrual cycle, or occurs at irregular intervals, the clinical picture becomes much more obscure and may fall into the realm of *chronic pelvic pain*. This syndrome requires an intensive evaluation, oftentimes multidisciplinary.

## OTHER CAUSES OF PELVIC PAIN

Some gynecologic and nongynecologic disorders causing pelvic pain, especially those with relatively acute onset of pain, require a timely diagnosis and prompt surgical intervention (Tables 15–3 and 15–4). A delay in diagnosis may not only result in significant short-term morbidity, but it also may have a lasting impact on the woman's reproductive potential. For example, an undue delay in the diagnosis of tubal pregnancy may result in surgery and removal of a fallopian tube, whereas early diagnosis would have allowed medical treatment with methotrexate, possibly avoiding surgery altogether.

### *Miscarriage (Spontaneous Abortion)*

Miscarriage occurs in approximately 50% of pregnancies detected with a sensitive pregnancy test, but it complicates only 25% of clinically evident pregnancies. Once fetal cardiac activity is detected on ultrasound, only 5% of pregnancies will subsequently be lost.

**TABLE 15-3**

| Gynecologic Causes of Pelvic Pain |
|---|
| Uterine |
|   Miscarriage |
|   Fibroid tumors (especially pedunculated with torsion or prolapsing) |
|   Infection |
|   Retroflexion (uncommon) |
| Adnexal |
|   Ectopic pregnancy (tubal, uterine, or ovarian) |
|   Torsion of tube or ovary or both |
|   Ovarian cyst |
|     Physiologic |
|     Hemorrhagic |
|     Endometroid |
|     Neoplastic (especially dermoid cyst) |

TABLE 15-4

### Nongynecologic Causes of Pelvic Pain

Gastrointestinal
    Appendicitis
    Inflammatory bowel disease
    Gastroenteritis
    Functional bowel disorders
    Constipation
    Bowel obstruction
    Diverticular disease
    Neoplasm
    Helminthiasis
    Pelvic or abdominal adhesions
    Meckel's diverticulum
    Intussusception
Urologic
    Urethritis, cystitis, and pyelonephritis
    Interstitial cystitis
    Calculi
    Neoplasm
Other
    Musculoskeletal disorders
        Chronic back pain
        Radiculopathy
        Spondylolisthesis
    Sickle-cell crisis
    Porphyria
    Somatization disorders

Following a period of amenorrhea, vaginal spotting and cramping occur (*threatened abortion*). Physical findings are often nonspecific, consisting of bloody discharge in the vaginal vault, a closed cervix, and mild lower abdominal and uterine tenderness. The presence of tissue in the cervix (*incomplete abortion*) requires referral for suction curettage. If all placenta and fetal tissues are passed spontaneously (*complete abortion*), expectant management may be considered. Blood type and antibody testing are required and Rh immune globulin should be administered if indicated.

## Ectopic Pregnancy

*Ectopic pregnancy* is defined as implantation of the conceptus outside the uterine cavity. The fallopian tube is the most common site of ectopic gestation; other sites include the uterine cornua, ovary, cervix, and abdominal cavity. Ectopic pregnancy occurs in approximately 16 of 1000 pregnancies and is the second most common cause of maternal death in the United States. Risk factors for ectopic pregnancy include pelvic inflammatory disease, in which the risk is increased six fold, previous ectopic pregnancy (with a ten fold increased risk), increased age, prior sterilization procedure, and conception via assisted reproductive technologies (in vitro fertilization). The most common symptoms include abdominal pain, amenorrhea, and abnormal bleeding. With tubal rupture and heavy intra-abdominal bleeding, shoulder pain due to irritation of the diaphragm may occur. The abdomen may be tender to palpation and distended with significant intraperitoneal bleeding. In addition, the uterus is slightly enlarged and may be mildly tender, and there may be unilateral or bilateral adnexal tenderness.

The diagnosis of ectopic pregnancy is fairly straightforward. Using sensitive serum assays, $\beta$hCG can be detected as early as 5 days after conception. In a woman with suspected ectopic pregnancy, a quantitative $\beta$hCG should be followed at 2-day intervals. During early pregnancy, the $\beta$hCG should increase by approximately 66% every 48

probe testing has supplanted culture of the cervix for *N. gonorrhoeae* and *C. trachomatis*. A bimanual exam should be performed to detect signs of upper tract infection such as uterine tenderness, adnexal tenderness, or pain with cervical motion.

Treatment of cervicitis should be delayed pending laboratory confirmation of a chlamydial or gonococcal infection, but empiric treatment is indicated for women whose partner has urethral symptoms or is known to have gonorrhea or chlamydia. Treatment recommendations are noted in Table 15–5. Women with gonorrhea should receive empiric treatment of *C. trachomatis* owing to the high incidence of coinfection with *N. gonorrhoeae* (approximately 60%).

## PELVIC INFLAMMATORY DISEASE

Pelvic inflammatory disease (PID), also known as endometritis-salpingitis-peritonitis, is a cause of significant morbidity in women. There are approximately 1 million cases of PID in the United States annually, and approximately 250,000 women require hospitalization. Approximately 15% develop tubo-ovarian abscess and about 1% to 3% require surgery during the initial hospitalization.

Most cases of acute pelvic inflammatory disease in the United States are due to the sexually transmitted pathogens *N. gonorrhoeae* (about 40%) and *C. trachomatis* (20%–30%). Both organisms can be recovered from approximately 10% of women with PID. Instrumentation of the uterus, such as dilation and curettage (D & C) or endometrial biopsy, are important risk factors for PID in women who are not infected with sexually transmitted pathogens. In addition to the sexually transmitted pathogens, it is common for other virulent bacteria often found in the lower genital tract to be recovered from the uterine cavity and peritoneal cavity of women with PID. These include aerobic and anaerobic gram-positive and gram-negative pathogens.

The symptoms of PID vary greatly. Many women will have only mild symptoms such as a nondescript lower abdominal discomfort or irregular bleeding; these are most commonly seen with chlamydial infections. Approximately 50% of women with asymptomatic chlamydial infection of the cervix will be culture-positive from the endometrial cavity. Other symptoms include more severe lower abdominal pain, cervical discharge, metrorrhagia (irregular bleeding), and fever.

The diagnostic criteria for pelvic inflammatory disease are listed in Table 15–6. These criteria are nonspecific; many other gynecologic and nongynecologic conditions can be misdiagnosed as PID. Prospective studies have indicated that up to 30% of women suspected to have PID turn out to have other gynecologic and nongynecologic conditions when laparoscopy is performed to confirm the diagnosis.

Laboratory testing for suspected PID is rather straightforward. All symptomatic women should be tested for *N. gonorrhea* and *C. trachomatis*, pregnancy must be excluded with a sensitive pregnancy test, and a complete blood count should be per-

**TABLE 15–6**

### Diagnostic Criteria for Pelvic Inflammatory Disease

*Major Criteria (All three must be present)*
Lower abdominal tenderness
Adnexal tenderness
Cervical motion tenderness

*Minor Criteria (At least one must be present)*
Oral temperature >38.3°C
Abnormal cervical or vaginal discharge
Elevated erythrocyte sedimentation rate
Elevated C-reactive protein
Laboratory documentation of cervical infection with *N. gonorrhoeae* or *C. trachomatis*

TABLE 15–7

## Treatment of Pelvic Inflammatory Disease

*Inpatient Treatment Options*
Regimen 1
1. Cefoxitin 2 g IV every 6 hours
or
Cefotetan 2 g IV every 12 hours
2. Doxycycline 100 mg PO or IV every 12 hours
Regimen 2
1. Clindamycin 900 mg IV every 8 hours
2. Gentamicin: Loading dose IV or IM (2mg/kg body weight) followed by maintenance dose of 1.5 mg/kg every 8 hours

*Outpatient Treatment Options*
Regimen 1
1. Cefoxitin 2 g IM
2. Probeneid 1 g PO in single dose concurrently
3. Doxycycline 100 mg PO every 12 hours for 14 days
Regimen 2
1. Ceftriaxone 250 mg IM
2. Doxycycline 100 mg PO every 12 hours for 14 days
Regimen 3
1. Ofloxacin 400 mg PO every 12 hours for 14 days
2. Metronidazole 500 mg PO every 12 hours for 14 days
Regimen 4
1. Ofloxacin 400 mg PO every 12 hours for 14 days
2. Clindamycin 450 mg PO 4 times daily

---

• ▬▬

*All patients with PID and a positive pregnancy test are considered to have an ectopic pregnancy until proven otherwise.*

formed. A urinalysis is helpful to rule out symptomatic urinary tract infection or calculi. Surgical consultation is recommended when the diagnosis is uncertain or when there is a suspicion for appendicitis or other gastrointestinal conditions. Laparoscopy should be considered for those patients whose diagnosis is uncertain or who do not show prompt clinical improvement with the initiation of therapy.

Indications for hospitalization include systemic toxicity, significant leukocytosis, and nausea and vomiting that preclude the completion of outpatient therapy. All patients with PID and a positive pregnancy test are considered to have an ectopic pregnancy until proven otherwise. Patients with tubo-ovarian abscess or those in whom a satisfactory pelvic exam is not possible should be admitted for parenteral therapy. Table 15–7 lists treatment regimens recommended by the Centers for Disease Control.

A few women will require surgical intervention during the initial hospitalization. Indications for surgery include inadequate clinical improvement in spite of parenteral therapy or imminent or suspected rupture of a tubo-ovarian abscess. Consultation with a gynecologic or general surgeon is indicated in this circumstance. Total abdominal hysterectomy and bilateral salpingo-oophorectomy was previously the treatment of choice in women requiring surgery for acute tubo-ovarian abscess. The current tendency is to employ more conservative surgical approaches, such as drainage of the tubo-ovarian abscess or removal of the affected adnexal structures.

Several large retrospective studies have shown that up to 30% of women with PID will require surgery at a time remote from the first infection, most often because of chronic infection, persistent pelvic mass, adhesive disease, and chronic pain. In vitro fertilization is an option for women who retain some reproductive capacity. In addition, approximately 5% to 10% of women with tubo-ovarian abscess will conceive naturally.

## POSTMENOPAUSAL PELVIC ABSCESS

In the woman of reproductive age, pelvic abscess is usually due to a community-acquired infection such as PID. The same cannot be said for the postmenopausal

**TABLE 15–8**

### Conditions Associated with Postmenopausal Pelvic Abscess

Genital malignancy
   Cancer of the cervix
   Cancer of the endometrium; uterine sarcomas
Radiation therapy of pelvic malignancies
Colorectal cancer
Diverticular disease of the colon

woman. Although tubo-ovarian abscesses in younger women usually respond to parenteral therapy, postmenopausal women usually require prompt surgical intervention for a pelvic abscess. Such women may present with an acute abdomen with generalized peritonitis or, more often, vague lower abdominal discomfort. Gastrointestinal symptoms are common. Many abscesses are incidental findings detected during an evaluation of abdominal pain or a change in bowel habits. There may be a history of instrumentation of the uterus (D & C, endometrial biopsy, or radiation therapy of a genital neoplasm).

Evaluation of a postmenopausal woman with a suspected pelvic abscess consists of a thorough abdominal and pelvic exam and a rectovaginal exam. Any or all of the exams may suggest an inflammatory condition or pelvic mass. Pelvic ultrasound is helpful in delineating the characteristics of a suspected pelvic mass, and consultation with a surgeon early in the evaluation is most helpful. Colonoscopy and radiologic studies can be performed to further assess the gastrointestinal tract. Consultation with a gynecologist may also be needed to rule out endometrial or cervical carcinoma.

The underlying condition causing the abscess will determine the surgical approach. Following initial treatment with systemic antibiotics, surgical intervention is required to treat the associated conditions and the pelvic abscess. Most postmenopausal pelvic abscesses are due to genital tract cancers or gastrointestinal (GI) cancers or are a complication of diverticular disease of the colon. The latter usually involve the left adnexae (Table 15–8).

*Most postmenopausal pelvic abscesses are due to genital tract cancers, gastrointestinal tract cancers or diverticulitis.*

Critical to the patient's well-being is the diagnosis and treatment of genital tract and GI cancers or their exclusion. Antibiotic therapy is indicated for acute pelvic infection, but the long-term management is surgical, and early consultation with a surgeon is advised.

### *When to Call the Surgeon about Pelvic Pain*

- Acute pelvic pain where diagnosis is unclear
- Chronic pelvic pain where diagnosis is unclear
- Incomplete abortion
- Ectopic pregnancy
- Adnexal torsion
- Pelvic abscess (especially in postmenopausal women)

## RECOMMENDED READING

Dysmenorrhea and Chronic Pelvic Pain. Obstetrics and Gynecology, ed 2. Beckman, CRB, et al (eds). Williams & Wilkins, Baltimore, 1995, pp 271–278.

Adelson, MD, and Adelson, KL. Miscellaneous benign disorders of the upper genital tract. In Copeland, LJ (ed): Textbook of Gynecology. WB Saunders, Philadelphia, 1993, pp 857–870.

Beckman, CRB, et al: Health Care For Women: Obstetrics and Gynecology as Specialty and Primary-Preventive Health Care: Obstetrics and Gynecology, ed 2, 1995, pp 1–18.

Centers for Disease Control: 1993 Sexually transmitted diseases treatment guidelines. MMRW, 1993.

Centers for Disease Control: Summary of Notifiable Diseases, United States 1995. MMWR 44:53.0, 1996.

Herbst, AL, et al (eds): History and Examination of the Patient: Comprehensive Gynecology, ed 2. Mosby, St. Louis, 1992, pp 143–160.

McNeeley, SG: Gynecologic infections. In Hajj, SN, and Evans, WJ (eds): Clinical Postreproductive Gynecology Appleton & Lange, Norwalk, Connecticut, 1993, pp 271–284.

McNeeley, SG, and Ransom, SB: Genital tract infections. In Ransom, SB, and McNeeley, SG (eds): Gynecology for the Primary Care Provider. WB Saunders, New York, 1997.

Smith, RP, and Ling, FW: Gynevision. Obstetrics and Gynecology. 78:708, 1991.

Steege, JF: Chronic Pelvic Pain and Dyspareunia. In Seltzer, VL, and Pearse, WH (eds): Women's Primary Health Care. McGraw-Hill, New York, 1995, pp 241–247.

# Hernias

## DAVID FROMM, MD,
## and REBECCA GLADHU, MD

A *hernia* is an abnormal protrusion of tissue through an opening, or defect, in the fascia. The majority of hernias of the torso occur through the anterior abdominal wall and most are located in the groin. Most hernias are associated with a sac in continuity with the parietal peritoneum. Inguinal, femoral, umbilical, and incisional hernias constitute more than 95% of abdominal wall hernias.

Most uncomplicated, symptomatic hernias are relatively easy to diagnose because symptoms are usually localized to the hernia site and thus direct the examiner's attention to that area. However, lack of awareness of proper examination, potential hernia sites, manifestations of hernias, and postoperative complications leads to not only misdiagnosis and unnecessary studies but also mistreatment.

The mere presence of a hernia is sufficient reason to consult a surgeon. Most hernias present the potential threat of development of simple or strangulating bowel obstruction. Repair relieves pain and prevents intestinal obstruction. Delaying repair adds an additional problem because most hernias enlarge over time, making repair more difficult.

The time-honored approach to treating hernias involves repairing even asymptomatic hernias in patients suited for operation. Repair avoids pain and prevents intestinal obstruction. In time, even asymptomatic small hernias enlarge. Most eventually become symptomatic, and hernias are second only to adhesions as the most common cause of intestinal obstruction. Accurate estimates of the chance of obstruction are difficult to obtain, however, because most hernias are repaired prophylactically. Definition also plays a role. For example, "troublesome" incisional hernias were found to develop obstruction in one study. Most hernia repairs are associated with a very low morbidity and mortality (less than 0.01% for an elective inguinal herniorrhaphy) and a satisfied patient. The morbidity and mortality associated with a bowel obstruction (especially a strangulated one) are many times greater than those of an elective herniorrhaphy.

A misconception is that the smaller the hernia defect, the less danger there is of a

*Most hernias present a potential threat of the development of simple or strangulating bowel obstruction.*

*Most hernia repairs are associated with a very low morbidity and mortality.*

complication. However, most strangulating obstructions due to a hernia are associated with small fascial defects.

## Symptoms

Although many hernias are either asymptomatic or associated with mild symptoms that are not elicited prospectively, the diagnosis of a symptomatic hernia is usually suggested by the patient's history. However, the symptoms will vary with the location of the hernia and state of its contents. The patient may relate the appearance of the hernia to a specific episode of strenuous activity, the history may be one of gradual onset of symptoms, or the patient may be asymptomatic.

The main symptom of a *simple hernia* (one not associated with incarceration or obstruction) is a frequently visible bulging or a sensation of bulging at the hernia site. This symptom is usually intermittent and associated with minimal discomfort (i.e., not enough to require medication). Patients are not always aware of a bulging sensation but may complain more of a gnawing or dragging sensation in the vicinity of the hernia. Such symptoms are straightforward and easily confirmed by physical examination, but others may be more deceptive. For example, intestinal obstruction may be the first sign of a hernia. New-onset constipation may be due to a sliding left inguinal hernia (discussed later), in which the sigmoid colon and its mesentery make up the lateral wall of the hernia. Knee pain may be a symptom of an obturator hernia. On occasion, the patient's symptoms are not convincing in the presence of a hernia associated with a low risk of complications (e.g., a high epigastric hernia occurring after a median sternotomy). From the patient's point of view there may be cosmetic indication for repair. Patients may even fear that their hernia will burst through the skin, but this is extraordinarily rare.

*Patients with a simple hernia are not always aware of a bulging sensation.*

## Diagnosis

Diagnosis is most often made by examination. If a hernia is evident on physical examination, radiologic confirmation of its presence is unnecessary. If the patient's history suggests a hernia but none is evident at the time of examination, re-examination at a future date is frequently helpful. Plain abdominal radiographs may suggest a hernia, but computed tomography (CT) in the appropriate setting is better for questionable cases. However, examination with the patient both upright and recumbent, relaxed and during increasing intra-abdominal pressure nearly always reveals either a visible or easily reducible palpable bulge or a palpable fascial defect. There are some pitfalls in examination that are peculiar to the specific hernia site; these are discussed in the sections dealing with specific hernias.

## Management of Incarceration and Obstruction

Bowel obstruction associated with a hernia is always preceded by incarceration of the intestine in the fascial defect. Most cases of incarceration of a palpable hernia are associated with an acute increase in pain at the hernia site. If the hernia is palpable, incarceration is diagnosed by the examiner's inability to reduce the hernia. If incarceration is allowed to persist untreated, edema ensues. This leads to bowel obstruction and progression to venous and finally arterial thrombosis, resulting in a strangulating obstruction. It is difficult to make a diagnosis of strangulation in the absence of overlying skin erythema, septic shock, or peritonitis. Operation obviously is desirable before irretrievable intestinal necrosis occurs.

*If incarceration of the intestine is allowed to persist untreated, edema ensues.*

Quite often, the examining practitioner can manually reduce an incarcerated hernia, but there are a few caveats to consider before an attempt at reduction is made. If the hernia cannot be reduced, one must assume that strangulation is present. A frequent error is to assume that an acute appearance of an irreducible hernia not associated with overt symptoms of intestinal obstruction consists of incarcerated omentum. An early bowel obstruction can be very deceptive in its manifestations. Do not attempt to reduce an incarceration associated with cellulitis of the overlying skin, because this is a sign of infarction.

A rare but devastating complication of manual reduction is reduction en masse. It most often results from forcible manual reduction of the hernia. Even though the hernia mass is reduced, the incarceration or strangulation is not relieved because the neck of the sac causing it remains intact. Diagnosis is made by a history indicating either manual or spontaneous reduction of an incarcerated mass without relief of intestinal obstruction, or a painful, difficult reduction. Thus, it is important to ensure that symptoms of obstruction are indeed relieved after reduction and to warn the patient about the development of new symptoms.

Irreducible incarceration with or without overt symptoms of obstruction, failure of reduction to give relief, and development of new symptoms after reduction are indications for emergent operation. In general, incarcerations that have been reduced will recur.

*Do not attempt to reduce an incarceration associated with cellulitis of the overlying skin, because this is a sign of infarction.*

*An irreducible incarceration, the failure of reduction to give relief, or the development of new symptoms after reduction are indications for emergent operation.*

## Classification of Hernias

Hernias are classified by a number of descriptive terms: location (e.g., umbilical or inguinal); the state of its contents (reducible, incarcerated, strangulated); its relationship to the peritoneum (sliding); and terms or eponyms that say something about its etiology or specific location (incisional, Spigelian). The contents of a hernia are variable. In part, they are related to the location of the fascial defect, and almost any intra-abdominal or extraperitoneal organ or tissue can be involved.

### HERNIAS OF THE GROIN

There are three types of groin hernias: indirect inguinal, direct inguinal, and femoral. An *indirect inguinal hernia* is one that involves herniation through the internal inguinal ring (Fig. 16–1). The internal inguinal ring is located along a line drawn from the anterior superior iliac spine to the pubic tubercle and is situated at a point two-thirds of the distance from the spine to the tubercle. The fascial defect of a *direct inguinal hernia* is medial to that of an indirect one and involves Hesselbach's triangle, which is bound inferiorly by the inguinal ligament, laterally by the inferior epigastric vessels, and medially by the lateral border of the rectus muscle (see Fig. 16–1). A *femoral hernia* involves a defect in the femoral canal just medial to the femoral vein. The canal exits posteriorly to the inguinal ligament in the upper thigh (see Fig. 16–1).

Inguinal hernias are far more common in men and femoral hernias occur more often in women. Of all groin hernias, 86% occur in men. Even though the most common type of hernia in women is an indirect inguinal hernia, women account for 84% of all femoral hernias.

Intestinal incarceration and strangulation can occur in both indirect inguinal and femoral hernias. A direct inguinal hernia is the least dangerous of groin hernias because it is rarely associated with intestinal complications. The reason is that Hesselbach's triangle is not usually associated with a fascial ring and the hernia occurs as a result of weakness of the deeper layer (transversalis) of fascia. Because direct inguinal hernias are so rarely associated with intestinal complications, some question the necessity for repair when the patient is asymptomatic. However, this question assumes that an accurate distinction can be made between the two types of inguinal hernias. One study found that the correct diagnosis was made in 77% of indirect and only 59% of direct hernias examined by surgeons. Furthermore, some patients have a combined hernia

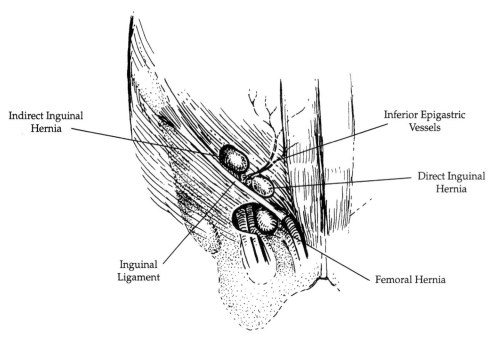

Indirect Inguinal Hernia

Inferior Epigastric Vessels

Direct Inguinal Hernia

Inguinal Ligament

Femoral Hernia

**FIGURE 16–1**
Anterior view of the groin, showing locations of indirect inguinal hernia, direct inguinal hernia, and femoral hernia, based on anatomic landmarks.

that has both a direct and an indirect component. Thus, most surgeons will repair any type of inguinal hernia.

A difficult differential can involve an incarcerated hernia and inguinal adenopathy with or without associated cellulitis. The presence of cellulitis could be due to strangulation or related to the adenopathy. In most patients, we see little point in doing an array of diagnostic studies to make a distinction and thus prefer to undertake operation. If the mass is not a hernia, at least lymph node tissue can be obtained for definitive diagnosis of the etiology.

*A difficult differential can involve an incarcerated hernia and inguinal adenopathy with or without associated cellulitis.*

### Diagnosis of an Inguinal Hernia

Any visible and reducible bulge at or between the level of the internal inguinal ring and pubic tubercle is a reliable sign of a hernia. Indirect inguinal hernias lie in the inguinal canal, which is just superior and parallel to the inguinal ligament. In men, enlargement of the hernia permits its passage through the external inguinal ring and down into the scrotum. A mass in the scrotum is not necessarily a hernia, but the diagnosis becomes evident from the history and examination indicating reducibility or acute symptoms of intestinal obstruction. The presence of bowel sounds over a scrotal mass and lack of transillumination distinguish a hernia from a hydrocele. Smaller hernias are detected by invaginating the scrotum and passing the index finger (with the pulp of the finger facing the pubic tubercle) superiorly along the spermatic cord and through the external inguinal ring—which lies just lateral to the pubic tubercle—and entering the inguinal canal. With straining or coughing a bulge will be evident. In women, the external inguinal ring is found by placing the examining finger just medial and inferior to the pubic tubercle.

An enlarged or dilated external inguinal ring that is not associated with an impulse at the level of the internal inguinal ring or within the inguinal canal does not signify the presence of a hernia. Neither is a large external ring necessarily associated with a hernia.

*A large external ring is not necessarily associated with a hernia.*

### Sliding Inguinal Hernia

A *sliding inguinal hernia* is an indirect hernia in which a viscus forms a portion of the hernia sac. The visceral component of the sac does not lie free within the peritoneal cavity, nor is it bound by adhesions within the sac (Fig. 16–2). The cecum is most frequently involved on the right and the sigmoid colon on the left. There are no precise signs or symptoms to distinguish a sliding hernia from an ordinary indirect inguinal hernia, but it is not essential to make this distinction preoperatively.

### Should a Truss Be Prescribed?

Wearing a truss to control an inguinal hernia is generally considered to be an antiquated practice. Most patients find a truss uncomfortable, and a truss does not control the hernia in the majority of patients. Trusses are believed to increase the probability of complications, such as testicular atrophy, incarceration, ilioinguinal or femoral neuritis, iliac vessel thrombosis, and atrophy of fascial margins, which can make subsequent repair more difficult.

### Femoral Hernia

A palpable femoral hernia presents as a mass inferior to the inguinal ligament and just medial to the femoral vein (see Fig. 16–1). Herniation limited to the femoral canal may be associated with a femoral venous thrill. This is elicited by palpation over the femoral vein (which is just medial to the femoral artery) and asking the patient to cough while in the supine position. The femoral ring is rigid superiorly, inferiorly, and medially. Coughing transmits intra-abdominal pressure through the hernia sac laterally and impinges on the femoral vein, causing temporary stenosis and hence a palpable thrill.

FIGURE 16–2
Sliding left inguinal hernia involving sigmoid colon.

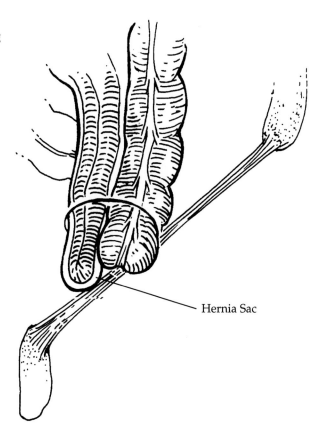

Hernia Sac

Detection of a femoral venous thrill in the upright position (Cruveilhiers's sign) does not distinguish between a proximal varix and a femoral hernia.

Occasionally, a large femoral hernia may protrude through the fossa ovalis in the proximal thigh, and the sac may even dissect superiorly, presenting above the inguinal ligament and leading to the misdiagnosis of an inguinal hernia. Even if the type of hernia is erroneously diagnosed, it should be repaired.

## UMBILICAL HERNIA

Umbilical hernias in adults differ from those in children. This umbilical defect normally closes spontaneously over the first 4 to 5 years of life. Spontaneous closure does not occur in adults. About 10% of adults have a childhood history of an umbilical hernia.

The fascial defect most often lies just superior to the umbilicus and is best observed by having the patient standing, leaning forward, and straining.

The patient with ascites poses a difficult problem. The misconception is that ascites prevents the development of incarceration. Neglected umbilical hernias in patients with cirrhosis can be associated with maceration of the thin overlying skin and eventual infection or an ascitic leak. These hernias can be repaired under local anesthesia, but repair does not necessarily prevent a postoperative ascitic leak through the suture line. Thus, aggressive attempts at reducing the ascites should be made preoperatively in an elective situation.

## INCISIONAL HERNIA

The incidence of incisional hernia is generally higher than most expect. When carefully sought, nearly 8% of patients develop an incisional hernia within a year of operation. The incidence is about 11% when carefully looked for over a 10-year period. Thus, most incisional hernias occur within a year of an abdominal operation, but about 6% of patients are found to have a hernia between 2.5 and 5.5 years after operation. Another study found that 86% were diagnosed by 5 years.

Most incisional hernias (63%) are asymptomatic. Male sex, obesity, postoperative chest infection, postoperative abdominal distention, and wound infection are common precursors, but this is not a uniform finding.

A prospective randomized trial showed that within a year of operation, a midline incision, which goes through the linea alba, was followed by a 9% incidence of hernia—about 10 times the 1% incidence with a paramedian incision, which goes through the anterior and posterior rectus sheaths. Nevertheless, most surgeons use a midline abdominal incision because of its convenience.

*Sometimes a hernia will appear lateral to an incision.*

Confusion sometimes occurs because the hernia lies lateral to the incision. This may happen because the hernia sac has dissected laterally, or the hernia may result from a far laterally placed suture that has cut through the rectus sheath.

Another type of incisional hernia involves sites that contain a drain. When most drains are removed from the peritoneal cavity, the fascial defect is allowed to close spontaneously without suture. Hernias occurring high in the epigastrium following a median sternotomy are technically not epigastric hernias; they are incisional.

### Parastomal Hernia

A *parastomal hernia* is an incisional hernia related to an intestinal stoma on the abdominal wall (Fig. 16–3). The incidence of such hernias varies from 2% to 20% and is higher for colostomies than ileostomies. There are three types of such hernias: (1) *interstitial*, in which the sac lies within the muscular layers of the abdominal wall; (2) *parastomal* (the most common type), in which the hernia sac lies between the bowel and its abdominal wall aperture and protrudes into the subcutaneous tissue; and (3) *peristomal*, which can occur if a space is left between the lateral abdominal wall and the bowel as

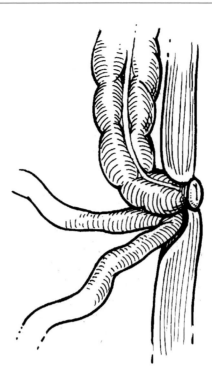

FIGURE 16-3
Parastomal hernia involving a colostomy.

it exits the peritoneal cavity. Interstitial and peristomal hernias present as a partial or complete bowel obstruction or as a small-bowel obstruction, which, if treated late, is often associated with strangulation of the herniated small intestine. A parastomal hernia is not generally associated with pain but can be a source of considerable morbidity, as it may interfere with the wearing of an appliance.

Indications for operation include small-bowel obstruction, interference with the satisfactory wearing of an appliance, and in appropriate patients, cosmesis. However, many surgeons are reluctant to undertake repair of a parastomal hernia with cosmesis as the sole indication because of the high incidence of recurrence. If just the fascia is repaired, a contemporary series reports a 76% recurrence rate, but this decreased to 33% with relocation of the stoma. Repair of the fascial defect using prosthetic material may be more effective in the treatment of recurrent parastomal hernias.

## EPIGASTRIC HERNIAS

Hernias occurring spontaneously anywhere in the linea alba (except the umbilicus) are referred to as *epigastric hernias* because most occur superior to the umbilicus. The fascial defect is often small and multiple. Symptoms usually consist of focal pain or discomfort, and a defect or mass is evident. Incarceration usually consists of properitoneal fat (the fatty layer of tissue just on top of the peritoneum). Epigastric hernias are an important source of pain that is often attributed to some other condition.

## RICHTER'S HERNIA

A *Richter's hernia* does not refer to a specific site but rather to a particular configuration of the hernia. This type of hernia involves incarceration of only a portion of the intestinal wall (Fig. 16–4). It occurs when the hernia ring is small. Most (82%) are associated with femoral hernias, and 16% are associated with indirect inguinal hernias. Even though only a portion of bowel is incarcerated, 50% of Richter's hernias are associated with obstruction of the small intestine due to kinking or twisting of adjacent bowel. Necrosis and perforation occur in 35% of such cases, with few, if any, antecedent

*Necrosis and perforation occur in 35% of Richter's hernias with few, if any, antecedent symptoms.*

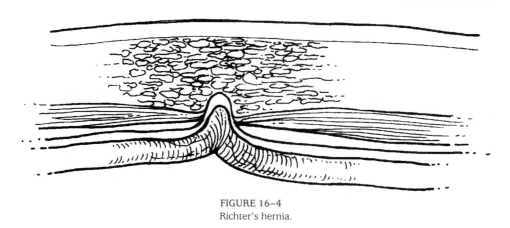

FIGURE 16–4
Richter's hernia.

*An increasing incidence of Richter's hernia occurs after laparoscopic procedures.*

symptoms. An enterocutaneous fistula occurs in 15% and is generally preceded by focal pain or abscess. An increasing incidence of Richter's hernia occurs after laparoscopic procedures associated with incomplete closure of the laparoscopic port sites.

## OBTURATOR HERNIA

A hernia occurring through the obturator canal is relatively rare. Most frequent in elderly women, these hernias are difficult to diagnose and are associated with a high mortality because of the delay in diagnosis.

Classically, this type of hernia is associated with the Howship-Romberg sign: pain along the medial aspect of the thigh extending to the knee that is aggravated by abduction, extension, or internal rotation of knee and is a result of hernial compression of the nerve passing through the obturator canal. Flexion of the thigh usually relieves the pain. Unfortunately, the Howship-Romberg sign occurs in fewer than 65% of patients, and it can be chronically intermittent and misinterpreted as being due to arthritis.

The obturator foramen is formed by the rami of the ischium and pubis and lies on the anterolateral pelvic wall inferior to the acetabulum (Fig. 16–5). The obturator canal is 2 to 3 cm long and 1 cm in diameter. Normally, the space around the obturator vessels and nerve passing through the foramen is closed by the obturator membrane, which is continuous with the periosteum of the encircling bone and the tendinous attachments of the obturator muscles. A hernia mass in the medial, upper third of the thigh, between the extensor and flexor muscle groups, is evident in only a few patients. The optimum position for palpation is with the patient lying supine with the thigh flexed, adducted, and rotated outward. Rectal or pelvic examination may on occasion reveal a tender, palpable mass.

An obturator hernia is often of the Richter type. Ninety percent of patients present with a small-bowel obstruction, which varies in severity. About one-third have had previous obstructive symptoms, the intermittent nature of which is due to spontaneous reduction of the hernia. This, in addition to the lack of external signs and absence of the Howship-Romberg sign in many patients, leads to a delay in diagnosis, which accounts for the high mortality in patients with an obturator hernia. Intestinal resection rates vary from 25% to 100%. Mortality varies from 12% to 70%, but is lower (about 6%) when attention is paid to the diagnosis.

If a patient presents with a small-bowel obstruction (especially in the absence of prior abdominal surgery), its cause should be confirmed in the operating room; radiographic confirmation is not needed. However, a CT scan of the pelvis is the most accurate means of making the diagnosis; it can show a mass containing an air density located between the pectineus and obturator muscles.

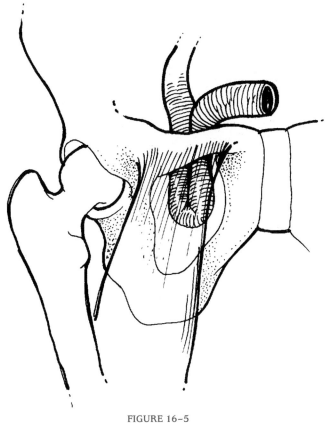

FIGURE 16-5
Obturator hernia.

## SPIGELIAN HERNIA

The spigelian, or semilunar, line is the depression at the lateral margin of the rectus muscle and marks the transition from muscle to aponeurosis in the transversus abdominis muscle (Fig. 16-6). The line runs from the costal arch to the pubic tubercle. Spigelian hernias lie superior to the inferior epigastric vessels located in Hesselbach's triangle, and 90% lie between a transverse line drawn between the anterior superior iliac spines and umbilicus. Although any hernia occurring along the semilunar line is technically a *Spigelian hernia*, most occur near the intersection of the semilunar line and the semicircular line of Douglas (see Fig. 16-6). The semicircular line of Douglas is situated inferior to the umbilicus and represents the site where the internal oblique aponeurosis no longer splits into two layers but form the posterior and some of the anterior parts of the rectus sheath. The internal oblique aponeurosis contributes only to the anterior rectus sheath beginning at the semicircular line and ending in the groin. The junction of the musculoaponeurotic elements of the internal oblique and transversus abdominal muscles varies and can lead to a fascial defect and a hernia. This defect can be difficult to detect on physical examination, not only because it can be quite small but also because the hernia sac lies just beneath the external oblique aponeurosis.

Pain is the most common symptom of a Spigelian hernia. It is quite variable and often difficult for the patient to localize, but it is aggravated by a Valsalva's maneuver. A distinct point of tenderness is frequently noted over the hernia site even if the hernia defect is not palpable when the abdominal muscles are tensed. Hyperesthesia of the abdominal wall medial to the hernia orifice occurs if the hernia causes irritation of the corresponding intercostal nerve.

Only 5% of patients present with a subcutaneous mass and 21% present with in-

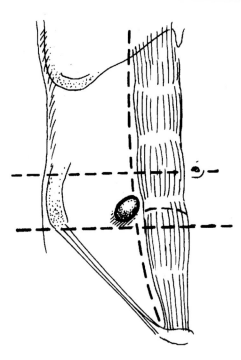

FIGURE 16–6
Spigelian hernia.

carceration. The diagnosis is most often made when there is a mass. The differential diagnosis includes an abscess, seroma, and hematoma. Because such a mass may be a hernia, it is unwise to pass a needle for diagnosis, lest contamination occur. Incarceration or Richter's type herniation can be confused with other intra-abdominal conditions such as appendicitis or colon cancer. CT scan or ultrasound has been anecdotally reported to be useful in difficult cases.

## PERINEAL HERNIA

Hernias of the perineum are rare. They occur most often after abdominal perineal resection of the rectum and even more rarely after pelvic exenteration. The diagnosis is made by observing a perineal bulge on straining. Symptoms include pain, intestinal or urinary obstruction, and impending skin breakdown.

## LUMBAR HERNIAS

There are two types of lumbar hernias: Petit's and Grynfeltt's, both occurring in triangular defects in the lumbar region. The base of Petit's triangle consists of the iliac crest, the medial limb is the lateral edge of the latissimus dorsi, and the lateral limb is the medial edge of the external oblique (Fig. 16–7). The more superiorly located Grynfeltt's triangle (which is inverted) has as its base the 12th rib and serratus posterior; the medial limb is the lateral border of the quadratus lumborum; and the lateral limb is the medial edge of the internal oblique (see Fig. 16–7).

The most frequent physical finding is a reducible mass in one of the triangles. About 10% of Petit's hernias present with incarceration. Twenty percent of lumbar hernias are congenital and are usually associated with other congenital anomalies. About 26% of lumbar hernias are traumatic. Most of these are Grynfeltt's hernias caused by direct trauma, penetrating wound, abscess, or a flank incision. The most frequent symptoms are a sensation of lumbar heaviness and back pain.

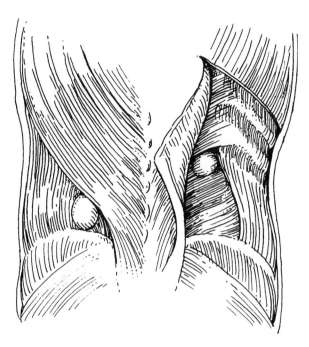

**FIGURE 16–7**
Typical locations of Petit's hernia (inferior lumbar hernia) and Grynfeltt's hernia (superior lumbar hernia).

Inferior Lumbar
Hernia

Superior Lumbar
Hernia

## Complications of Herniorrhaphy

Complications occurring after repair of an abdominal-wall or lumbar hernia, aside from recurrence, are about the same as those occurring after any operation. The most common complication of any repair is recurrence.

### RECURRENCE

Aside from technical issues relating to the hernia repair, chronic cough, chronic constipation, and chronic straining on urination are believed to be factors that contribute to recurrence.

Several series report a high incidence of recurrence following repair of an incisional hernia. For example, in a veteran population, almost 25% of hernias recurred after repair; this figure increased to about 42% after the second repair. Some instances of recurrence are not strictly a recurrence at the repaired site. Hernias occur adjacent to the repair because intra-abdominal pressure is redistributed to additional sites along the incision that were not recognized as incipient hernias at the time of operation. Incisional hernias less than 4 cm have been reported to have a lower recurrence rate (28%) than larger defects (41%).

Recurrence is the most common complication of inguinal hernia repair. Direct hernias recur more frequently than indirect hernias. Indirect hernias tend to recur as indirect and direct hernias as direct, but in some instances recurrence is due to an overlooked hernia or true development of a new hernia. The incidence of recurrent inguinal hernias is mostly in the range of 5% to 10% but varies. Almost one-third to one-half of the recurrences are noted within a year of repair, 77% to 80% are apparent by 5 years, an additional 16% are found between 5 to 10 years, and nearly all are manifest by 25 to 30 years. Recurrence is generally higher after a repair for a recurrent hernia and ranges from about 3% to 33%.

An immediate postoperative recurrence is a rare complication caused by intense straining (Valsalva's maneuver) with rupture of sutures on anesthetic extubation of the patient.

## LATE INFECTION RELATED TO PROSTHETIC MATERIAL

- *If prosthetic mesh was used to repair a hernia, bacterial contamination can cause sinus tracts that erode through the skin.*

If prosthetic mesh was used to repair a hernia, bacterial contamination can cause sinus tracts that erode through the skin. These tracts may spontaneously heal, but they recur, becoming chronic. If no fatty tissue (e.g., omentum) or peritoneum lies between the mesh and intestine, the intestine can erode through the mesh, resulting in an enterocutaneous fistula. Chronically draining sinus tracts or an abscess frequently precedes the obvious appearance of a fistula. Complications related to prosthetic material can appear years after its placement. Treatment involves removing the infected mesh.

## COMPLICATIONS SPECIFICALLY RELATED TO INGUINAL HERNIORRAPHY

### Urinary Retention

In a prospective study of patients with a mean age of 54 years, 15% developed urinary retention in the immediate postoperative period. The incidence ranges from 3% to 25%. Overzealous intravenous fluid administration, benign prostatic hypertrophy, groin discomfort, and narcotic medication are believed to be contributing factors.

### Wound Swelling

- *Postoperative swelling of an inguinal incision does not signify recurrence of the hernia.*

Swelling of an inguinal incision is common postoperatively and may last for a few weeks. Swelling during this period does not signify recurrence of the hernia and spontaneously subsides. Treatment consists of reassurance of the patient.

### Ecchymosis

Ecchymosis of the scrotum is due to blood gravitating through areolar tissue from the site of repair into the scrotum and is rarely associated with a palpable hematoma. Ecchymosis is alarming to the patient but clears spontaneously without sequela.

### Scrotal Swelling

A hernia repair may aggravate a hydrocele but is generally believed not to cause it. Dependent edema of the scrotum or accumulation of blood can occur and spontaneously subsides. Edema causing discomfort is frequently relieved by a scrotal support.

### Pain

- *The most common cause of groin pain after inguinal herniorrhaphy is muscle strain from exertion.*

Abdominal muscle strain, nerve entrapment, neuroma, and periostitis of the pubic tubercle are among the common causes of groin pain after inguinal herniorrhaphy. The most frequent type of pain results from muscle strain related to exertion and subsides spontaneously with lessened activity.

### Nerve Injury

Nerve injury following repair of a groin hernia is rare but potentially can be very debilitating. It has been reported more frequently with laparoscopic repairs. The resulting neuralgia is not easily controlled with pain medication and tends to be chronic. Anesthetic block of the affected nerve is diagnostic but rarely provides permanent relief. Nerve resection is effective if the nerve block caused temporary relief of the pain and the symptoms began in the immediate postoperative period. There are also anecdotal reports of slow, spontaneous improvement in symptoms, as well as relief occurring after early removal of an offending suture or surgical clip. The most frequently involved nerve is the ilioinguinal nerve. Other nerves injured include the iliohypogastric nerve, the femoral nerve, and the genital branch of the genitofemoral nerve.

## Ischemic Orchitis and Testicular Atrophy

Ischemic orchitis is associated with fever in the setting of a painful, swollen testicle and spermatic cord. The testicular abnormality does not become apparent until 2 to 3 days after operation. The pain may last for several weeks, but the testicular swelling tends to last for months. The ischemia may resolve completely or progress to testicular atrophy; testicular gangrene occurs only rarely. Testicular atrophy is progressive and is usually apparent within a few months of operation, at which time the testicle is no longer painful. The spermatic cord can become foreshortened in some cases, causing the testicle to retract. Testicular atrophy secondary to ischemic orchitis does not place the patient at greater risk for testicular malignancy.

The incidence of atrophy is about 0.5% in primary repairs and as high as 5% in recurrent repairs. The etiology of this complication is poorly understood, but it is generally held that ischemic orchitis is related to closing the internal inguinal ring too tightly, causing compression of the pampiniform plexus. Anomalous blood supply to the testicle may also be a factor. There is no specific treatment other than relief of pain with medication and scrotal support once symptoms appear.

## Vas Deferens Transection

Injury to the vas deferens is generally not apparent but may be noted on the operative report.

## Sexual Dysfunction

Sexual function and inguinal herniorrhaphy are not related. Such complaints are functional, and treatment generally consists of reassurance.

*Sexual function and inguinal herniorrhaphy are not related.*

## Femoral Thrombosis

Thrombosis of the femoral vein can either be spontaneous or a result of injury during the herniorrhaphy.

## Visceral Injury

Visceral injury is generally manifest by fever, an undue amount of wound swelling, ileus, peritonitis, or fistula. The urinary bladder, intestine, or ureter may be inadvertently injured during the course of the operation. In addition, ischemic intestine released from an incarcerated hernia, which initially was judged to be viable, may go on to necrose.

# Return to Activity after a Herniorrhaphy

Advice about postoperative activity varies among surgeons. A frequent instruction given to patients after repair of an abdominal-wall or groin hernia is to not engage in heavy activity for 6 weeks. This recommendation is mostly based on the observation that the most rapid return of wound strength occurs during the first 6 weeks of repair, although strength is even greater at 12 weeks. However, at least two reports indicate that normal physical activity can be resumed within 3 to 4 weeks of inguinal herniorrhaphy without increasing the incidence of recurrence, although recurrence was only followed for 1 year. Some surgeons advocate unrestricted postoperative activity, basing their safety judgments on long-term observation.

Patient factors also play a role in the healing process. In a case-control comparison of open inguinal herniorrhaphy, it was found that the median number of days to being pain-free after operation was 27 days for patients with workers' compensation and 7.5

days for patients with commercial insurance. Patients who engage in heavy or physically active work take a significantly longer time (median, 40 to 44 days) before they consider themselves having regained full capacity to work than those with sedentary occupations (median, 17 to 21 days).

Psychological factors relating to an incision rather than laparoscopic port sites or the enthusiasm for the laparoscopic approach may also play a role. This may account for the observation in a prospective randomized study done by a single surgeon that the duration of postoperative discomfort and the need for narcotic medication were the same for open and laparoscopic inguinal herniorrhaphy, but the time until return to full-time work was significantly greater for open (mean, 11.8 days) than for laparoscopic (mean, 7.5 days) repair. However, other prospective randomized studies have found significantly less pain following the laparoscopic approach, although selection bias may have played a role. The reported benefits of laparoscopic repair remain controversial. Any benefits such as earlier return to full activity may be canceled out by an increased early recurrence rate.

### *When to Call the Surgeon about a Hernia*

- *Every hernia should be seen by a surgeon.*
- An irreducible incarceration, the failure of reduction to give relief, or the development of new symptoms after reduction are indications for *emergent* operation.
- The cause of any small-bowel obstruction should be confirmed in the operating room.
- Chronically draining sinus tracts, an abscess, or a fistula at a site where a hernia was repaired with prosthetic mesh, even years previously, may indicate a late infection and requires surgical consultation.

## RECOMMENDED READING

Brooks, DC: A prospective comparison of laparoscopic and tension-free open herniorrhaphy. Arch Surg 129:361–66, 1994.

Cheek, CM, et al: Trusses in the management of hernia today. Br J Surg 82:1611–13, 1995.

Kozol, RA, et al: A prospective randomized study of open vs. laparoscopic inguinal hernia repair. Arch Surg 132:292–95, 1997.

Law, NW, and Trapnell, JE: Does a truss benefit a patient with inguinal hernia? Brit Med J 304:1092, 1992.

Lichtenstein, IL, et al: Twenty questions about hernioplasty. Amer Surgeon 57:730–33, 1991.

Mudge, M, and Hughes, LE: Incisional hernia: A 10-year prospective study of incidence and attitudes. Br J Surg 72:70–71, 1985.

Salcedo-Wasicek, MC, and Thirlby, RC: Postoperative course after inguinal herniorraphy. Arch Surg 130:29–32, 1995.

Stoker, DL, et al: Laparoscopic versus open inguinal hernia repair: Randomized prospective trial. Lancet 343:1243–45, 1994.

Wantz, GE: Complications of inguinal hernia repair. Surg Clin NA 64:287–98, 1984.

# Chapter 17

# Anorectal Problems

ROBERT A. KOZOL, MD,
and CHARLES DRISCOLL, MD

## *Examining the Patient*

Anorectal disorders are annoying, commonplace problems, yet they are often difficult to investigate because of the embarrassment they cause for patients. The appearance of rectal bleeding or serious discomfort can also be quite frightening, and the distraught patient will not always be a good historian. For these reasons, Professor JC Goligher, a noted authority writing on anorectal pathology, concluded that the physical exam will make more diagnoses in this area than will the history. A careful history, however, should not be neglected and may offer some clues to the cause of the anorectal complaint.

The practitioner should put the patient at ease by conducting the interview in a relaxed, unhurried manner. Critical elements of the history include travel outside the United States; a past history of inflammatory bowel disease; HIV status; bowel habits; presence, frequency, and nature of any bleeding; and sexual history. Pain is best localized with the patient pointing to the area during the physical examination.

The physical exam begins with inspection. This may be done with the patient in the lateral "knee-to-chest" position or with the patient kneeling on an adjustable table suited for anorectal exams. On inspection the perianal skin may offer clues to some disorders (see pruritis ani below). Other problems may be immediately identifiable on inspection. These include thrombosed external hemorrhoids; prolapsed, incarcerated internal hemorrhoids; and fissures. The external opening of a fistula-in-ano may be readily apparent. Skin tags at the anal verge are markers for internal anorectal pathology (often internal hemorrhoids).

A digital rectal examination is important. The patient should be positioned as described earlier and advised that the exam may be uncomfortable. The examiner should wear rubber or latex gloves and lubricate an index finger. If the patient has pain or tenderness, prelubrication of the anus with lidocaine (Xylocaine) 2% jelly may be helpful. With the palpating finger in the anal canal, examine the prostate gland (anterior)

*If the patient has pain or tenderness, pre-exam lubrication of the anus with lidocaine (Xylocaine) 2% jelly may be helpful.*

**181**

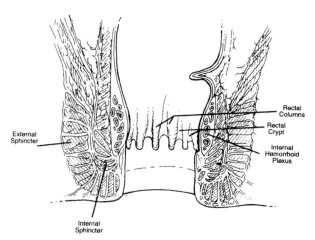

**FIGURE 17-1**
Anatomy of the anorectal region.

in males for nodules and for size. The rectal mucosa is soft, smooth, and redundant, so palpation for internal hemorrhoids is unreliable. Any nodules, masses, or areas of firm irregularity are abnormal and require anoscopic examination. Stool in the rectal vault allows for guaiac card testing for occult blood. At the conclusion of the digital examination, ask the patient to "squeeze on the examining finger" to assess anal sphincter tone.

Anoscopy is a common office procedure that completes any thorough examination of the anus. As with digital examination, anoscopy should be performed in the lateral decubitus position or, preferably, with the patient kneeling on a proctologic exam table. A variety of anoscopes are available with attached light sources. Most are stainless steel and some have an open notch (side viewing) on one side, which is useful when performing minor anorectal procedures. If the patient is extremely anxious, sedation with midazolam (Versed), 1 to 3 mg IV is useful. To prevent painful pinching of the mucosa, the obturator should be replaced each time a side-viewing anoscope is turned during examination. Firm, constant pressure on the lubricated obturator will overcome sphincter spasm. Great force should not be used when inserting any scope.

The anal canal is about 1¼ inches long, extending from the perianal skin to the dentate or pectinate line (Fig. 17–1). The dentate line is visible as an undulating line formed by alternating rectal crypts and columns. Above the dentate line the mucosa is purple due to the underlying hemorrhoidal complexes. It has been commonly reported that the mucosa above the dentate line is insensate to pinprick or touch, but in many patients sensitivity of the mucosa extends several millimeters above the dentate line. This is of great practical importance when performing procedures such as rubber-band ligation of internal hemorrhoids. Prebanding testing with a gentle pinch of the grasping forceps will tell the examiner whether the ligator should be positioned higher within the rectum.

The anal crypts are believed to be a frequent source of infection. Small tears in a crypt may result in bacterial growth and migration in the submucosa, leading to perianal abscess formation. Beyond the anal sphincters, the anal canal is surrounded by fat, which frequently becomes the site of further extension of the abscess.

## Pain

The aspects of the history mentioned above may be helpful in evaluating the patient with anorectal pain. A commonly believed fallacy (promoted by television commercials) is that uncomplicated internal hemorrhoids cause pain. In many hemorrhoid patients, the hemorrhoids prolapse slightly during defecation. This may be manifested by red bleeding into the toilet water, red blood on the toilet tissue, or pain if a significant

*To prevent painful pinching of the mucosa, the obturator should be replaced each time a side-viewing anoscope is turned during examination.*

*In many patients sensitivity of the mucosa extends several millimeters above the dentate line.*

*A commonly believed fallacy is that uncomplicated internal hemorrhoids cause pain.*

mucosal erosion develops on the hemorrhoid. Pain from this complication occurs with each subsequent bowel movement. External hemorrhoids, in contrast, cause pain when thrombosis develops. They are seen as a firm purple or black lump just outside the anal canal. The time-honored treatment is incising the hemorrhoid under local anesthesia, thus releasing the thrombus. This offers immediate relief but is accompanied by a significant recurrence rate. The treatment rule for thrombosed external hemorrhoids is to *excise* rather than *incise*. Excision is performed under local anesthesia using 1% lidocaine (Xylocaine) with epinephrine. Additional hemostasis is achieved with electrocautery. The skin is not closed, and the wound is left to heal by granulation.

Perianal abscess (Fig. 17–2) presents with pain (often upon sitting) and is most often obvious on inspection. Some patients with perianal abscess will be febrile. The condition may cause systemic sepsis and should be considered an emergency in patients with diabetes, valvular heart disease, HIV infection, and other immunocompromised states. Neglected perianal abscess will frequently point to the skin and begin to drain pus spontaneously. Deep perianal abscesses (such as supralevator abscess), which cause pain during defecation but may not be visible to inspection, may be palpable on digital exam. Perianal abscess may result in aching discomfort in some patients and excruciating rectal pain in others. Perianal abscess requires incision and drainage. Most perianal abscesses can be drained by primary care providers. Local anesthesia with lidocaine or bupivacaine (Marcaine) is a must. Although it is true that anesthetic injection into an abscess offers no pain relief, circumferential injection around the abscess will provide adequate anesthesia. After injection, the provider should wait 3 to 5 minutes to allow the anesthetic to work. Remember that bupivacaine (Marcaine) takes longer to take effect than lidocaine but will offer longer pain relief. These anesthetics come mixed with 1:100,000 epinephrine, which affords improved hemostasis in all anorectal procedures. Large abscesses (>3 cm) or intersphincteric or suprasphincteric abscesses should be referred to a surgeon for drainage.

Pain in the perianal posterior midline suggests fissure. These lesions may be so acutely painful that the patient may not allow the examiner to spread the buttocks to perform any examination. In this situation, or when a patient cannot tolerate a digital exam, an examination under anesthesia is indicated, as discussed later. Fissures are probably caused by the passage of large or scybalous (hard, dry) stool, stretching the anoderm and perianal skin. Ninety percent of fissures occur in the posterior midline. Fissures appear as a split in the anoderm and the skin. This longitudinal rift may be l to 10 mm wide, and chronic fissures may be surrounded by a ridge of scar tissue. Pain is the predominant symptom of fissure, but minor bleeding may accompany the pain. Fissures not located in the posterior midline suggest inflammatory bowel disease, HIV infection, tuberculosis, Crohn's disease, trauma, or malignancy.

Fissures are exacerbated by anal sphincter spasm and heal with anorectal dilation. "Physiologic" dilation may be accomplished with fiber supplements to the diet. A high-

*The treatment rule for thrombosed external hemorrhoids is to* excise *rather than* incise.

*Circumferential injection around an abscess will provide adequate anesthesia.*

*Bupivacaine (Marcaine) takes longer to take effect than lidocaine but will offer longer pain relief.*

*Pain in the perianal posterior midline suggests fissure.*

FIGURE 17–2
Perianal abscess extending to the base of the scrotum. See color photograph in Color Section 2.

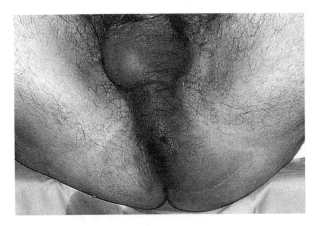

fiber diet or fiber supplements combined with daily hot baths may allow healing in some early cases. Surgical therapy involves either a lateral internal sphincterotomy or a four-finger dilation under anesthesia (Lord's procedure). Most surgeons have abandoned dilation owing to the higher complication rate (mostly hematomas) compared to sphincterotomy.

Pain in the coccygeal region or superior natal cleft indicates an infected pilonidal cyst. As the name "pilonidal" suggests, these are more common in hirsute individuals. Often a 1-mm pore can be identified in the skin over the cyst. Early infection with pain alone and no fluctuance, drainage, or significant erythema can be treated with hot soaks and oral antibiotics. Pilonidal abscess, with fluctuance, drainage, and in some cases fever, requires surgical drainage.

*Carcinoma of the anus may present with perianal or anal canal pain.*

Carcinoma of the anus may present with perianal or anal canal pain. The pain may be so severe that the patient may refuse digital examination. These patients warrant an examination under anesthesia.

### When to Call the Surgeon about Perianal Pain

- Patient unable to tolerate examination (requiring examination under anesthesia)
- Unclear diagnosis after examination
- An anorectal mass
- A large abscess (perianal or pilonidal)
- A large or deep fissure

## EXAMINATION UNDER ANESTHESIA

Patients who cannot tolerate digital rectal exam because of pain and tenderness should undergo examination under anesthesia. This may be done using local anesthesia, but spinal, epidural, or caudal blocks are excellent for this purpose. Often such an examination will reveal a deep perirectal abscess, which can be drained. Squamous cell carcinoma of the anus, which can present with severe pain and tenderness, is occasionally discovered during this examination. After inspection and digital rectal examination, the examiner should insert an anoscope and perform an anoscopy. This exam will usually define the problem, and fissures, abscesses, fistulas, and hemorrhoids can be treated at the same session.

## *Bleeding*

*The most common cause of red rectal bleeding is internal hemorrhoids.*

*Patients over 40 years of age with red rectal bleeding should have a complete evaluation of the colon whether they have hemorrhoids or not.*

*Mahogany-colored blood, blood interspersed with stool, or melena suggests more proximal bleeding sources.*

The most common cause of red rectal bleeding is internal hemorrhoids. Hemorrhoidal bleeding stains the toilet tissue and the toilet water red. Patients over 40 years of age with red rectal bleeding should have a complete evaluation of the colon by colonoscopy or flexible sigmoidoscopy plus barium enema whether they have hemorrhoids or not. Mahogany colored blood, blood interspersed with stool, or melena suggests bleeding sources more proximal than internal hemorrhoids (see Chapter 12). Treatment of bleeding internal hemorrhoids (confirmed by anoscopy) should begin with noninvasive treatment consisting of fiber or bulking agents combined with a change in defecatory habits. Patients should be discouraged from "straining at stool" or from spending lengthy periods on the toilet. These habits result in hemorrhoidal prolapse beyond the internal sphincter, which contributes to bleeding. If a 2- or 3-week trial of noninvasive treatment fails to eradicate bleeding with bowel movements, some form of invasive treatment is required. Rubber banding, injection therapy, infrared coagulation, laser ablation, and operative hemorrhoidectomy are all options. Except for operative hemorrhoidectomy, these are office procedures associated with minimal morbidity. Oper-

**TABLE 17–1**

## Treatment Options for Symptomatic Internal Hemorrhoids

| Grade | Description | Treatment Options |
|---|---|---|
| Grade I | Nonprolapsing (rarely bleed) | Bulking agents, dietary change, ointments, suppositories |
| Grade II | Prolapse with defecation, self-reducing | Above options, injection therapy, infrared or cryoablation, rubber banding |
| Grade III | Prolapse with defecation, digitally reducible | Above options or surgical hemorrhoidectomy |
| Grade IV | Always prolapsed, irreducible | Surgical hemorrhoidectomy |

ative hemorrhoidectomy is generally reserved for large, prolapsing hemorrhoids. Classification of internal hemorrhoids and treatment options are summarized in Table 17–1.

Occasionally prolapsing hemorrhoids will fail to reduce back into the anal canal. The discomfort often leads to sphincter spasm. This "incarcerates" the hemorrhoids outside the anal canal. They rapidly become engorged, edematous, and excruciatingly painful (Fig. 17–3). On inspection, a "rosette" of edematous hemorrhoids is visible. The unfamiliar practitioner may misdiagnose this as rectal prolapse. The edema and sphincter spasm prevent digital reduction of the incarcerated hemorrhoids. We recommend sedation (midazolam 2–3 mg IV) followed by circumferential anal block with 1% lidocaine (Xylocaine). The lidocaine is injected subcutaneously and into the sphincter muscles circumferentially. A volume of 10–15 mL is typically used. The sedation plus the anal block overcome the sphincter spasm so that 5 minutes later the previously incarcerated hemorrhoids are easily reduced with the gloved finger. This converts an emergency to an elective situation. An elective hemorrhoidectomy should be performed 1 to 2 days later, after the edema has resolved. If the hemorrhoidectomy is deferred, the condition is likely to recur. As an alternative to this approach, some authorities recommend a partial (one- or two-quadrant) hemorrhoidectomy as an urgent operation in the face of prolapsed, incarcerated internal hemorrhoids.

### *When to Call the Surgeon about Hemorrhoids*

- Massive hemorrhoidal bleeding
- Persistent bleeding after office treatment
- Large hemorrhoids (requiring surgery)
- Prolapsed, incarcerated hemorrhoids

FIGURE 17–3
Prolapsed, incarcerated internal hemorrhoids. See Color Section 2.

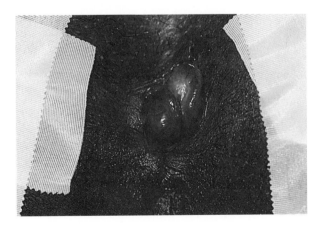

# Anal Discharge or Fecal Soiling

Anal discharge of mucus or pus may be due to a variety of conditions. Perianal abscess usually presents with pain and may be associated with discharge. The diagnosis is obvious on physical examination. Inflammatory bowel disease may present with a discharge of pus or mucus mixed with blood. This diagnosis is confirmed via sigmoidoscopy or colonoscopy.

Fistula-in-ano (Fig. 17–4) presents with fecal or purulent staining of underwear. This disorder most frequently develops after a bout with perianal abscess, whether the abscess was surgically drained or not. It may develop months or years after an abscess. Anal fistulas may also be a manifestation of inflammatory bowel disease. On physical examination the external orifice of a fistula is often visible. In addition, a fibrous tract may be palpable beneath the skin. Fistula-in-ano requires surgical therapy (fistulotomy) for cure. The search for the internal opening during fistulotomy is guided by *Goodsall's rule*, which states that a fistula with an external opening anterior to an imaginary horizontal line through the anus will have an internal (mucosal) opening straight ahead of the external opening. A fistula with a posterior external pore will have an internal opening in the posterior midline mucosa. The external opening and internal openings define the fistula. The fistula is surgically opened by sharply laying open the entire tract from external to internal opening (fistulotomy). The wound is allowed to heal via granulation. Fistulae that encompass both the internal and external anal sphincters require staged surgical therapy. These procedures should be performed in the operating room.

*Hidradenitis suppurativa* is a purulent infection of sweat glands. It occurs most commonly in the groin, axillae, and perineal regions. The presentation includes purulent drainage on underwear. Multiple draining pores and microabscesses are visible. This has been described as "waterspout perineum." The differential diagnosis includes complicated perianal Crohn's disease. Mild cases of hidradenitis may be treated with oral antibiotics. Recalcitrant and severe cases require surgical therapy. Initial therapy is directed towards control of infection. Ultimately, wide excision with skin grafting may be required.

Severe fecal incontinence may accompany rectal prolapse. *Rectal prolapse* is believed to be due to a loss of pelvic muscular support to the rectum. Predisposing factors include neurologic disorders, prior pelvic surgery, chronic constipation, and nulliparity. The condition is much more common in women. A Valsalva's maneuver may bring on the rectal prolapse, and significant prolapse may occur with each bowel movement. The condition is best revealed when the patient attempts to have a bowel movement. In some cases prolapse may be demonstrated with the patient in the lateral decubitus, knee-to-chest position (with Valsalva's maneuver). When the history suggests rectal prolapse but the condition cannot be reproduced in the office, a sigmoidoscopic ex-

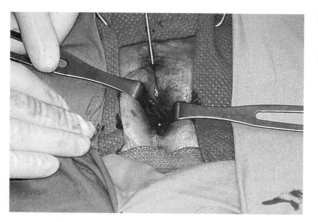

**FIGURE 17–4**

Fistula-in-ano as demonstrated by a metal probe through the fistula. See Color Section 2.

amination may help. Rectosigmoid ulceration (often solitary and often anterior) or areas of mucosal thickening, edema, and hyperemia, or all of these symptoms, may be compatible with rectal prolapse.

Some cases of rectal prolapse benefit from nonoperative therapy including dietary changes, pelvic muscle exercises, and electrical stimulation of the sphincter mechanism. Submucosal injection of sclerotherapy agents such as sodium tetradecyl will also benefit mild cases.

Severe, full-thickness prolapse requires surgical therapy. Many surgical procedures are available, reflecting the imperfect nature of any single procedure. Most procedures attempt to fix the rectum in the pelvis with sutures or prosthetic materials. Detailed descriptions of these procedures are beyond the scope of this chapter.

*Rectosigmoid ulceration and/or areas of mucosal thickening, edema, and hyperemia all may be compatible with rectal prolapse.*

### *When to Call the Surgeon about Fecal Soiling*

• • • • • • • • • • • • • • • • • • • • • • • • • • • • • • • • • • • • • • • •

- Fistula
- Hidradenitis suppurativa
- Significant rectal prolapse
- Unclear diagnosis

## Pruritus Ani

Severe anal itching is a very aggravating symptom. It occurs more commonly in men than in women (4:1) and may be caused by a myriad of conditions (Table 17–2). The history may offer clues to the cause and should include specific inquiry about chewing tobacco, anal intercourse, frequent use of enemas or suppositories, diarrhea, the use of deodorant sprays or perfumed toilet papers, foreign travel, vaginal discharge, and the existence of dermatologic conditions elsewhere on the body. Also, inquire about the frequent use of spicy seasonings in foods (e.g., hot peppers, chilies, Tabasco sauce). Any condition causing a moist perineum can result in pruritus. Excessive sweating, hirsutism, and poor anal hygiene may all contribute to this problem.

Physical examination includes inspection and anoscopy. This may reveal papillomas, anal lesions, condylomas, or other obvious causes. Occult diabetes should be ruled out by obtaining a serum glucose. The examiner can search for pinworms by pressing clear cellophane tape into the anal skin and putting it on a glass slide for microscopic

**TABLE 17–2**

| Common Causes and Treatment of Pruritus Ani | |
|---|---|
| **Cause** | **Treatment** |
| Pinworms | Mebendazole |
| Inflammatory bowel disease | Cortisol enema, sulfasalazine |
| Candida | Clotrimazole, fluconazole |
| Pediculosis, scabies | Lindane lotion |
| Prolapsing hemorrhoids | Banding or surgery |
| Anal papilloma or exophytic lesion | Surgery |
| Condylomas (HPV) | Podophyllin, cryosurgery |
| Food allergy, irritation | Dietary change |
| Tinea cruris | Clotrimazole, ketoconazole |
| Diabetes mellitus | Hypoglycemic agent |
| Fecal soiling, moisture | Talcum powder, improved hygiene |

HPV = human papillomavirus

exam. Commonly, the perianal skin is red and excoriated from scratching. If a specific cause can be pinpointed, treatment will be more effective (see Table 17–2). If a precise diagnosis cannot be reached (which is not unusual), then symptomatic therapy can be offered. Dietary changes should focus on elimination of any offending irritants, toilet paper should be white and nonscented, and cleansing pads with 50% witch hazel can be used after each bowel movement. Talcum powder may be used to decrease moisture, and the patient should avoid wearing tight underclothing made from synthetic material. Hydrocortisone cream (0.5%–1.0%) may be applied sparingly to reduce itching, but prolonged use may lead to fungal overgrowth, thus exacerbating the pruritis.

## Complications of Radiation Therapy

Anorectal complications of radiation therapy for prostatic or uterine malignancies are fairly uncommon but are being seen more often with the increased use of radiation therapy for prostate cancer. *Radiation proctitis* is the most frequently seen complication of radiation therapy. It presents with red rectal bleeding. On anoscopy or sigmoidoscopy, the endoscopist sees one of two common pictures. Early cases reveal erythematous, friable rectal mucosa with numerous bleeding petechia-like lesions. In chronic cases, the mucosa may be white and nonglistening, with scattered vascular ectasias or hemangioma-like lesions.

Radiation proctitis usually responds to steroid enemas. Sucralfate (Carafate) enemas have also been effective. Recalcitrant cases may be treated with topical formalin or laser therapy.

A second, rare complication of radiation therapy is *anorectal stenosis*. This presents with constipation or thin caliber stools or both. With this history, rectal cancer must be ruled out. The strictures are dense and the perianal tissue is "woody." These strictures do not dilate well. Treatment may require a plastic procedure such as flap anoplasty. The worst cases may require a permanent colostomy.

### RECOMMENDED READING

Corman, ML (ed): Colon and Rectal Surgery. ed 3. JB Lippincott, Philadelphia, 1993.

Goligher, J (ed): Surgery of the Anus, Rectum and Colon. ed 5. Bailliere Tindall, London, 1984.

# Chapter 18

# Low Back Pain

WJ KROMPINGER, MD,
and MARCUS PLESCIA, MD, MPH

The primary care provider will assess and treat low back pain more than any other disease entity except the common cold. More than 80% of the adult population will be temporarily disabled with low back pain for at least 2 to 3 days. Chronic low back pain may be one of the most frustrating clinical situations for the primary care provider. The cause is often poorly understood and causes may be multifactorial. Social and psychological issues frequently play a significant role. Fortunately, most episodes of low back pain are limited in duration and intensity; most resolve within 3 weeks. With such a favorable natural history, it is understandable that many treatment modalities have been given credit for relieving the pain and disability of low back pain. It can even be argued that specifically diagnosing the cause of low back pain in an individual may not be necessary and could lead to overtreatment. When low back pain does not resolve, however, further assessment and treatment become necessary.

The assessment of low back pain begins with an understanding of the patient's complaint. It is important to assess the origination point of the pain and the destination point of the pain. Aggravating factors such as coughing, sitting, or walking and alleviating factors (e.g., sitting) should be elicited. The examiner must assess the presentation of the pain in combination with any systemic complaints and should consider age-related conditions such as osteoporosis. A social history including potential occupational risk factors and screening for depression, abuse, or significant stress is extremely important early in the workup. From an assessment of all these parameters, an initial classification system can be applied.

The examiner can use the following three-group system to classify patients' pain (Table 18–1). Patients with pain radiating below the knee have *radicular* low back pain (sciatica). A patient is also placed in this category if the pain is in a buttock, thigh, or calf without the presentation of low back pain. Pain in the thigh in the absence of low back pain is often initially misdiagnosed as a hamstring strain when it is actually a manifestation of radicular low back pain. Patients with pain radiating from the back

**TABLE 18–1**

### Classification of Low Back Pain

Radicular
Referred
Central

into the buttock or to the thigh are classified as having *referred* low back pain. Pain that does not radiate is classified as *central* low back pain.

## Radicular Low Back Pain

Probably the best understood type of back pain is radicular low back pain. The primary cause of pain is mechanical or chemical nerve root irritation. The patient may initially have a severe episode of low back pain that rapidly evolves over days into leg pain. Frequently the back pain disappears with the onset of leg pain. Patients commonly have nerve root tension signs manifested by the presence of a positive straight-leg raise. This can also be accompanied by neurologic deficits, usually in the distribution of a single nerve root. Treatment efforts are directed at decreasing the inflammatory reaction around the root and minimizing mechanical pressure on the nerve root.

The most common cause of nerve root irritation is a disk herniation (Table 18–2). This commonly occurs in the 30- to 40-year age group. Disk herniation is often assumed to cause sciatica, but asymptomatic herniation is commonly diagnosed on computed tomography (CT) and magnetic resonance imaging (MRI) scanning, and the extent of disk protrusion and the degree of clinical symptoms often do not correlate. Herniation most commonly affects the L5-S1 or L4-L5 disk (Fig. 18–1). Patients with an acute L5-S1 disk herniation frequently have an absent ankle reflex (Table 18–3). This may also be accompanied by weakness in the gastrocnemius-soleus muscle group. Clinically this can be detected by having the patient repeatedly rise up on the toes for 8 to 10 repetitions. There may also be decreased sensation and a sense of numbness over the lateral foot. These findings characterize S1 radiculopathy. With nerve root irritation, a positive straight raise is generated at about 45°.

Patients with a disk herniation at L4-L5 will commonly have weakness in the ankle and big-toe dorsiflexors. More subtle weakness is detected by having the patient heel walk. There are usually no reflex abnormalities. Numbness is felt over the first web space of the foot or over the dorsum of the foot. These findings characterize L5 radiculopathy. As in a patient with an L5-S1 herniation, there will be a positive straight-leg raising test.

The third most frequent herniation is at the L3-L4 level. This will commonly lead to L4 root irritation and dysfunction. Patients will have weakness in the quadriceps and

**TABLE 18–2**

### Causes of Radicular Low Back Pain

Lumbar disk herniation
Spinal stenosis
Spinal tumor
Vascular disease
Piriformis syndrome

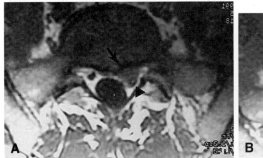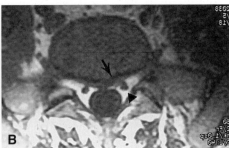

**FIGURE 18–1**
A 42-year-old with radicular low back pain. (*A*) The MRI demonstrates an L5-S1 disk herniation (*arrow*) with posterior deflection of the S1 root (*arrowhead*). The patient was treated conservatively. (*B*) Three months later, repeat MRI shows resolution of the disk protrusion (*arrow*). The S1 root is no longer deflected posteriorly (*arrowhead*).

may have a diminished knee reflex. Numbness may be detected over the medial foot. The L4 nerve contributes to the formation of the femoral nerve, which runs anterior to the hip joint. Given this anatomy, patients with L4 root irritation will have a negative straight-leg raise. If the patient is placed in a side position with the affected side up, however, nerve root tension can be detected by extending the hip, thereby stretching the femoral nerve.

Fortunately, lumbar disk herniation will resolve with conservative treatment in over 80% of patients. Initial treatment is directed toward reducing nerve root inflammation. The use of nonsteroidal anti-inflammatory medication can be very helpful, with or without narcotic pain medication. A period of bedrest of 2 to 3 days may be necessary. Longer periods of bedrest are now generally discouraged to avoid deconditioning. Patients are advised not to sit. Walking is allowed and encouraged. If leg pain persists after 2 to 3 weeks, an epidural steroid injection may be a useful treatment adjuvant. A back corset or brace may also be useful. With initial control of the more disabling aspect of the leg pain, a flexion exercise regimen may be instituted by a physical therapist. Extension exercises are introduced as long as leg pain is not exacerbated by lumbar extension or lying in the prone position. After the patient achieves a more normal range of motion, he or she can focus on cardiovascular conditioning, upper-body strengthening, and lumbar-extensor strengthening.

The primary care provider can monitor the patient's progress through resolution of nerve root irritation and overall rehabilitation. A patient's unresponsiveness to such a treatment regimen is a reason to consider further diagnostic studies and a surgical approach. The most urgent reason for early surgical intervention is severe nerve root

*Lumbar disk herniation will resolve with conservative treatment in over 80% of patients.*

*The most urgent reason for early surgical intervention is severe nerve root compromise or multiple nerve root compromise.*

**TABLE 18–3**

| Signs of Lumbar Herniation | |
|---|---|
| **Site** | **Signs** |
| L5-S1 | Absent ankle reflex |
| | Weak gastrocnemius-soleus |
| | Numbness of lateral foot |
| L4-L5 | Weak ankle dorsiflexors |
| | Numbness of anterior foot |
| L3-L4 | Absent knee reflex |
| | Weakness of quadriceps |
| | Positive tension signs with hip extension |

*Patients with bowel and bladder symptoms need an urgent assessment, including a rectal examination.*

*The most common reason for surgical diskectomy is disabling leg pain.*

compromise or multiple nerve root compromise. The latter condition, called *cauda equina syndrome*, can be caused by a massive central disk herniation and will involve the sacral roots. The clinical presentation will be of perineal numbness (saddle anesthesia), inability to void or incontinence, and diffuse lower-extremity weakness. Patients with bowel and bladder symptoms need an urgent assessment, including a rectal examination. The presence of rectal tone and perianal sensation should be assessed. If sacral root involvement is suspected, an urgent MRI or myelogram should be performed, followed by surgical decompression. Another reason for early surgical intervention is severe involvement in a single root distribution. The presence of an acute foot drop may be an indication for urgent decompression of the L5 root. The third reason for early surgical intervention is the development of a rapidly progressive neurologic deficit: A patient who develops numbness followed by a progressively increasing weakness of the ankle dorsiflexors may be a candidate for earlier surgical assessment.

The most common reason for surgical diskectomy is disabling leg pain. Such patients feel that the pain is significant and has intolerably damaged the quality of their lives. Commonly, these patients are not responding to conservative treatment. They can only ambulate short distances and cannot sit for more than 30 minutes at a time. They can no longer exercise. If these symptoms persist for 6 to 8 weeks, a CT scan or MRI should be considered. In general, a CT scan is indicated when bony pathology is suspected and the neurologic level is well defined by the patient's clinical presentation. In less clear presentations, an MRI allows better tissue resolution and may provide more definitive information.

Concurrently, referral to a spine specialist should be considered. The patient may still be a candidate for conservative treatment, but referral at this stage allows the surgeon to develop a relationship with the patient and better understand the patient's disability. This understanding leads to better treatment decisions. In this scenario, it generally is rare to consider surgery before 12 weeks have passed since the development of radicular symptoms.

The success rate of lumbar surgery is closely correlated with appropriate patient selection. Of patients with a disk herniation documented on neuroradiographic studies (CT, MRI, myelogram) who have a clinical exam consistent with the lesion demonstrated on these studies, 85% can be expected to achieve significant symptom improvement. Clinical successes tend to be fewer and return-to-work percentages tend to be lower in cases associated with compensation. Most series report a recurrence rate of 7% to 12% and a reoperation rate of 10% for all complications. The decision to proceed with disk surgery must take into account the risk of failure, the complications, and the possibility of significant spontaneous improvement over time. Saal and others have documented resorption of extruded disk fragments in a significant percentage of patients who have not had surgery. When the patient has clinically plateaued at an unacceptable level of pain and dysfunction, however, lumbar diskectomy can be exceptionally gratifying to the patient and treating practitioners.

In the age group over 50, *spinal stenosis* and *atherosclerotic claudication* become the major disease entities causing leg pain. Commonly, the pain with spinal stenosis is only aggravated by walking and is rapidly relieved by sitting or lying supine. Patients find relief of the pain when bending forward. They find that walking is significantly improved by leaning on a grocery cart. These patients with neurogenic claudication should be differentiated from those with vascular disease, in whom the pain generally does not change with positional changes. Elderly patients may have both vascular and neurogenic claudication, however, making treatment decisions difficult. These patients will require vascular studies and spinal imaging. The primary care provider is in a position to monitor the patient's status. Patients will begin to complain of leg pain that comes with progressively shorter walking distances. These patients may be helped with a flexion-based exercise regimen in conjunction with nonsteroidal anti-inflammatory medication. Patients with resting leg pain in a single root distribution may be amenable to epidural steroid injections. At some point, however, conservative treatment may be unsuccessful in improving the patient's status. When the patient's quality of life is significantly impeded, surgical intervention should be considered.

As for patients with lumbar disk herniation, patient selection is the key factor in determining the success of surgery. In patients with single root pain, radiographic stenosis must be demonstrated at the clinically involved root. In patients with claudication, central stenosis must be documented with radiographic studies. Surgical success rates of 80% to 90% can be expected with appropriate patient selection.

Patients presenting with rest pain and night pain symptoms that are not clearly vascular in origin require radiographs of the spine to rule out spinal tumor and infection. Tumors about the conus can mimic nerve root irritation from disk herniation or stenosis. Also, resting leg pain may be an indicator of advanced vascular disease with impending ischemic changes to the extremity (see Chapter 20).

Another disease entity causing radicular pain is *piriformis syndrome*. Patients with this disease commonly are under 40 years of age. They frequently give a history of falling onto a buttock, which results in a local hematoma. With resolution of the inflammatory response, there is shortening of the hip external rotators. With piriformis shortening and fibrosis, the sciatic nerve is compressed underneath the tendon or muscle belly. Leg pain can be aggravated by forced adduction and internal rotation of the extremity. The diagnosis is further clarified by a CT through the piriformis fossa, revealing asymmetry of the muscle belly when compared to the uninvolved side. If symptoms of leg pain do not improve with physical therapy directed to stretching the hip extensors, surgical piriformis release can be a very gratifying procedure.

*Patients presenting with rest pain and night pain symptoms require radiographs of the spine to rule out spinal tumor and infection.*

## Referred Back Pain

Patients with pain radiating from the back to a buttock or proximal thigh are characterized as having *referred back pain*. Referred pain patterns are commonly caused by structural abnormalities of the spinal motion segment (Fig. 18–2, Table 18–4). Each vertebral element articulates with the one above and the one below through the disk and two facet joints. At each segment of motion, these two facets and the disk are referred to as the *spinal motion unit*, or *three-joint complex*. Abnormalities of the spinal motion unit lead to referred patterns of back pain.

FIGURE 18–2
A 52-year-old with referred low back pain. Flexion radiograph indicates forward slippage of L4 in reference to L5 (*arrow*).

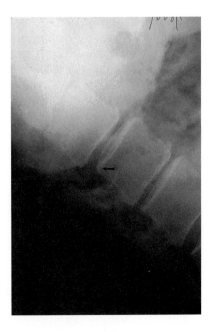

**TABLE 18-4**

| **Disease Entities Causing Referred Low Back Pain** |
| --- |

*Annular Low Back Pain*
Spondylolisthesis
Degenerative disk disease
Internal disk derangement

*Facet Pain*
Facet arthritis

*Sacroiliac Pain*
Traumatic disorders
Spondyloarthropathies

Common disease entities causing referred pain include spondylolisthesis, degenerative disk disease, and internal disk derangement. The pain from these entities probably emanates from the internal structure of the disk. The patient may have *annular low back pain*. Disease entities can also affect the facet joint. *Facet arthritis* can be localized to an individual facet and cause a unilateral referred pain complex. A third anatomic area to consider in referred pain patterns is the *sacroiliac (SI) joint*. The SI joint can be the source of pain in traumatic injuries to the joint and in the spondyloarthropathies.

Patients with abnormalities of the spinal motion segment have pain with examination of spinal mechanics. Typically the pain is exacerbated by lumbar extension. Spinal extension compresses the facet articular cartilage. If the disk is significantly degenerated, it will bulge posteriorly. If the motion segment is significantly impaired, translational abnormalities will be appreciated on radiographs, using lateral flexion/ extension films. Typically, patients have a totally normal neurologic assessment and have negative tension signs manifested by a normal straight-leg raise. The one exception to this is the patient with an *isthmic spondylolisthesis*. This condition is commonly associated with bilateral tight hamstrings.

Patients with referred pain are initially treated with nonsteroidal anti-inflammatory medication and muscle relaxants, as are patients with radicular low back pain. The institution of a mobilization program is very important. Physical therapy is started with the introduction of back stabilization exercises. The patient is instructed in pelvic tilts and learns to find the neutral position of the pelvis, in which back and leg pain is minimized. Referred pain is a mechanical process modulated by a biochemical environment of inflammation. The combination of a mechanical therapy program and nonsteroidal anti-inflammatory drugs (NSAIDs) can be effective in controlling the disability from referred pain.

*Surgical intervention for referred pain is reserved for the patient for whom conservative treatment over at least 6 months has failed.*

Surgical intervention for referred pain is reserved for the patient who has failed conservative treatment over at least 6 months. These patients feel that their quality of life has deteriorated, with an adverse effect on activities of daily living. Surgery is an option for the patient with pain and disability who has an abnormality detected on diagnostic studies (Fig. 18–3). The diagnostic studies include provocative examination of the spinal structural unit. Flexion-extension radiographs are helpful in assessing abnormal translational motion. The MRI, frequently in combination with diskography, can identify painful disk segments. After such studies, the patient is commonly treated with a period of brace immobilization to reduce forces in the painful motion segment. The corrective surgery generally consists of forms of lumbar fusion (see Figure 18–3B). Surgery for patients with referred pain generally has the highest failure rate. The selection of patients for lumbar fusion is probably the most critical factor in whether there will be clinical success. The surgeon must assess the patient's pain, reaction to dis-

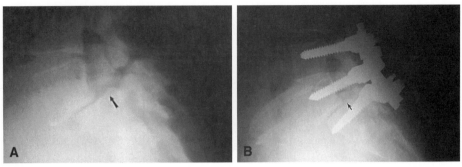

**FIGURE 18-3**
A 47-year-old woman with spondylolisthesis. (*A*) L5 is translated forward in reference to S1 (*arrow*). (*B*) The patient underwent fusion with internal fixation. The slippage of L5 has been reduced (*arrow*).

ability, psychosocial status, secondary gain, and expectations before deciding whether to offer him or her a surgical solution. An open dialog between the primary care provider and the treating surgeon greatly facilitates decision making in this situation.

## Central Back Pain

Most patients present to their primary care provider with localized back pain without significant radiation. Typically the pain is related to activity and is commonly associated with localized muscular spasm. The cause of this complex is not well understood. The pain may be secondary to strain of the musculoligamentous supporting structures. It also could be secondary to localized injury to the disk annulus without violating the overall mechanical function of the disk. Whatever the cause, this syndrome commonly responds to short periods of rest with use of anti-inflammatory medication and possibly narcotic pain medication. After 5 to 7 days, most patients are significantly improved. If the pain does not respond within this time period, further assessment may be necessary.

Osteoarthritis is the most common cause of low back pain in the elderly (Table 18–5). In the elderly patient with nonresponding central back pain, however, the diagnosis of a compression fracture should be considered. The diagnosis can be made with plain radiographs. To establish the age of a compression fracture and to rule out associated lesions, a bone scan may be helpful. This is especially important if the pain

*Osteoarthritis is the most common cause of low back pain in the elderly.*

**TABLE 18-5**

### Causes of Central Back Pain

Musculoskeletal disorders
    Muscle spasm
    Compression fracture
    Osteoarthritis
Infection
Osteomyelitis
Diskitis
Myeloma
Metastatic disease
Visceral disease
Vascular conditions
Inflammatory arthritis

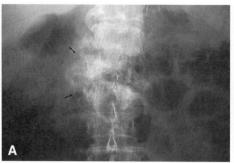
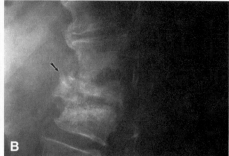

**FIGURE 18–4**
(*A*) Anteroposterior and (*B*) lateral radiographs of 69-year-old with osteomyelitis of the upper lumbar spine. Arrows point to areas of bony hypertrophy and sclerosis secondary to the infectious process.

*Back pain may be secondary to organ system disease.*

does not resolve within 3 to 4 weeks. The possibility of pathological fracture secondary to tumor must be ruled out. The workup also should include a serum protein electrophoresis, calcium, phosphate, alkaline phosphatase, acid phosphatase, prostate-specific antigen, and routine blood work. In some instances, a needle biopsy of the fracture site might be required to establish a definitive diagnosis. Other diagnostic entities commonly encountered in the elderly include infections such as osteomyelitis and diskitis (Fig. 18–4). These conditions typically occur after episodes of bacteremia associated with genitourinary conditions.

Back pain may be secondary to organ system disease. Pancreatitis, prostatitis, ulcer disease, and kidney disease can all mimic forms of low back pain, but they can be distinguished from musculoskeletal causes through a detailed history. Vascular conditions such as abdominal aortic aneurysms can cause acute low back pain. The astute primary care provider can save a patient's life by making an early accurate diagnosis for these entities.

For patients with central back pain that does not respond to conservative modalities, the examiner should consider a bone scan to rule out the possibility of occult tumor, fracture, or infection. Also, the presence of a spondyloarthropathy should be considered in the patient under age 40 with central back pain and morning stiffness. In this situation, blood work should include antinuclear antibodies (ANA), rheumatoid factor, sedimentation rate, HLA-B27 (human leukocyte antigens), and Lyme titers to rule out an inflammatory arthritis.

### When to Call the Surgeon about Low Back Pain

- Multiple nerve root compromise (cauda equina syndrome)
- Profound neurologic deficit
- Progressive neurologic deficit
- Disabling, nonresponding leg pain (failure of conservative therapy)
- Night pain
- Disabling resting leg pain in patient over 50 years of age

### RECOMMENDED READING

Deyo, RA, et al: What can the history and physical examination tell us about low back pain? JAMA 268:760–765, 1992.

Quebec Task Force on Spinal Disorders: A scientific approach to the assessment and management of activity-related spinal disorders: A monograph for clinicians. Spine 12(suppl 7):S22–S30, 1987.

Rainville, J, et al: Low back and cervical spine disorders. Ortho Clinics NA 27:729–746, 1996.

Rothman, RH, and Simeone, FA (eds): The Spine, ed 3. WB Saunders, Philadelphia, 1992.

Saal, JA, et al: The natural history of lumbar disc extrusions treated non-operatively. Spine 15:683–686, 1990.

Waddell, G, et al: Non-organic physical signs in low back pain. Spine 5:117–125, 1980.

Weber, H: Lumbar disc herniation: A controlled prospective study with ten years of observation. Spine 8:131–140, 1983.

Weinstein, JN, et al (eds): Essentials of the Spine. Raven Press, New York, 1995.

# Leg Pain
# and Vascular Disease

MARK S. FRIEDLAND, MD

As with most diagnostic problems in medicine, the cause of lower extremity pain usually can be determined by a careful history and examination. Conditions causing lower extremity pain arising from the hip, knee, ankle, or foot are covered elsewhere in this text. Aside from musculoskeletal injury resulting in contusion or fractures, vascular pathology is the most common cause of this pain. Benign and malignant tumors of the lower extremity are rare and will not be discussed in this chapter.

This chapter therefore focuses on peripheral vascular causes of leg pain. Some of the disease processes discussed here are common and may coexist in patients presenting to primary care providers' offices for other reasons. All too frequently patients with complications of diabetes or cardiac disease have not had a lower extremity examination with documentation of arterial pulses. It is my feeling that the most sensible method of documenting a pulse is as present (p), weak (w), detectable by Doppler only (d), or absent (O). If uncertainty of arterial insufficiency remains, noninvasive testing in the vascular surgery laboratory will usually confirm the suspected diagnosis.

Some problems mentioned in this chapter require surgical intervention and should be referred to the appropriate surgical specialist. Other problems can be managed nonoperatively, and the need for referral is based on the primary care provider's comfort with managing that problem. If an intervention such as a bypass or angioplasty is indicated, then an arteriogram should be obtained. Arteriography is not part of the diagnostic evaluation and should not be obtained unless intervention is indicated and planned. Any bypass done in the lower extremity has a finite long-term patency and will require surveillance, usually again by history and physical as well as noninvasive testing. Again, referral to a vascular surgeon will depend on the primary care provider's preference to perform this routine surveillance and an understanding of the indications for intervention.

*Arteriography is not part of the diagnostic evaluation and should not be obtained unless intervention is indicated and planned.*

# Color Plates 9–15

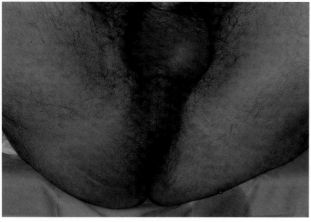

FIGURE 17–2
Perianal abscess extending to the base of the scrotum.

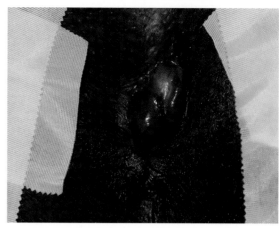

FIGURE 17–3
Prolapsed, incarcerated internal hemorrhoids.

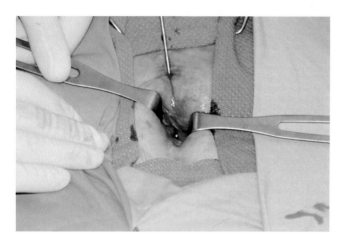

FIGURE 17–4
Fistula-in-ano as demonstrated by a metal probe through the fistula.

FIGURE 22–1
(A) Verruca vulgaris. (B) Perineal wart (condyloma).

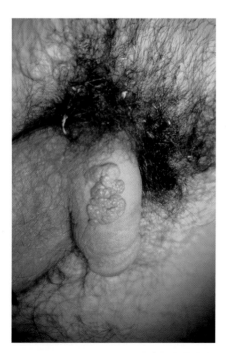

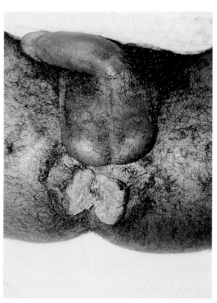

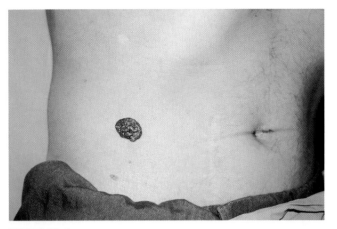

FIGURE 22–2
Seborrheic keratosis.

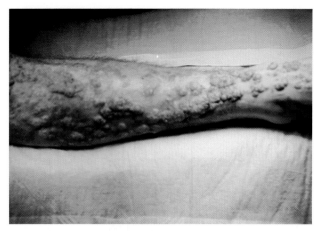

FIGURE 22–3
Linear nevus.

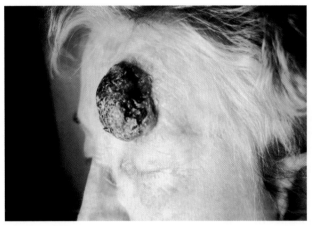

FIGURE 22–4
Keratoacanthoma.

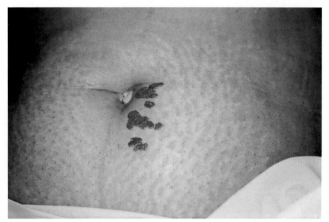

FIGURE 22–5
Common melanocytic nevi.

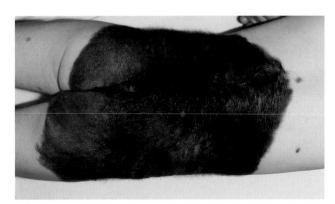

FIGURE 22–6
Giant hairy cell nevus.

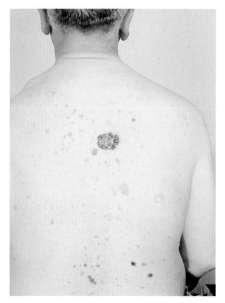

FIGURE 22–7
Halo nevus.

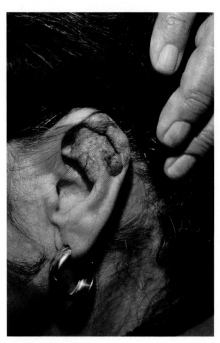

FIGURE 22–8
Nevus sebaceous of Jadassohn.

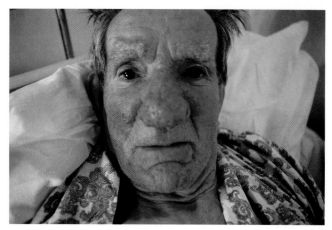

FIGURE 22–9
Rhinophyma.

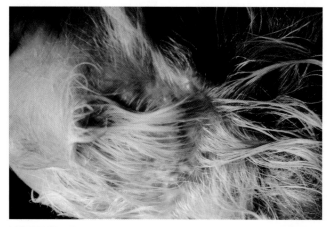

FIGURE 22–10
Cylindroma.

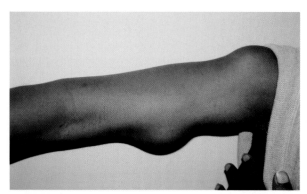

FIGURE 22–11A
Neurofibroma. von Recklinghausen's disease.

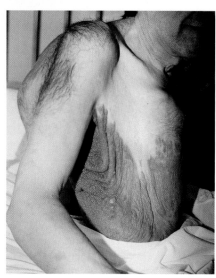

FIGURE 22–11B
Plexiform neurofibroma.

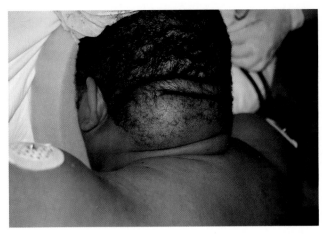

FIGURE 22–12
Lipoma.

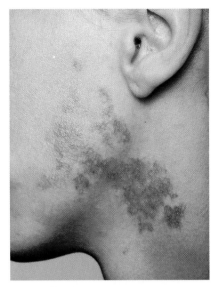

FIGURE 22–13
Port-wine stain.

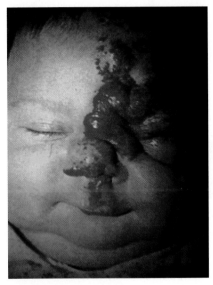

FIGURE 22–14
Hemangioma.

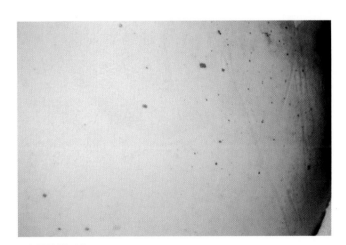

FIGURE 22–15
Senile angioma.

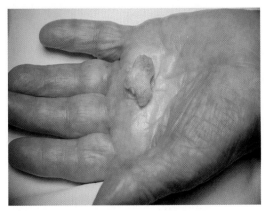

FIGURE 22–16
Pyogenic granuloma.

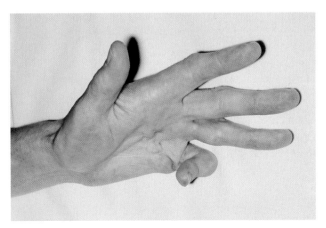

FIGURE 22–17
Dupuytren's contracture.

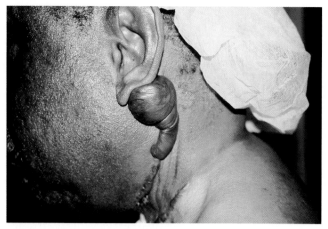

FIGURE 22–18
Keloids.

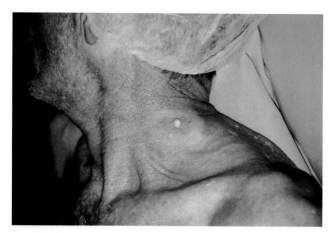

FIGURE 22–19
Epidermoid cyst.

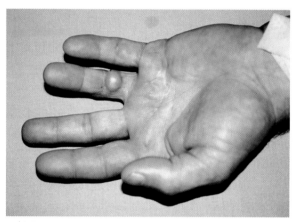

FIGURE 22–20
Epidermal inclusion cyst.

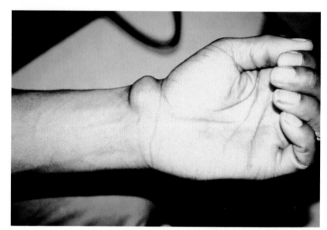

FIGURE 22–21
Wrist ganglion.

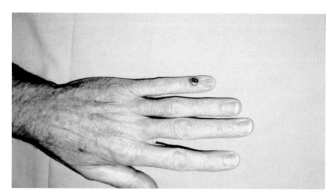

FIGURE 22–22
Digital mucous cyst.

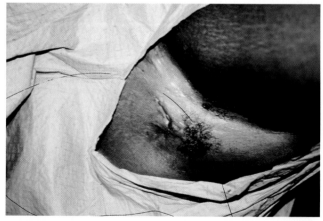

FIGURE 22–23
Hidradenitis.

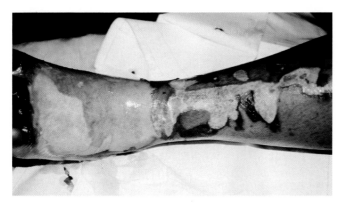
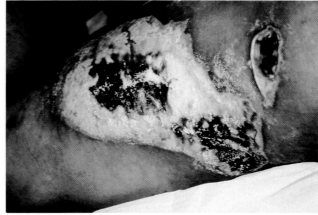

FIGURE 22–24
Thermal injuries. (A) _____ . (B) _____ .

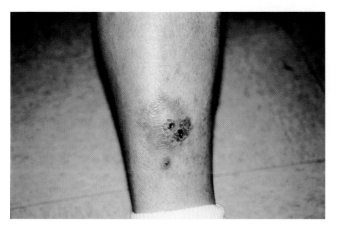

FIGURE 22–25
Bowen's disease.

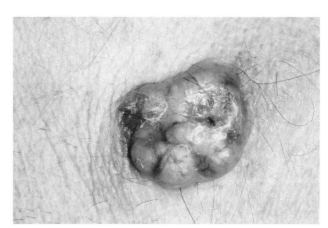

FIGURE 22–26
Basal cell carcinoma.

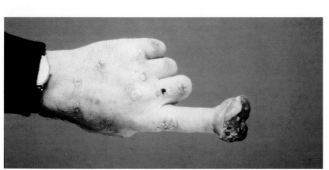
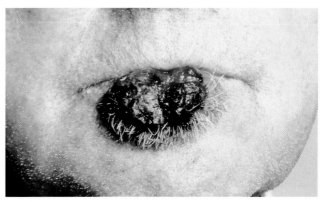

FIGURE 22–27
Squamous cell carcinoma. (A) _____ . (B) _____ .

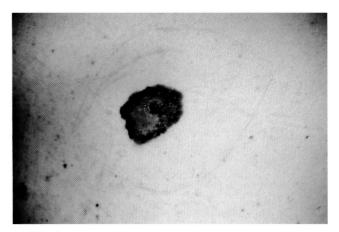

FIGURE 22–28A
Superficial spreading melanoma.

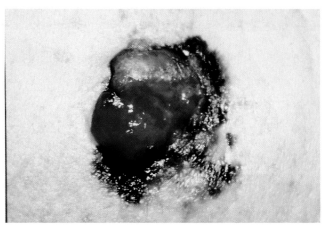

FIGURE 22–28B
Nodular melanoma.

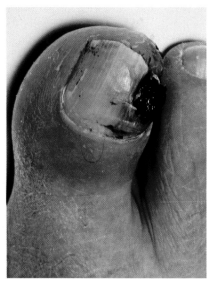

FIGURE 22–28C
Subungual melanoma.

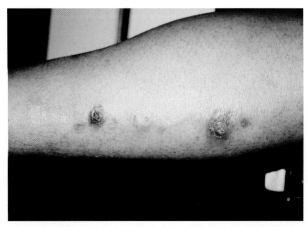

FIGURE 22–29
Kaposi's sarcoma.

FIGURE 22–30
Tumor metastatic to skin. Adeno carcinoma
from lung to arm.

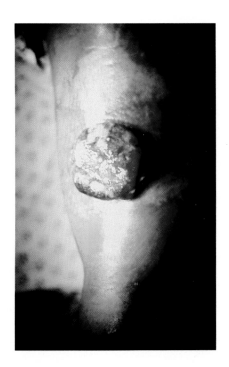

# Arterial Occlusive Disease (Chronic)

Arterial occlusive disease of the lower extremity can be asymptomatic or may manifest as intermittent claudication, rest pain, foot ulcers, or gangrene. The simple absence of a palpable pulse on its own is not an indication for intervention in most patients. All that is required is careful documentation; no referral is needed. In other patients, however, the history will reveal leg pain on ambulation or at rest, or the physical examination may demonstrate an ulcer or frank gangrene.

*Intermittent claudication* is a reproducible ache or tightening of the calf, thigh, or buttock muscle with ambulation, which is relieved with standing or rest. The walking distance that brings on claudication in a patient tends to be consistent and should be documented. The pain is brought on earlier by increased muscle work. Therefore, carrying groceries or walking up an incline will result in claudication pain sooner than walking only. The anatomic level of claudication depends on the level of arterial occlusive disease. Aortoiliac occlusive disease will frequently present with claudication symptoms involving the buttocks and thighs as well as the calf region. These patients may also complain of impotence. Buttock claudication plus impotence due to aortoiliac occlusion is known as *Leriche's syndrome*. In severe or long-standing cases, the lower extremity muscles may be atrophied.

On examination these patients typically have diminished or absent femoral pulses, but because of the extensive collateral network in the pelvis this is not always the case. The Doppler examination is very helpful, as the femoral Doppler wave form will have a diminished amplitude and loss of the normal triphasic appearance. The typical patient with calf claudication will have a palpable or weak femoral pulse and a weak or absent popliteal, dorsalis pedis, and posterior tibial artery pulse. Patients with proximal arterial occlusive disease may continue to have palpable distal pulses.

Claudication is generally a benign condition. Most patients do not proceed to tissue loss or require surgery. A simple rule to remember is the rule of thirds: roughly a third of patients will show improvement, a third will be stable over time, and a third will have progression of their symptoms. The initial treatment should include controlling all risk factors, including tobacco use. Patients should follow a daily program of walking up to the point of pain, followed by brief rest. Most will note improvement after following these steps. If progress is limited, the examiner may consider prescribing pentoxifylline, which will produce some improvement in about half of the patients. It will generally take several weeks to start working. The patient should then be evaluated in 2 to 3 months for improvement in symptoms. If no significant improvement is noted, the drug should be discontinued.

*Claudication is generally a benign condition. Most patients do not proceed to tissue loss or require surgery.*

Patients to consider for referral to a vascular surgeon are those with severe symptoms who have significant limitations that affect lifestyle or employment or any young patient with these symptoms, who may have popliteal artery entrapment syndrome or cystic disease of the arterial wall. If it is unclear whether the symptoms are caused by arterial occlusive disease, an exercise lower extremity Doppler exam can be performed. Worsening of distal Doppler waveform or pressures following a 5- to 10-minute walk on a treadmill at 10° of elevation is consistent with symptoms due to arterial occlusive disease.

The symptoms of *neurogenic claudication* mimic ischemic symptoms. Symptoms are caused by venous congestion and spinal cord or nerve root compression. Pain in the involved extremity may or may not be radiating. Pain symptoms are reproducible by standing or ambulating a short distance, and usually the patient must sit or recline to relieve the symptoms. Claudication due to arterial disease, on the other hand, is relieved by simply standing at rest (Table 19–1).

Rest pain suggests more serious occlusive disease and is usually intolerable. Typically patients describe rest pain as a constant ache or burning in the toes, the base of the toes, or the foot, which may be relieved by placing the foot in a dependent position. Patients may describe the need to hang their foot over the edge of the bed at night or

TABLE 19–1

| A Comparison of Vascular and Neurogenic Claudication | | |
|---|---|---|
| Disorder | Pain | Relief |
| Vascular Claudication | Requires muscular work | Any rest, including standing |
| Neurogenic Claudication | May be induced by standing | Requires sitting or lying down |
| | May radiate | |

to get up and walk to relieve the pain. Although these are classic descriptions, many patients with rest pain have an atypical presentation not relieved by dependency. In addition, persons with diabetes and peripheral neuropathy may have severe occlusive disease without significant pain. Peripheral neuropathy in alcoholic or diabetic patients can also produce a burning sensation, frequently on the plantar surface of the foot. Other history and objective findings on exam or on Doppler analysis must be used to determine the need for surgical intervention. Patients with neuropathy and abnormal pressures on Doppler examination should be referred for evaluation of the need for vascular reconstruction.

Patients may present with an ulcer that does not heal or gangrene, usually involving the toes. Ulcers may develop following nail care or a superficial injury and can also appear over pressure points or on the heel. Owing to the severity of arterial occlusive disease, these ulcers will not heal without surgical intervention. Patients with significant gangrene involving a toe or portions of the foot will require some form of amputation. If significant proximal arterial disease is present, surgical intervention (bypass grafting) may be required to improve inflow to allow the amputation wound to heal. Those with sepsis and severe foot infection may require an initial emergent open amputation to control the sepsis, followed by a staged formal amputation. It is recommended that any patient with tissue loss and arterial occlusive disease be referred for a vascular surgical consultation. Patients with significant neuropathy symptoms may have strong pedal pulses and excellent blood supply but develop pressure ulcers, usually on the plantar surface of the foot over the metatarsal heads. If a good blood supply is present, these will only require an evaluation for infection and an appropriate protective shoe.

## *Arterial Occlusive Disease (Acute)*

The patient who presents with a complaint of sudden onset of unrelenting pain in an extremity may have an acute arterial occlusion. This may be due to thrombosis or embolus. Patients may have risk factors for embolism, such as atrial fibrillation, and left ventricular or aortic aneurysms. Other patients may have risk factors for thrombosis such as a history of long-standing peripheral vascular disease due to atherosclerosis. These patients will have a cool, numb extremity without palpable pulses at or below the femoral artery. Cases of acute arterial occlusion are often associated with the six Ps: pain, pallor, paresthesias, paralysis (weakness), poikilothermy, and pulselessness. These cases require emergency referral for surgical evaluation. Embolization or thrombosis related to aortic, femoral, or popliteal artery aneurysms may produce gangrene in one or more toes, and this finding should prompt an arteriogram or an ultrasound evaluation of proximal arteries.

*Cases of acute arterial occlusion are often associated with the six Ps: pain, pallor, paresthesias, paralysis (weakness), poikilothermy, and pulselessness.*

Anticoagulation with IV heparin is generally instituted in cases of acute arterial occlusion regardless of the cause. This helps to maintain any available collateral blood flow. If the vascular surgeon suspects arterial embolism, an embolectomy is performed in the operating room. If acute thrombosis is suspected, the patient may be treated with thrombolytic therapy via the angiogram catheter. Clinical improvement with this therapy may allow elective bypass surgery for high-grade stenotic lesions.

## Popliteal Aneurysms

About one-third of patients with popliteal artery aneurysms are symptomatic. They may have pain from nerve compression or venous compressive symptoms. More frequently, they present with symptoms related to thrombosis, which include claudication, rest pain, gangrene, or acute, limb-threatening ischemia. Most of these aneurysms are found when the patient is asymptomatic. Elective repair of these aneurysms should be considered before symptoms develop. Surgical treatment of popliteal aneurysms is much more successful in asymptomatic patients than in symptomatic ones. About 45% of these aneurysms are bilateral, and they frequently have associated femoral or aortic aneurysms. Ultrasound of the aorta and the femoral and popliteal arteries is indicated when a popliteal or femoral aneurysm is discovered. Conversely, the incidence of popliteal or femoral artery aneurysm in a patient with an aortic aneurysm is low, and no screening study is indicated unless directed by findings on the physical exam.

## Compartment Syndrome

Patients who suffer lower extremity ischemia or trauma can develop increased leg compartment pressure resulting in *compartment syndrome* even if the event seems trivial, such as ischemia with strenuous exercise or lying on a limb for a prolonged period. Early diagnosis and a high index of suspicion are crucial to successful treatment. Compartment syndrome is a limb-threatening emergency! Initial symptoms are neurologic because nerves are most sensitive to ischemia. These include pain and tenderness of the muscle compartment, which may feel tense; pain on passive extension; decreased sensation; loss of two-point discrimination; and loss of vibratory sense. Loss of a palpable pulse distally is a very late finding, so its absence should not be used to exclude this diagnosis. Measurements of compartment pressures may be helpful if the diagnosis is questionable or the patient is unable to communicate. These measurements should not delay emergent referral and are best performed by those who will be performing the fasciotomy. Early fasciotomy may prevent permanent deficits or even limb loss.

*Compartment syndrome is a limb-threatening emergency!*

### When to Call the Surgeon about Arterial Disease

- Severe limiting claudication
- Rest pain
- Wounds or ulcers not healing
- Gangrene
- Surveillance following bypass
- Popliteal artery aneurysm
- Acute arterial occlusion
- Compartment syndrome

## Venous Disorders

*Deep venous thrombosis (DVT)* frequently presents with unilateral calf and ankle edema. Homan's sign (calf pain upon dorsiflexion of the foot) is unreliable for diagnosis. Patients may complain of leg pain or tightness in the calf. Risk factors include stasis (i.e., during long car or airplane rides), obesity, pregnancy, history of DVT, and malignancy. The diagnosis is confirmed with venous duplex studies or venography. First-line treatment is anticoagulation with IV heparin or low molecular weight heparin. Some patients with deep venous thrombosis require surgical intervention. Placement of a vena cava filter should be considered for any patient with a DVT who cannot be treated with heparin and warfarin (Coumadin) owing to a contraindication or complication of anticoagulation or who experiences progression of venous thrombosis or develops a pulmonary embolus (PE) while receiving adequate anticoagulation. Prophylactic filters are frequently placed in patients who are at high risk of PE, such as trauma patients facing prolonged immobilization.

Patients with iliofemoral venous thrombosis with severe venous hypertension can develop ischemic changes and require venous thrombectomy. Current randomized trials are studying thrombolytic therapy for DVT in an attempt to maintain valve function and reduce the risk of venous claudication and ulcer formation. Patients with isolated iliac or common femoral vein thrombosis or both are the best candidates for thrombolytic therapy and should be referred immediately because most protocols require the therapy to begin less than 2 to 4 weeks after onset. Long-term follow-up of these studies is not complete, but advocates believe this therapy may prevent the postphlebitic syndrome. These studies have also demonstrated a 5% to 10% rate of bleeding complications, which must be discussed with the patient and weighed against the possible benefit.

Repeated episodes of DVT can damage venous valves and render them incompetent. This results in chronic venous insufficiency. Patients with nonhealing venous stasis ulcers or symptomatic venous insufficiency should be considered for surgical referral. Symptoms from varicose veins include a dull ache (which usually develops over the course of the day), bleeding, and ankle ulceration. Pain or discomfort due to venous insufficiency may be relieved with leg elevation. Although most venous stasis ulcers are due to deep venous insufficiency, some patients with these ulcers have incompetent valves in the saphenous vein or incompetent perforating veins. Ligation of the saphenofemoral junction or saphenopopliteal junction, vein stripping, or ligation of perforating veins will usually allow the ulcer to heal and will relieve symptoms. The cause of venous insufficiency can best be determined by duplex examination, specifically looking for insufficiency in the saphenofemoral system, saphenopopliteal system, perforating veins, or deep venous system. Patients with chronic venous insufficiency deal with their problem daily. Successful treatment of venous insufficiency often requires elevation of the legs above the chest at night, appropriate use of compression stockings on rising in the morning, liberal use of skin moisturizer, and meticulous skin care. Methodical personal attention toward these general measures may prevent skin breakdown. Malleolar ulcers are not uncommon, and once established they have difficulty healing. An Unna's paste boot changed two to four times a week often results in healing of ulcers over several months. Ulcers developing secondary infections with surrounding cellulitis require antibiotic therapy.

Patients with cosmetic complaints of telangiectasias or "spider veins" are frequently treated with sclerotherapy. Because a wide range of specialists are performing sclerotherapy, the results vary. These patients should be referred to a clinician with demonstrated interest and knowledge in the treatment of venous disease.

*Successful treatment of venous insufficiency often requires elevation of the legs at night, use of compression stockings, use of skin moisturizer, and meticulous skin care.*

### When to Call the Surgeon about Venous Disease

- Symptomatic varicose veins
- Nonhealing venous stasis ulcers
- DVT with
    —Complication or contraindication to anticoagulation
    —Failure of anticoagulation
    —High risk for pulmonary emboli
    —Recurrent pulmonary emboli

## RECOMMENDED READING

Kozol, RA, et al: Dependent rubor as a predictor of limb risk in patients with claudication. Archives of Surgery 119:932–935, 1984.

Moore, WS (ed): Vascular Surgery, A Comprehensive Review. WB Saunders, Philadelphia, 1993.

Semba, CP, and Dake, MD: Catheter-Directed Thrombolysis for Iliofemoral Venous Thrombosis. Seminars in Vascular Surgery. 9:26–33, 1996.

Strandness, ED, and Van Breda, A (eds): Vascular Diseases, Surgical and Interventional Therapy. Churchill Livingstone, New York, 1994.

# Chapter 20

# Hip and Knee Pain

SAM NASSER, MD, PhD

The proper diagnosis and treatment of musculoskeletal conditions is vitally important to the primary care provider. Over half of all emergency room visits are related to musculoskeletal complaints. Hip and knee problems are particularly common in young, active patients, making knee arthroscopy the most common surgical procedure performed in North America over the last 5 years. Because musculoskeletal injuries among sports figures are highly publicized, the general public is widely aware of the nature of common knee injuries. Arthritis and other degenerative conditions of the joints are particularly common in older patients. Consequently, total knee arthroplasty has become the most frequent major surgical procedure in the United States, followed closely by total hip replacement surgery.

One may ask why the hip and knee are considered together. These joints are linked not only anatomically, being at the proximal and distal ends of the femur, but also mechanically and functionally. For example, the same nerves supply both joints, making referred pain of hip pathology to the knee a frequent finding. As the largest joints in the body, with extreme muscle forces across them, each is subjected to many times a person's body weight with even simple activity. It is now understood that even subtle alterations in knee rotation may ultimately result in hip pathology.

Because of the complexity of these joints, problems with the hip and knee may pose diagnostic dilemmas for the primary care provider. The history is often complicated, with multiple, difficult-to-isolate symptoms. Hip pain may mean different things to different patients. The patient may grasp the fleshy area over the iliac wing or point to the lower midline when describing ''hip'' pain. Furthermore, with referred pain, the symptoms may not localize the condition. Often the patient with a hip or knee injury is difficult to examine, especially after acute trauma, and underlying conditions such as degenerative disk disease or vascular insufficiency may mask hip and knee problems.

An additional factor making diagnosis difficult for the primary care provider is the difficulty in imaging both the hip and knee. Plain film radiographs have the advantage of being rapid and inexpensive. They are often available in a primary care office. However, many practitioners find details of the musculoskeletal system difficult to interpret, particularly in children. In addition, although plain films are adequate for bony details, they do not adequately image soft tissues. Computed tomography (CT) shows bony detail but at considerable added expense. Furthermore, CT is limited in its availability and often requires expert interpretation. Magnetic resonance imaging (MRI) has the advantage of showing soft tissue detail but also at significant added expense and limited availability. MRI requires specialist interpretation and poses particular difficulty in assessing bony details in the hip and knee.

Problems involving the hip and knee can usually be divided into four categories: traumatic injuries, degenerative conditions, inflammatory disorders (infectious and noninfectious), and neoplasms.

## Trauma

Hip and knee trauma presents in many ways, from the simplest soft-tissue contusion to the most severe fracture. *Fractures* are defined as any breech in the cortical envelope of a bone. Midshaft femoral fractures are, fortunately, relatively rare. In reality, fractures involving the proximal and distal epiphyseal and metaphyseal regions of the bone—that is, the hip and knee—are much more common. In orthopedic terminology, a *sprain* is a disruption of one or more of the ligaments surrounding a joint. Such injuries are particularly common at the knee. When the ligamentous injury is severe enough, a partial loss of joint integrity may occur. This is known as a *subluxation*. If the injury is so severe that complete loss of joint integrity results, the condition is referred to as a *dislocation*. Dislocation implies disruption of the ligamentous envelope surrounding a joint.

### FRACTURES

Fractures involving the hip and knee are among those most commonly treated in any large emergency department. The history will often suggest the nature of the injury. For example, after a fall, pain along the anterior groin and anterior thigh usually points to a femoral neck fracture in the elderly patient. An unrestrained passenger in a high-speed motor vehicle accident may sustain an acetabular fracture, whereas a pedestrian hit by an automobile may suffer injury about the knee. All such injuries should be sought in the unconscious or confused patient.

#### Hip Fractures

Hip fractures are most common in the elderly population. The most frequent type of hip fracture is the intracapsular or femoral neck fracture (Fig. 20–1). Such injuries are usually associated with osteoporosis. Physical examination will show pain in the groin and thigh with range of motion, and may also demonstrate the characteristic deformity associated with hip fractures: shortening, abduction, and external rotation of the hip. Plain film radiographs are usually adequate for diagnosis. Numerous grading systems and classification schemes have been developed to describe femoral neck fractures, but in most cases it is easiest to distinguish them on the basis of displacement—that is, displaced versus nondisplaced. An orthopedic consultation should be obtained when the fracture is diagnosed. Surgery is contingent on appropriate medical clearance. Frequently patients with hip fractures are discovered hours, if not days, after the injury, when their families finally notice their absence. As a result, these patients are often dehydrated and have not taken their medications for some time. The treatment of the fracture must, therefore, follow appropriate medical management. The use of pre-operative traction is somewhat controversial. In general, most surgeons feel that if

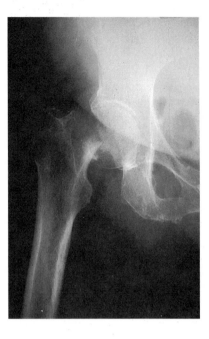

**FIGURE 20–1**
An anteroposterior radiograph of a typical intracapsular hip fracture. Osteoporosis is a common associated problem in patients with such fractures.

*If preoperative traction provides pain relief it should be continued; otherwise it is unnecessary.*

preoperative traction provides pain relief it should be continued; otherwise it is unnecessary.

The second major type of hip fracture is that of the intertrochanteric region (Fig. 20–2). These injuries are more often associated with arthritic conditions than with osteoporosis. Unlike the fracture of the femoral neck, this injury is generated by a fall and is associated with significant bleeding. Because this injury is not contained by the hip capsule, the volume of hemorrhage may dictate transfusion.

A third and much less common type of hip fracture is the subtrochanteric fracture, which is usually seen in patients slightly younger than those sustaining the previously mentioned fractures (Fig. 20–3). These patients are usually healthier and able to undergo surgery much earlier. However, because these injuries are more often associated with more severe trauma, a thorough physical examination should always be undertaken to detect associated injuries. Acetabular fractures are also the result of high-energy or high-speed injuries. Motor vehicle accidents are the most frequent cause, but such injuries are also seen after falls from heights, industrial accidents, and even such unusual incidents as rollover accidents involving horses. The most important feature of acetabular injuries involves injuries to the surrounding soft tissues, particularly the

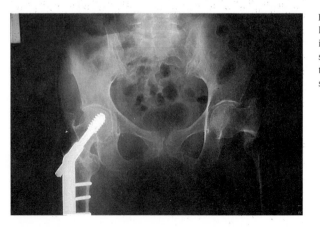

**FIGURE 20–2**
Intertrochanteric fractures generally involve more bleeding than intracapsular fractures. As with all hip fractures, the patient must be medically stabilized before surgery.

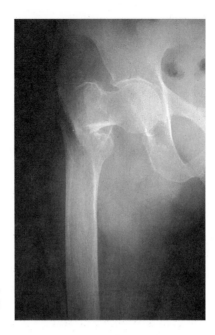

**FIGURE 20–3**
Patients sustaining subtrochanteric fractures are usually younger than patients with other types of hip fractures, and the injuries involve higher energy.

sciatic nerve, and even intrapelvic and visceral organs. Therefore, patients with acetabular fractures should be thoroughly examined for associated problems.

## Knee Fractures

The most common fracture associated with the knee is the tibial plateau fracture (Fig. 20–4). This type of injury is intra-articular and requires orthopedic reconstruction to avoid long-term problems such as post-traumatic arthrosis. Other fractures about the knee include supracondylar and intracondylar fractures of the femur and fractures of the patella. Fractures about the knee are generally nonemergent, but all require orthopedic evaluation and thorough examination for associated injuries such as damage to

**FIGURE 20–4**
A lateral radiograph of a comminuted fracture of the tibial plateau. Neurologic evaluation for possible peroneal nerve injury is essential.

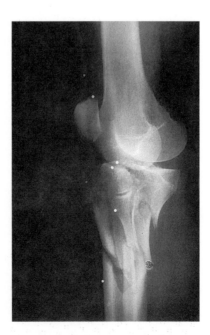

the popliteal artery. The documentation of the neurologic status should be detailed because tibial and peroneal nerve injuries are common with these fractures as they are with knee dislocations.

### "Occult" Fractures

"Occult" fractures involving the hip and knee are particularly difficult to diagnose. Patients sustaining these may be sent home from the emergency room having had "normal" x-rays, only to present in the primary care provider's office days or weeks later with continued pain. In the hip, these usually result from a nondisplaced or "incomplete" femoral neck fracture. They occur most often in elderly female patients with a history of aching pain in the groin and anterior thigh. The patient has mild discomfort with range of motion and pain when bearing weight. Radiographs taken at the time of the initial presentation are usually negative, but 3 to 4 weeks after the injury a small amount of bony callus is often visible along the medial side of the femoral neck. The definitive diagnostic test for this condition is a technetium bone scan. This can be done within a few days of the injury. A "hot" scan indicates a fracture, and an orthopedic consult is in order.

Occult tibial plateau fractures may present in a similar manner. Usually there is a history of force applied to the side of the knee, often after relatively minor trauma such as a slip and fall in an elderly patient or a motor vehicle "bumper" injury in a younger patient. Examination shows a painful, swollen knee but radiographs may be read as normal. Diagnosis should be based on the examination of the fluid aspirated from the knee. A bloody aspirate always implies tissue damage, which may have any number of causes. However, if fat globules appear in a joint aspirate, or if a layer of fat appears on the surface of blood allowed to sit for a time, the diagnosis of fracture is confirmed. Orthopedic consultation is appropriate and surgery is usually indicated to prevent collapse of the fracture (Fig. 20–5).

### Open Fractures

Open fractures are always considered an orthopedic emergency. The classification system is based on the size of the opening and the amount of associated soft-tissue injury. A grade I injury has an associated wound of less than 1 cm in size. This is often the

> *If fat globules appear in a joint aspirate or if a layer of fat appears on the surface of blood allowed to sit for a time, the diagnosis of fracture is confirmed.*

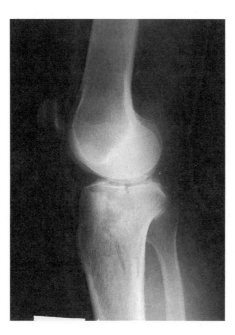

**FIGURE 20–5**
A minimally displaced tibial plateau fracture may be missed on initial radiographic evaluation. Marrow fat in the blood aspirated from the knee is a sure sign of an occult fracture.

result of an "in-and-out" or "poke-hole" type of wound, in which the jagged bone end penetrates the skin and then retracts back into the soft tissues. Emergency room treatment of this type of fracture may be appropriate in the upper limb or even in the ankle, but it is usually not appropriate for the hip or knee due to the amount of associated soft-tissue damage required to penetrate through the envelope around both of these major joints. Almost all "grade I" fractures actually involve much more soft-tissue damage than initially suspected.

In a grade II injury, the wound is 1 to 10 cm in length, with an associated increase in the amount of soft-tissue damage. These injuries always should be evaluated by the orthopedic surgeon on call and generally require hospital admission with operative debridement and intravenous antibiotics. In addition, fixation is usually necessary to stabilize the bones and prevent further injury.

Grade III injuries involve major soft-tissue damage or contamination. These wounds are usually more than 10 cm in size and may also involve arterial or neurologic injuries. As with grade II open fractures, these require hospital admission, operative debridement, fracture fixation, and intravenous antibiotics.

When evaluating open fractures, a safe rule is to overreact. It is much preferable to treat a grade I fracture as a grade II than to assume that a small "poke hole" is the full extent of the soft-tissue injury involved. About the hip and knee, these types of injuries often involve lacerations of the patellar or quadriceps tendon, major vascular or neurologic injury, or penetration of the open fracture into the joint. All of these are appropriate for emergency orthopedic consultation.

*Almost all "grade I" fractures actually involve much more soft tissue damage than suspected.*

*When evaluating open fractures, a safe rule is to overreact.*

## DISLOCATIONS

Dislocations of the hip and knee are both considered orthopedic emergencies and require immediate surgical evaluation (Fig. 20–6). Hip dislocation is usually the result of a very high-energy injury and, as with acetabular fracture, is often associated with internal abdominal injuries, thoracic injuries, and injuries to the soft tissues about the hip. Laceration of major vessels or nerves of the lower limb are not uncommon. Emergency orthopedic consultation should be made as soon as such an injury is suspected. If the surgeon is not immediately available, reduction of the dislocation should be undertaken as soon as neurologic status is documented and the injury confirmed on radiographs. This is vitally important because a hip left dislocated for more than a few hours has a rate of avascular necrosis approaching 100%. Furthermore, a dislocated hip may apply pressure on the sciatic nerve or the blood vessels about the hip, resulting in severe injury or even paralysis if allowed to persist. The treatment should therefore not be delayed for the orthopedic evaluation. The hip should be reduced under sedation by applying traction to the femur, then bringing the hip into flexion and adduction with

*Dislocations of the hip and knee are considered orthopedic emergencies.*

**FIGURE 20–6**
The anteroposterior pelvis film dramatically shows an inferior dislocation of the hip. This is an orthopedic emergency and must be reduced as soon as possible following neurovascular assessment.

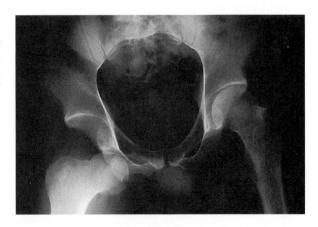

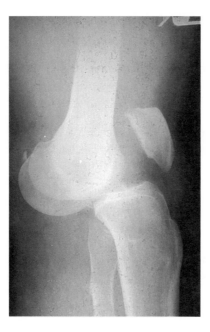

**FIGURE 20–7**
An anterior dislocation of the knee. As with hip dislocations, these injuries are orthopedic emergencies and must be reduced as soon as possible following neurovascular assessment. Because of a high incidence of popliteal artery injury after knee dislocations, an arteriogram is usually indicated.

*Dislocation of the knee is also a surgical emergency, but timing may require treatment prior to arrival of the specialist.*

the pelvis stabilized. Successful reduction is usually accompanied by an audible "pop" as the hip slips back into place. This is usually followed by substantial pain relief. With associated fractures of the acetabulum, it may be necessary to place the affected limb in skeletal traction in order to maintain reduction of the hip. Postoperative radiographs should be obtained as soon as possible to confirm the reduction and to identify associated fractures.

Dislocation of the knee is also a surgical emergency (Fig. 20–7). The dislocation should be reduced as soon as possible to prevent further damage to the popliteal artery and injury to the tibial and peroneal nerves. Because the blood supply to the lower limb across the knee is tenuous, the potential for loss of the limb is very high if knee dislocation is not appropriately treated. After emergency reduction, the knee should be splinted, and an arteriogram is usually indicated. An emergency consultation is indicated, but timing may require treatment prior to arrival of the specialist.

Patellar dislocations, unlike dislocations of the hip joint or the tibiofemoral joint of the knee, are not limb threatening and are infrequently associated with substantial soft-tissue injury. These dislocations are relatively rare in adults and may be associated with a previous injury to the knee. Reduction of the dislocation is performed with direct manipulation, after sedation, followed by immobilization. Once this is done, pain relief is dramatic and the patella is usually stable. An emergency orthopedic consult is not necessary, but it is advisable that the patient be seen by an orthopedic surgeon within a week or so because the dislocation invariably ruptures the capsule of the knee and this may require surgical repair. Furthermore, the patellofemoral joint is particularly vulnerable to osteochondral fractures and may require arthroscopic debridement.

## SPRAINS AND OTHER LIGAMENTOUS INJURIES

Sprains are uncommon about the hip but are very common about the knee. Five different structures give stability to the knee: the anterior and posterior cruciate ligaments, the medial and lateral collateral ligaments, and the quadriceps mechanism made up of the quadriceps muscles and tendon, the patella, and the patellar tendon. All are vulnerable to injury and in fact may be more prone to damage because of the great strength of the muscles that cross the knee. The pull of the quadriceps, hamstring, and gastrocnemius muscles may actually aggravate the sprain and increase the amount of damage that is sustained during the injury.

The anterior cruciate ligament (ACL) is commonly ruptured in athletes participating in professional and college sports. This type of injury is relatively well known to the general public and is often overdiagnosed. The usual mechanism of injury is a twisting fall or a fall involving a fixed ankle. Because of the type of ski boots that are commonly used today, this type of injury is common in downhill skiing. Diagnosis of ACL rupture can be difficult in the acute phase because of the pain that follows most knee injuries and the reflex overpull of the muscles across the knee. Physical findings include swelling and hemarthrosis with positive anterior drawer and pivot shift tests. If suspected, evaluation under anesthesia may be necessary to provide a definitive diagnosis. Once the acute phase of the injury has passed, physical examination is much more reliable, with positive Lachman's and anterior drawer tests providing more definitive information. Unfortunately radiographic evaluation is unreliable. Plain films are usually negative, although this injury may be associated with other injuries about the knee that do show certain types of avulsion fractures. However, isolated ACL rupture has no plain radiographic features other than a distended joint capsule. CT is also unreliable. MRI examination is frequently ordered to diagnose this problem, but it too is not reliable. Often minor problems with the ligaments will be misinterpreted as ruptures when in fact the ligament is relatively normal. MRI evaluation should, therefore, be left up to the treating surgeon rather than be ordered as a screening test.

Treatment of ACL rupture is somewhat controversial. Twenty-five years ago there was no satisfactory method of surgical augmentation or repair of the ligament. Numerous operations were developed to try to reduce the instability that followed ACL rupture, but none was entirely successful. With the introduction of more aggressive surgical treatment, including the successful replacement of the ruptured tendon, orthopedic surgeons became convinced that early, aggressive treatment of the injury was necessary. It is now known, however, that this type of treatment is both unnecessary and unwise. Current treatment recommendations for suspected ACL injury include immobilization for comfort and an orthopedic consult for the patient within 2 to 3 weeks after the injury, once the acute phase has started to resolve and the physical examination is much easier and more reliable. The amount of guarding is much decreased and the hemarthrosis is less tense, allowing better evaluation of the joint. Diagnosis of an ACL rupture should be made on the basis of physical examination. Additional radiographic imaging should be used primarily to identify additional soft-tissue injuries, not the ACL tear itself.

The need for surgical treatment of the injury depends on the patient's age and activity level. Patients who have already developed signs of degenerative arthritis are not usually candidates for surgical reconstruction. Often patients do well with simple rehabilitation and physical therapy rather than operative intervention.

Posterior cruciate ligament (PCL) ruptures are much more difficult to treat than ACL tears. The usual mechanism of injury is a blow to a fixed knee such as would be sustained in a sporting competition or a twisting fall. Again, as with ACL injuries, diagnosis may be difficult in the acute phase because of pain and reflex overpull of the muscles. Physical findings usually show hemarthrosis and swelling, with a positive posterior drawer test. Plain films are again usually negative. MRI is more reliable with PCL injuries than with ACLs, but is not usually indicated in the acute phase. The treatment plan again is immobilization and an orthopedic consult within 2 to 3 weeks after the injury.

Unfortunately, the track record of surgical treatment of PCL ruptures is worse than for ACL injuries. Even the best series report only 50% improvement over the preoperative condition—in other words, a 50% failure rate.

Collateral ligament injuries are graded by the extent of the damage to the ligament. A type I injury consists of a "stretch" without tearing of the ligament. Type II injuries are a partial tear with some portion of the ligament still intact, and type III injuries involve a complete tear or an avulsion of the ligament from its bony anchor. Collateral ligament sprains may or may not be associated with meniscal injuries.

Examination demonstrates swelling and hemarthrosis with tenderness directly over the area of the ligamentous injury. Force at the ankle with the knee fixed results in pain at the site of injury and may cause the knee to "gap open" if the injury is severe. Radiographs may be positive for an avulsion fracture but are often negative. As with ACL injuries, an MRI is often unreliable and generally not indicated unless associated soft-tissue injuries are suspected.

Treatment of collateral ligament injuries consists of immobilization, with bracing of types I and II. Orthopedic consultation should be made if any problems persist after the first few weeks. Type III collateral ligament injuries usually require more urgent orthopedic consultation because operative treatment may be necessary. This is especially true if a portion of the ligament has avulsed a fragment of bone. Operative treatment may be desirable to reanchor the bone and ligament. Without appropriate treatment of type III collateral ligament injuries, chronic instability may be a long-term result.

Ruptures of the quadriceps tendon are usually due to hyperextension of the knee during a fall. The reflex action of the quadriceps literally pulls the tendon apart. This is a typical "stepping off the curb" type injury and is often seen in individuals who have tried to stop a fall down a flight of stairs. This type of rupture may be associated with diabetes and is not uncommonly seen in patients undergoing hemodialysis for chronic kidney disease. In these patients, bilateral quadriceps ruptures are not uncommon. Diagnosis is based on a high index of suspicion. Pain superior to the patella following a hyperextension injury should call attention to the problem. Pain and swelling over the area is seen on examination, and usually a palpable defect can be identified. If the rupture is complete, an extensor lag will be seen (the patient will be unable to fully extend the knee against gravity). Radiographs are usually negative but may show a large soft-tissue deficit in some cases. *Patella baja*, an unusually low-riding patella, may be identified on radiographs if the rupture is complete and there is no force holding the patella in place. Another finding may be a small rim of avulsed patella on the edge of the quadriceps tendon. Treatment should consist of immobilization followed by early orthopedic consult. Surgical repair should be undertaken early to prevent retraction of the muscles for ease of repair if the patient's medical condition allows. Immobilization followed by physical therapy may be sufficient for minor tears.

Most patellar fractures require surgical treatment. As with quadriceps rupture, an early orthopedic consult should be obtained and appropriate medical management instituted to prepare the patient for surgery. On rare occasions, excision of the patella may be necessary to treat very comminuted fractures. However, because of the morbidity that usually accompanies patellectomy, it should be avoided if at all possible.

Patellar tendon ruptures usually follow the same hyperextension type injury as quadriceps tendon ruptures, although they may also follow forced flexion of the knee. The physical findings usually include a palpable patellar defect and extensor lag. These injuries are often missed and an entire field of orthopedic surgery involves the late repair of missed patellar tendon injuries. Again, a high index of suspicion should accompany examination of the knee. Radiographs usually show a *patella alta*—an abnormally high patella that does not move appropriately with flexion of the knee. A soft-tissue defect is often visible on radiograph. Treatment should consist of early surgical repair. Late repair of the patellar tendon may be successful but is never as satisfactory as early treatment.

## OTHER SOFT-TISSUE INJURIES

### Meniscal Tears of the Knee

Meniscal tears are among the most frequently encountered injuries to the knee. Usually classified by location of the tear in the meniscal body, they can be radial, longitudinal, horizontal, or in the anterior and posterior horns. Longitudinal tears need orthopedic treatment most often because they may displace, resulting in a "bucket handle" tear.

The mechanism of injury of meniscal tears is quite variable. They can occur with twisting injuries to the knee and in this respect are often associated with ACL injuries. They may result from lateral force with the knee fixed; this type of meniscal injury is often associated with medial collateral ligament sprains. Most common are "degenerative" injuries, which occur with minimal trauma and are often difficult to identify.

Symptoms of meniscal tears include nagging toothache-type pain, particularly at or near the joint line. There is usually pain with range of motion, particularly when going up and down stairs. The classic symptom of "locking" is actually quite rare in meniscal injuries and is indicative of a displaced bucket-handle type of tear. Physical findings include joint line tenderness and a positive MacMurray's test, which places pressure on the meniscus. Meniscal injuries may also become painful with varus and valgus force on a fixed knee, which may stretch the collateral ligament and pull the meniscus through its attachment to the ligament.

*The classic symptom of "locking" is actually quite rare in meniscal injuries.*

Radiographic examination is unreliable in the diagnosis of meniscal injuries. Arthrography accurately diagnoses the problem but is difficult to interpret and is rarely done in this age of noninvasive testing. Unfortunately the noninvasive substitute, MRI, results in many false positives. A high index of suspicion followed by an adequate physical examination is usually all that is required, and if the patient does not experience locking, treatment is usually uncomplicated.

Operative treatment for meniscal tears is infrequently necessary. Total meniscectomy is rare today. Most meniscal tears are peripheral and will heal given enough time. The healing time depends primarily on the available blood supply. Very peripheral tears in the vascularized portion of the meniscus may heal in a few weeks, whereas those on the edge of the vascularized zone of the meniscus may take up to 6 months. Symptoms usually resolve gradually, and often the patient cannot remember when the symptoms stopped. An emergency orthopedic consult is necessary only if the knee is locked. Otherwise the patient may be followed for at least a month or two by the primary care provider. If improvement does not occur, orthopedic consultation is appropriate.

*Most meniscal tears are peripheral and will heal given enough time.*

## Acetabular Labral Tears of the Hip

An acetabular labral tear of the hip is a relatively uncommon injury. The largest series described consisted of only 50 patients. Nevertheless, it is becoming more widely understood. It is roughly analogous to a meniscal tear in the knee. Sometimes there is a history of a twisting injury, but in other patients repeated subacute injury may be involved, particularly in young women who are dancers or athletes. It is difficult to diagnose because of the rather enigmatic nature of the pain, which often presents only at the extremes of motion, especially in the flexed, abducted, and externally rotated position. Physical examination is often unreliable and may be quite confusing if other findings cloud the diagnosis. Radiographic examination is usually negative, although a small avulsion fragment on the acetabular rim may be identified. Arthrogram or CT arthrogram is diagnostic. The injection of a small amount of local anesthetic aids in diagnosis; it should completely relieve the symptoms of the acetabular labral tear. If it does not, the diagnosis is highly suspect. A small amount of corticosteroid injected with the local anesthetic may be helpful in reducing synovial irritation and in healing. An MRI scan is unreliable, is confusing, and should not be obtained.

Treatment for acetabular labral tears is somewhat controversial. Approximately half of the patients respond to strict nonweightbearing with crutches for 8 weeks and do not have symptoms again. If no improvement is seen after 8 weeks on crutches, an orthopedic consult should be obtained because surgical debridement of the joint may be necessary.

## Patellar Tendinitis

Post-traumatic patellar tendinitis is a rather frustrating condition to diagnose and treat. It is usually seen as a "dashboard injury" sustained in an automobile accident. Often the amount of trauma is unrelated to the magnitude of symptoms. The diagnosis is primarily one of exclusion. Only after other possibilities such as fracture, sprain, or occult meniscal tear have been eliminated should a diagnosis of patellar tendinitis be made.

Most of these injuries are very slow to recover and it may take months to see an improvement in symptoms. Oral corticosteroids and corticosteroid injections should be avoided because neither is effective and both may be associated with significant morbidity. Nonsteroidal anti-inflammatories and symptomatic treatment with either heat or ice is the preferred treatment.

## Degenerative Conditions

### OSTEOARTHROSIS

Osteoarthrosis is the most common degenerative condition affecting the hip and knee. This disease affects most people over the age of 50 and is nearly universal by the eighth decade. The general public recognizes such terms as "wear and tear arthritis" far better than the medical terminology.

In the hip, osteoarthrosis usually follows some other type of pathological condition. Some studies have shown that a detailed history will reveal some type of pathologic condition during childhood in well over 70% of the patients developing osteoarthrosis of the hip. These include developmental (congenital) dysplasia, Legg-Calvé-Perthes disease, or slipped femoral capital epiphysis of the hip (Fig. 20–8). This illustrates the need for timely diagnosis and treatment of these childhood conditions. Osteoarthrosis may also result from old trauma to the hip or knee, in which case it is termed *post-traumatic arthrosis*. Fortunately, with improved methods of diagnosis and treatment of fractures about the hip and knee, especially intra-articular fractures, this condition should decrease somewhat in frequency.

Early symptoms of osteoarthrosis include joint stiffness, pain when beginning an activity with gradual improvement as the activity progresses, and pain relieved by aspirin or other nonsteroidal anti-inflammatory drugs (NSAIDs). As the condition progresses, there is loss of range of motion, crepitus, pain with weightbearing and pain with activity. In the hip this may be very difficult to differentiate from claudication caused by vascular insufficiency and may also be difficult to differentiate from the symptoms of spinal stenosis. In the advanced stages of the disease the pain is worse as activity increases and eventually becomes refractory to NSAIDs, so that narcotics are required for pain control.

Physical findings show progressive loss of range of motion. In the hip, flexion and extension are often preserved, but internal and external rotation are lost early and abduction contractures are common. Loss of full flexion of the knee (i.e., flexion >100°)

- ▬

*A detailed history will reveal some type of pathologic condition during childhood in well over 70% of the patients developing osteoarthrosis of the hip.*

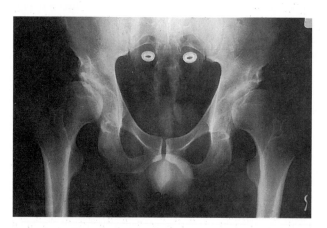

**FIGURE 20–8**
The late sequelae of bilateral developmental (congenital) dysplasia of the hip are evident in this anteroposterior pelvic radiograph. Shallow acetabulae with uncovered femoral heads have resulted in early degenerative changes including loss of joint space and large osteophytes.

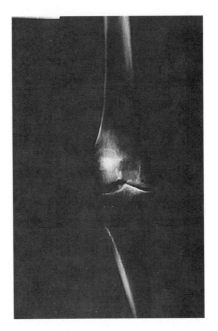

**FIGURE 20-9**
Early degenerative changes of the knee often include isolated loss of medial joint space, as shown here. Early referral to an orthopedic surgeon ensures that all surgical options can be considered.

is the most common finding; flexion contractures of the knee appear later. Crepitus about the hip and knee, especially of the patellofemoral joint, is a common physical finding.

Radiographic evaluation should be performed early on patients in whom osteoarthrosis is suspected. Plain film radiographs are diagnostic. Early changes include asymmetric joint space thinning. This is characteristically seen in the acetabular dome of the hip and the medial compartment of the knee. Small osteophytes, bone spurs, are also seen early in the course of the disease (Fig. 20-9). Late radiographic changes include loss of the joint space, which is circumferential in the hip and tricompartmental in the knee. Large osteophytes, subchondral sclerosis, and often subchondral cysts can be seen in the bone (Fig. 20-10).

**FIGURE 20-10**
Once the process of osteoarthritis becomes this advanced, with complete loss of joint space and large subchondral cysts, a total arthroplasty (a "total hip") becomes inevitable.

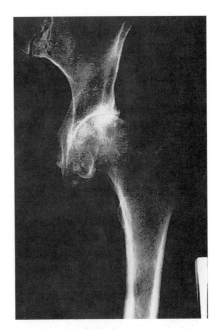

Radionucleotide studies such as [99]technetium scans are unnecessary and may, in fact, cloud the clinical picture. MRI is not diagnostic because it cannot visualize the joint space effectively, nor can it evaluate cortical bone changes well. CT is not useful in most cases, although it may be informative if post-traumatic arthritis is suspected.

Early treatment of degenerative arthrosis includes weight loss, activity modifications, and the use of NSAIDs. In some cases of arthrosis of the knee, bracing to unload a portion of the joint may be effective in relieving pain. Early orthopedic evaluation should be considered when patients present with symptoms of osteoarthrosis. Optimally the evaluation should be made before range of motion is lost, before contractures develop, before muscle weakness ensues, and before there is total loss of joint space on radiographs, thus allowing the full surgical armamentarium to be considered. Surgical treatment options in the early stages of osteoarthrosis of the hip and knee include observation, debridement, osteotomy, arthrodesis, or even joint replacement. When the patient with hip and knee arthrosis is referred to the surgeon late in the course of the disease, the surgical options are usually limited to arthrodesis in the young patient or joint replacement in the more elderly, sedentary patient. Many of the late complications of osteoarthrosis, including joint contracture, limb malalignment and other deformities, and loss of muscle strength about the joint, make surgery and postoperative rehabilitation more complicated and the surgical outcome less predictable.

## AVASCULAR NECROSIS

Other degenerative conditions include *avascular necrosis*, also known as osteonecrosis or aseptic necrosis. This condition follows loss of blood supply to cancellous bone. For reasons still not completely clear, this condition is particularly common at both ends of the femur and more common in the hip. The varied causes of avascular necrosis are so diverse that they include trauma (fracture of the femoral neck is typical) and nitrogen narcosis (the bends). Other pathologic conditions include Gaucher's disease, sickle-cell anemia, and other red blood cell abnormalities.

In general practice, the most common causes of avascular necrosis are the use of oral steroid medications and ethanol abuse. The physiologic link between the use of these chemicals and the development of avascular necrosis is unclear, but it appears to be related to alterations in fat metabolism. The common pathway may be clogging of the venous return from the bone, caused by release of fat from the marrow space. This link remains unproven, however, and at least one-third of all cases are never clearly related to any causative factor.

Symptoms and physical findings of avascular necrosis are similar to early osteoarthrosis, but the pain is much more severe. Radiographic analysis should start with plain film radiographs, even though these are generally negative until fairly late in the disease process. Their purpose is to rule out other conditions. The most sensitive and reliable imaging modality for osteonecrosis is MRI. MRI is indicated in the patient with severe hip or knee pain with normal radiographs, particularly if one of the previously described causative factors is present. Both hips or both knees should be viewed simultaneously, not only to provide a comparison, but also to identify preclinical lesions in the asymptomatic joint.

If the scan shows a change in signal within the cancellous bone of the femur, surgical referral should be made rapidly in order to preserve as much of the bone as possible. The best surgical results are associated with early diagnosis and treatment. Late diagnosis, after collapse of the cortical bone has begun, is associated with generally poor results. Nonsurgical options include observation or the use of crutches in the mildest cases of the disease. Surgical decompression of the bone has been shown to improve the condition in some patients, and decompression with grafting—both vascularized and nonvascularized—may be required. If the avascular necrosis is found late, after the cortex of the bone is involved, then osteotomy or joint replacement may be necessary.

## *Inflammatory Disorders*

### SEPTIC ARTHRITIS

Inflammatory disorders of the hip and knee can generally be divided into two categories: infectious (septic) and noninfectious. *Septic arthritis* of the major joints is relatively common in children, owing to the unique physiology and anatomy of growing bone. Fortunately, this condition is quite uncommon in adults, except in individuals with untreated primary gonorrhea, which can secondarily infect the major joints, most commonly the knee. (Gonorrhea actually means ''runny knee.'') Bacterial infections of the hip and knee are almost unheard of in the healthy adult, in the absence of trauma. When such infections are identified, immune system suppression or intravenous drug use must be considered as contributing factors. The most commonly isolated bacterial organisms from hip and knee include *Neisseria gonorroheae* and *Staphylococcus aureus*.

With infection related to immune system suppression, *Mycobacterium tuberculosis* has become more common. Unusual organisms include *Salmonella*, which should be suspected in the patient with sickle-cell disease. Lyme disease should also be considered as a possible cause of joint pain in those areas where the parasitic vectors are found. Fungal infections of the hip and knee are extremely rare outside the immune-suppressed patient and usually involve direct inoculation of the fungal agent into the joint.

Diagnosis of the infected knee is fairly simple. The patient usually presents with a characteristic history of rapid progression and a swollen, tender, erythematous joint. Because of its location deep within the body, diagnosis of the septic hip may be more difficult; it can be confused with such conditions as a psoas abscess, inguinal hernia, and even ureteral stones. Pain with even minimal rotation of the hip in a flexed position that relaxes pressure on the psoas is indicative of intra-articular pathology.

Laboratory studies will usually show an elevated white count and left shift in the differential. Again, it is important to remember that septic joints are rare in the normal host, and immune system suppression may complicate the picture. Radiographs are not specific unless the disease is late in its course and destruction of the joint is already present. Radionucleotide scans are usually not indicated because they may delay identification of the problem.

A definitive diagnosis of septic arthritis is made on the basis of aspiration with cell count and culture of the fluid. If purulent, antibiotics should be started immediately based on a Gram stain of the fluid. Orthopedic surgery consultation should follow immediately. In general, treatment of the septic joint consists of proper diagnosis rapidly followed by surgical debridement, either open or arthroscopic, and appropriate antibiotic therapy. Treatment with antibiotics alone without debridement may often result in continued destruction of the joint. The technique of ''multiple aspiration'' is not an effective alternative to surgery because it will not effectively remove viscous or loculated fluid from the joint.

*With septic arthritis, treatment with antibiotics alone without debridement may often result in continued destruction of the joint.*

### THE INFLAMMATORY ARTHRITIDES

Noninfectious causes of hip and knee arthritis include the vast array of the *inflammatory arthritides*, including rheumatoid arthritis, juvenile rheumatoid arthritis, gout, pseudo-

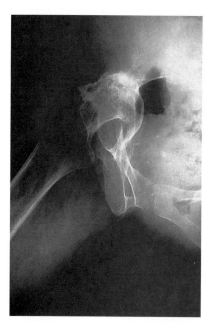

**FIGURE 20–11**
Severe protrusion of the femoral head is sometimes associated with advanced inflammatory arthritis. This patient had been wheelchair-bound for over a year before she was referred for an orthopedic evaluation. She experienced unnecessary pain, and the reconstruction of the pelvis was unnecessarily complicated.

gout (calcium pyrophosphate disease), ankylosing spondylitis, and related conditions. Each has its own features, and appropriate medical management is essential.

Given good medical management, the timing of surgical evaluation in patients with inflammatory arthritis of the hips and knees is somewhat controversial. Some rheumatologists suggest that the consultation be delayed until symptoms are quite severe and medical management is no longer effective. Unfortunately this often leads to the development of severe bone loss, ligamentous and muscular contractures, and loss of range of motion that cannot be corrected by surgery (Figs. 20–11, 20–12). Therefore, most orthopedic surgeons prefer early consultation to avoid these complications of the disease process. Joint replacement is not the only treatment for these conditions. If the

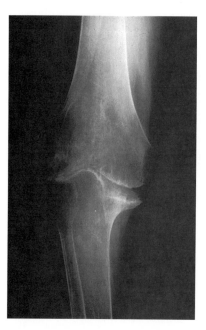

**FIGURE 20–12**
Destruction of the medial compartment is evident in this rheumatoid knee. Because of a severe flexion contracture, full activity could not be achieved after a total knee replacement. Earlier referral would have resulted in a much more independent patient.

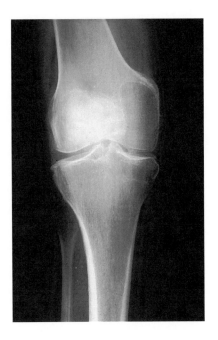

**FIGURE 20–13**
Early changes of inflammatory arthritis are often subtle, as in the mild, nearly uniform loss of joint space seen in this knee. As with osteoarthritis, referral early in the course of any inflammatory joint disease ensures that all the possible surgical options are open.

patient is referred early, surgical management may consist of simple arthroscopic debridement or arthroscopic synovectomy. Therefore, consultation should be made early in the course of the disease rather than late (Fig. 20–13).

## Neoplasms

The proximal femur is an especially common location for the development of neoplasms. Tumors in this area often present as aching pain in the thigh or groin and are missed by the primary care provider, being discovered only after fracture has occurred through the weakened bone. The diagnosis can usually be made on the basis of a simple plain film radiograph, which shows the lesion.

More than 90% of tumors of the femur are metastases from other sites. The most common primary tumors occur in the breast, lung, kidney, and thyroid in women; and lung, prostate, thyroid, and kidney in men. In most cases the lesion is lytic (radiolucent), but those from prostate cancers frequently present as a blastic (radiodense) lesion. Patients with a lesion should receive an immediate orthopedic evaluation. Because most lesions of bone are metastatic, it is not uncommon for the orthopedist to receive a request for "bone biopsy" to identify the primary tumor. Usually there are other more accurate and less invasive ways to identify the primary tumor.

The treatment of metastatic tumors of the bone is based on treatment of the primary tumor with appropriate chemotherapy, radiotherapy, or both. Orthopedic intervention is based on the potential for fracture through the lesion because prophylactic treatment of the lesion before fracture may prevent significant morbidity. The need for prophylactic treatment is based on the size of the lesion, with large lesions usually warranting fracture fixation.

Of the 10% of lesions in the skeleton that are not metastatic, 90% are of myeloid origin. As with metastatic lesions, an early orthopedic consult is appropriate if the lesions in the femur are large enough that they might cause a pathologic fracture.

Less than 1% of bone tumors are actually musculoskeletal in origin. The three most common of these—osteogenic sarcoma (osteosarcoma), chondrosarcoma, and malignant fibrous histiocytoma—vary significantly in their presentation and clinical course. The opinion of an orthopedic surgeon should be obtained as early as possible when

*Less than 1% of bone tumors are actually musculoskeletal in origin.*

these conditions are suspected. With the rarity of these neoplasms and the specialized approach needed for effective treatment, most orthopedic surgeons will refer patients with sarcomas to a specialist in orthopedic oncology for definitive care.

### *When to Call the Surgeon about Hip and Knee Pain*

- Fractures around the knee
- Suspicion of occult fractures of the hip or knee
- Any open fracture
- Dislocation of the hip or knee
- Ligamentous trauma where pain persists more than a few weeks
- Avulsion fracture of the patella
- Fracture of the body of the patella
- Locked knee
- Osteoarthritis of the hip or knee (early in its course to explore treatment options)
- Avascular necrosis
- Sepsis of the hip or knee joint
- Inflammatory arthritides (early in their courses)
- Bone tumors

## RECOMMENDED READING

Dieppe, P: Management of hip osteoarthritis. BMJ 311:853–857, 1995.

Handy, JR: Osteoarthritis in elderly knees. Southern Medical Journal 89:1031–1035, 1996.

NIH Consensus Conference: Total hip replacement. NIH Consensus Development Panel on Total Hip Replacement. JAMA 273:1950–1956, 1995.

Norman-Taylor, FH, et al: Quality-of-life improvement compared after hip and knee replacement. J of Bone & Joint Surgery—British volume 78:74–77, 1996.

Orthopaedic Knowledge Update: Hip and Knee 1996, American Academy of Orthopaedic Surgeons.

Ries, MD, et al: Improvement in cardiovascular fitness after total knee arthroplasty. J of Bone & Joint Surgery—American volume 78:1696–1701, 1996.

# Foot and Ankle Problems

## GREGORY POMEROY, MD,
## and CHARLES EATON, MD, MS

Foot and ankle problems are common presenting complaints in primary care, and if not properly diagnosed and treated they can lead to significant costs and morbidity. A working knowledge of the anatomy and biomechanics of the foot and ankle are very helpful in diagnosing and treating ankle and foot problems effectively.

## *Anatomy*

### BONES, JOINTS, AND LIGAMENTS

The ankle is a classic hinge joint and is responsible for dorsiflexion and plantarflexion of the foot (Fig. 21–1).

The foot is a complex structure that allows for the stabilization of weight with minimal muscular energy (energy conservation) and also provides for the push-off necessary for locomotion. It has 26 bones (Fig. 21–2).

### NERVES AND VASCULAR SUPPLY

The nerves supplying the foot and ankle are branches from more proximal nerves. Two main arteries supply the foot. The *dorsalis pedis artery* is a continuation of the anterior tibial artery and primarily supplies the dorsum of the foot via its many branches. The largest branch is the deep plantar artery, which runs between the first and second metatarsals and terminates in the plantar arch. The *posterior tibial artery* divides into both medial and lateral plantar branches. The larger lateral branch joins with the deep plantar artery to form the plantar arch.

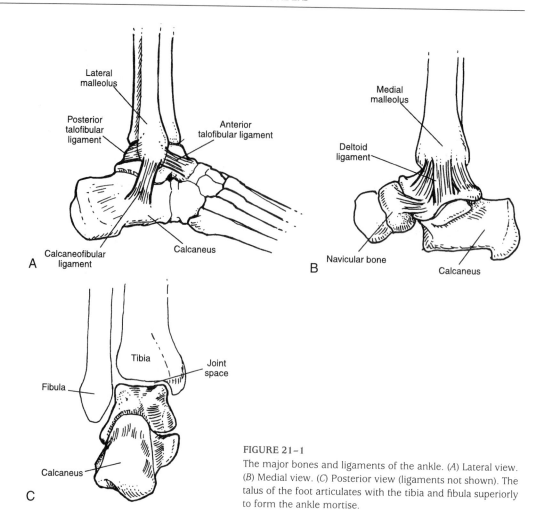

**FIGURE 21–1**
The major bones and ligaments of the ankle. (*A*) Lateral view. (*B*) Medial view. (*C*) Posterior view (ligaments not shown). The talus of the foot articulates with the tibia and fibula superiorly to form the ankle mortise.

## *Biomechanics*

### DEFINITIONS

Various postures of the foot have important biomechanical implications that lead to foot and ankle pathology. A uniform definition of these anatomic variations is shown in Fig. 21–3. The heel is said to be in *equinus* (*A*) when the ankle is plantarflexed and in *calcaneus* (*B*) when the ankle is dorsiflexed. When the calcaneus is more medial than the talus, the hindfoot viewed from behind is said to be in *hindfoot* or *calcaneal varus* (*C*). When the calcaneus is more lateral than the talus, the hindfoot viewed from behind is said to be in *hindfoot* or *calcaneal valgus* (*D*). This is also referred to as an *overpronated* foot.

If the forefoot is adducted toward the midline relative to the hindfoot, it is said to be in *metatarsus adductus* (*E*). If the forefoot is abducted away from the midline relative to the hindfoot, it is said to be in *metatarsus abductus* (*F*). If the forefoot is supinated, it is said to be in *forefoot varus* (*G*), whereas if it is pronated, it is said to be in *forefoot valgus* (*H*).

### BIOMECHANICS OF GAIT

Walking involves a cyclic pattern of integrated movements that are designed to minimize energy requirements. Prerequisites for normal gait include stance stability, nor-

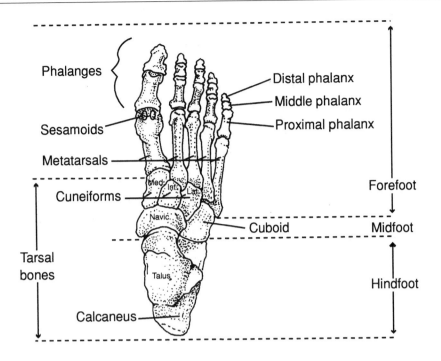

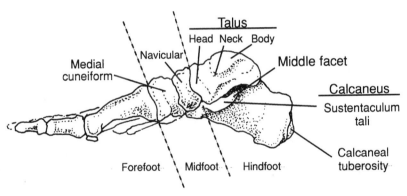

**FIGURE 21-2**
The bones of the foot. The foot can be divided into the hindfoot, midfoot, and forefoot.

mal clearance in swing, preposition of the foot in terminal swing, and adequate stride length. Walking requires that one foot be in contact with the ground at all times, while running requires that both feet be off the ground at the same time during some point in the gait cycle. The vertical load on the forefoot is greater than bodyweight at times and during running may be equal to four to five times the runner's bodyweight.

## Examining the Foot and Ankle

### INSPECTION

As the patient ambulates, the examiner should inspect the appearance and condition of the shoes and feet. In most cases, the shoe will deform to the deformity of the foot. Examples of this include excessive wear on the lateral border of the sole with toeing in and scuffing of the shoe from scraping the floor in swing phase with a dropped foot.

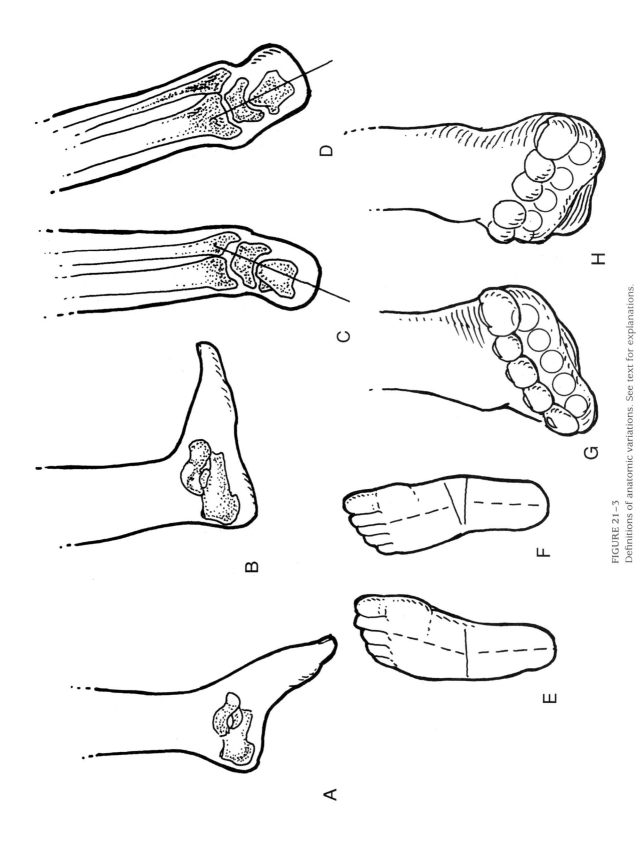

FIGURE 21–3
Definitions of anatomic variations. See text for explanations.

The clinician should examine both feet, and as the patient sits, the feet should adopt a plantarflexed and inverted posture. The skin should be thickened at the heel, lateral border and plantar to the first and fifth metatarsal heads. Increases in the thickness in these areas or in other areas of the foot may suggest that some areas are carrying excess weight. The examiner should also inspect both feet for swelling. Bilateral swelling may indicate systemic problems; unilateral swelling might indicate residual edema secondary to trauma or deep venous thrombosis.

*Bilateral swelling of the feet may indicate systemic problems; unilateral swelling may indicate residual edema secondary to trauma or deep venous thrombosis.*

## PALPATION

Palpation and knowledge of the relevant anatomy are the keys to the diagnosis of the common foot and ankle complaints. The first metatarsophalangeal (MTP) joint is a common site for gout, bunion deformities, and arthritis. Pain with palpation along the medial aspect of that joint suggests bunion, whereas pain with palpation along the dorsal aspect of the joint, especially with dorsiflexion, is more consistent with arthritis. The medial aspect of the first metatarsal head is also a common site of gout. Deposits of urate crystals (tophi) can mimic the pain and deformity of a bunion. Pain with palpation of the plantar aspect of the first MTP joint may indicate a medial or lateral sesamoiditis or fracture. Palpation of the plantar metatarsal heads or MTP joints will duplicate pain from synovitis of these joints. This must be distinguished from pain with palpation in the web spaces, which is more indicative of a neuroma. The fifth metatarsal is also a common site of problems. At its base, pain with palpation may be a sign of an avulsion fracture or insertional tendinitis of the peroneus brevis, whereas pain along the lateral border of the fifth MTP joint may indicate a bunionette deformity, also known as a tailor's bunion.

In the hindfoot, palpation of the insertion point of the plantar fascia into the calcaneus commonly reproduces the pain of true plantar fasciitis; more proximal pain with palpation of the heel fat pad may discount plantar fasciitis as the reason for heel pain. In the lateral hindfoot, the anterior talofibular ligament is often torn with ankle sprains and is painful with palpation. Much less commonly, the calcaneofibular ligament is involved, and even more rare is involvement of the posterior talofibular ligament. Just anterior to the lateral ankle ligaments is the sinus tarsi. Deep tenderness to palpation here may reflect a fracture of the anterior process of the calcaneus, a problem in the subtalar joint complex, or spastic flat foot. Posteriorly, the gastrocnemius and soleus muscles join to form the Achilles tendon. Palpation in this region can help the examiner detect a defect when the tendon is ruptured. To test the continuity of the Achilles tendon, the examiner should squeeze the calf musculature of the prone patient. If the tendon is intact, the foot should plantarflex. With rupture, plantarflexion will be absent or markedly diminished. Tendinitis of the Achilles tendon often manifests itself as a palpable nodule within the substance of the tendon itself. Usually this nodule is located 2.5 to 5 cm above the point of insertion of the Achilles tendon, where the blood supply is poorest. This is usually the area of maximal tenderness to palpation.

*To test the continuity of the Achilles tendon, squeeze the calf musculature of the prone patient. If the tendon is intact, the foot should plantarflex. With rupture, plantarflexion will be absent or markedly diminished.*

## *Diagnosis and Management*

### HALLUX VALGUS (BUNION)

*Hallux valgus* is a deformity defined by lateral deviation of the great toe and medial deviation of the first metatarsal. Often a bony exostosis develops over the medial eminence of the first metatarsal head and is the cause of pain associated with this deformity. In addition to the bony exostosis, hypertrophy of the bursa overlying the medial eminence may further add to the discomfort. The hallux valgus deformity occasionally is hereditary, but the vast majority of bunions are acquired. The hallux valgus deformity becomes painful in populations in the world that wear shoes, and it is shoes that are

*The hallux valgus deformity occasionally is hereditary, but the vast majority of bunions are acquired.*

mainly responsible for the development of bunions. Of inherited bunions, juvenile hallux valgus deformities are more notorious for their familial tendencies. There is also a higher incidence of hallux valgus deformities in patients with pes planus (flatfoot), especially those with neuromuscular disorders.

The evaluation of the patient with hallux valgus should include a careful history regarding footwear. The physical examination should include palpation of the medial eminence as well as documentation of the range of motion at the first MTP joint. Often there will be numbness caused by pressure over the dorsomedial sensory nerve to the great toe. If the deformity is severe, often the patient will complain of pain under the plantar second MTP joint, secondary to increased weightbearing because of loss of weightbearing at the first MTP joint. The presence of pes planus as well as any neuromuscular imbalances should be documented. The bunion deformity is usually exacerbated with weightbearing and the patient should be examined standing. Standing radiographs are essential to properly documenting the severity of the deformity. The conservative treatment of the patient with a hallux valgus deformity, as well as prevention of the problem in the first place, starts with the patient choosing a shoe with adequate height and width in the toe box. "Adequate width" implies that the shoe does not exert pressure over the medial eminence. In addition, the shoe should not have a seam over the medial eminence. Generally, soft leather shoes are best. The sole of the shoe should be made of either soft crepe or rubber. In more severe cases, stretching of the leather and relieving pressure points may be helpful. In the most severe cases, custom shoes can sometimes prevent the need for surgical intervention. Bunion pads and posts, night splints, and other such devices usually give little if any relief.

When conservative care fails, a surgical consultation is appropriate. Over 100 surgical procedures to correct the hallux valgus deformity have been described, indicating that no single procedure is adequate in all cases. Patients can have some residual stiffness or deformity following surgery, and often the foot is not significantly reduced in size. The patient who desires bunion surgery because he or she wants to wear a small shoe after surgery is not a surgical candidate. Because recurrences are more likely in adolescents treated for a bunion deformity, surgery should be put off if possible until the patient is more mature. The other group of patients for whom surgery should be delayed is professional athletes or dancers. Bunion surgery in this group should only be performed when the pain is keeping them from performing. The rate of recurrence following bunion surgery ranges between 1% and 10%, but in properly selected patients it can give long-lasting, satisfying results.

> • ▬▬
> *Over 100 surgical procedures to correct the hallux valgus deformity have been described, indicating that no single procedure is adequate in all cases.*

> • ▬▬
> *The patient who desires bunion surgery because he or she wants to wear a small shoe after surgery is not a surgical candidate.*

## LESSER TOE DEFORMITIES

Lesser toe deformities are very common and can occur by themselves or in conjunction with other deformities of the foot. The definitions of the various conditions have become somewhat confusing because the terms have been used interchangeably, but in reality they are quite simple. A *mallet toe* (Fig. 21–4) is present when the distal interphalangeal (DIP) joint is flexed. A *claw toe* (Fig. 21–5) is present when the proximal interphalangeal (PIP) joint is flexed and the MTP joint is in extension. Both of these conditions are acquired and, as with the hallux valgus deformity, are much more common in populations that wear shoes. It appears that placing the foot in a shoe with a narrow toebox causes the toes to buckle, leading to a propensity for these deformities. The incidence of each deformity appears to increase with age, and all are relatively rare in young people. Mallet toes tend to develop in the second toe—probably because the second toe is usually the longest. The toe becomes plantarflexed at the DIP joint because of pressure from the shoe. Another deformity, *hammertoe* (extension of the MTP and DIP with flexion of the PIP), also develops because of abnormal pressure from the shoe, but it tends to develop more slowly. Hammertoes also can develop in patients with neuromuscular diseases (secondary to a muscular imbalance), diabetes mellitus, and rheumatoid or psoriatic arthritis. Hammertoes may be flexible or rigid, a factor

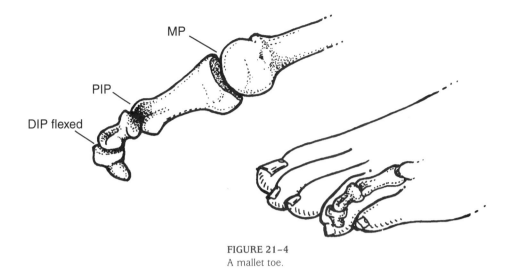

**FIGURE 21–4**
A mallet toe.

that is important when attempting conservative treatment. Claw toes can also be associated with neuromuscular diseases, diabetes, and arthritis. Regardless of the cause, the claw toe exists when there is an imbalance between the intrinsic and extrinsic musculature; they are usually multiple.

The treatment of lesser toe deformities hinges on whether they are flexible or rigid. If the deformity is flexible, the toe can be corrected passively, and thus is often amenable to the use of an appliance that will hold it in a corrected position. On the other hand, if the deformity is rigid and cannot be passively corrected, any attempt to correct it with an appliance will fail and can even cause the toe to ulcerate secondary to pressure from the appliance. For most patients with a flexible deformity, the treatment should be conservative. The first step is to place the patient in a well-fitting shoe, with enough width and depth in the toe box to accommodate the foot. This will avoid direct pressure against the deformity and help prevent painful callosities. Donut-shaped cushions or other similar devices may relieve pressure over the PIP joint. If there is pain under the metatarsal heads, orthotics with a metatarsal pad proximal to the affected joints can be added for further comfort. In severe cases, such as in patients with serious rheumatoid arthritis or diabetes, custom extra-deep, extra-wide shoes with plastizote insoles are useful to distribute pressure equally along the plantar aspect of the foot.

*For most patients with a flexible deformity, the treatment should be conservative.*

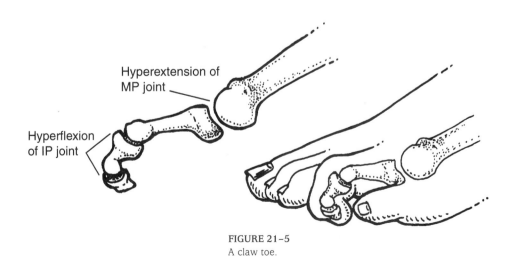

**FIGURE 21–5**
A claw toe.

Despite adequate conservative care, however, these deformities will often progress and become fixed, necessitating a surgical consultation.

### When to Call the Surgeon about Toe Deformities

• Failure of conservative therapy for hallux valgus
• Failure of conservative therapy for a flexible toe deformity
• Rigid toe deformities

## ARTHRITIDES

The major categories of arthritis that affect the foot and ankle are osteoarthritis, rheumatoid arthritis, the seronegative spondyloarthropathies, and crystal-induced arthritis.

### Osteoarthritis

Osteoarthritis usually affects middle-aged and elderly people, but younger patients with earlier trauma, obese patients, and heavy laborers can also be affected. Loss of function is the final result as structural integrity is lost with progression of the disease. Pain occurs not only at the affected joints but also at surrounding joints because of increased stress secondary to altered gait. Symptoms are generally worse in the morning and are aggravated by prolonged walking and standing. The affected joint will be tender on examination and often will be warmer to the touch. Radiographic examination reveals "squaring" of the joint surfaces, loss of joint space, sclerotic joint margins, osteophyte formation, and subchondral cyst formation.

*The key to conservative management of osteoarthritis is to reduce the local stress at the affected joint.*

In general, conservative management includes anti-inflammatory medication and, rarely, selective local injections. The key is to reduce the local stress at the affected joint. This can be accomplished through several mechanisms. The patient should choose aerobic activities that do not unduly stress the foot and ankle, such as swimming, aquatic aerobic classes, and bicycling. Standing jobs should be modified to sedentary ones. Shoes should be altered so that they do not apply pressure over prominent exostoses. Often, rocker-bottom soles added to shoes in conjunction with extended steel shanks will reduce stresses across proximal and distal arthritic joints and allow increased comfort with activity. In these conditions, rigid soles lessen the stress on the arthritic foot—especially the forefoot. Foot orthoses can also play a significant role in stress reduction. Only rarely should intra-articular steroid injections be contemplated; their benefit will vary. In osteoarthritis of the foot and ankle, surgical options should be limited to removing bony spurs (cheilectomy) and isolated fusions. Total joint replacements or Silastic implants do not have a proven track record of success and longevity, so they should be avoided.

### Rheumatoid Arthritis

Rheumatoid arthritis begins in the feet in about 17% of cases. The forefoot is the most common site. As with the hands, involvement is often bilateral and symmetric. Swelling is usually intra-articular. An effusion is generally present and perhaps erythema as well. Typically, forefoot involvement is at the level of the PIP and MTP joints. Rarely, if ever, are the DIP joints involved. Synovitis is usually the earliest hallmark of the disease, with deformity more prevalent later. The deformities that occur with rheumatoid arthritis tend to be dynamic and severe because the disease generally causes gradual joint destruction. In the forefoot, a hallux valgus deformity often develops. As it becomes more severe, weightbearing is transferred to the lesser toes, causing severe hammertoes or claw toes. As in the hands, the toes often drift, with frank subluxation or dislocation occurring at the MTP level. The plantar fat pad drifts distally with the toes, and eventually the plantar metatarsal heads are completely uncovered. Pressure calluses and occasional ulceration are the end result. In the midfoot, chronic synovitis causes eventual loss of joint space, followed by fibrous or bony ankylosis. Loss of the medial longitudinal arch is very common. Hindfoot involvement occurs in about one-third of patients with rheumatoid arthritis. The ankle is the least affected joint, but when it is involved the subtalar and midfoot joints are usually involved as well, resulting in severe dysfunction.

Conservative care is directed toward pain relief, prevention of deformity, correction of existing deformity, and restoration and preservation of function. Medical management is a keystone of treatment and is outside the scope of this chapter. Physical therapy is of limited usefulness in treating rheumatoid arthritis, but gentle stretching and range-of-motion exercises should be employed daily in all patients. Orthotic devices are very useful early in the disease. Metatarsal pads or bars can give significant relief from metatarsalgia and should be placed just proximal to the affected MTP joints. Foot orthotics that gently support the arch and keep the hindfoot in a neutral position can decrease stress across affected joints. Extra-deep, extra-wide shoes with plastizote insoles can relieve pressure and afford pain relief. New ones are required every 6 months to a year because of the dynamic nature of this disease. Canes can also be helpful. When used in the opposite hand, they can significantly reduce weightbearing stresses across the symptomatic foot. Often a light polypropylene ankle-foot orthosis can control moderate deformity in the hindfoot and therefore prevent ulceration and subsequent surgical intervention. The reasons for surgical intervention include an unbraceable deformity, an ulcer that will not heal secondary to increased bony pressure, a recurrent ulcer, or intractable pain.

*Gentle stretching and range-of-motion exercises should be employed daily in all patients with rheumatoid arthritis.*

## Seronegative Spondyloarthropathies

Several clinical and radiologic features separate the seronegative spondyloarthropathies from rheumatoid arthritis. In general, there is an absence of osteoporosis, a presence of ankylosis (which is rare in rheumatoid arthritis), and a presence of calcification about the periphery of the joints. Clinically, patients with one of the seronegative spondyloarthropathies often present with painful heel syndrome, Achilles tendinitis, or true plantar fasciitis.

### ANKYLOSING SPONDYLITIS

Ankylosing spondylitis usually affects the foot and ankle as an enthesopathy, usually in the hindfoot. The MTP joints can be affected, leading to bony ankylosis. The toes can drift similar to the deformity in rheumatoid arthritis, but subchondral sclerosis is more apparent than with rheumatoid arthritis and is a distinguishing feature.

### PSORIATIC ARTHRITIS

The arthritis in psoriatic arthritis precedes skin lesions in a significant number of patients. In the feet, the DIP joints are usually symmetrically involved, with classic changes in the nails. The typical radiographic appearance has been called the "cup and saucer"; it results from destruction of the proximal phalanges, forming sharp points. Patients complain of heel pain, though many of the cases are clinically indistinguishable from rheumatoid arthritis.

### REITER'S SYNDROME

The triad of conjunctivitis, urethritis, and arthritis constitutes Reiter's syndrome. The arthritis is asymmetric and usually involves the knees, feet, and ankles. The diagnosis should be suspected in a young male complaining of several lower extremity complaints—especially heel pain. There is usually tenderness with palpation and generalized swelling around the painful area. Radiographically there may be no significant findings at all, or there may be fluffy calcifications at the insertions of the ligaments and tendons. The treatment for most of the complaints of patients with seronegative arthropathies is conservative. Heel spur surgery and plantar fascia release rarely give significant relief of symptoms. Footwear modifications and orthotics are similar to those described for rheumatoid arthritis, and with appropriate anti-inflammatory medications they give some relief in a significant number of cases. Surgery should be reserved for end-stage joint destruction.

### Crystal-Induced Arthritis

Two types of crystal deposits cause arthritis: gout and pseudogout. *Gout* results from sodium urate crystal deposition, whereas *pseudogout* results from calcium pyrophosphate dihydrate crystal deposition. When viewed under a polarized microscope, sodium urate crystals are strongly negatively birefringent. Calcium pyrophosphate crystals are weakly positively birefringent.

Gout is caused by a malfunction in purine metabolism. It is more frequent in men than in women. Between 50% and 75% of initial attacks of gout occur in the first MTP joint, and in patients who have gout, 90% will have an attack in their toes during their lifetime. An acute gout attack affecting the toes causes the joint to become swollen, erythematous, and very painful. The overlying skin is often hyperesthetic. Each attack is self-limiting. Gout can also be the cause of plantar fasciitis and tenosynovitis. Radiographic findings of patients with gout range from no abnormalities to severe joint destruction. There can be proximal periarticular joint erosion. A radiographic hallmark of gouty arthritis is the presence of destructive bony lesions in areas removed from the joint surface.

*A radiographic hallmark of gouty arthritis is the presence of destructive bony lesions in areas removed from the joint surface.*

The acute attack is treated with elevation and rest of the affected extremity. An appropriate anti-inflammatory medication is begun immediately. With proper medical management, chronic tophaceous gouty deposits are rare. When present, these should be curretted, with subsequent application of wet-to-dry dressings. This usually prevents overgrowth. With local wound management and appropriate medical intervention, amputation is rarely required.

Pseudogout is also known as chondrocalcinosis. Symptoms begin when crystals are shed into a joint, causing a painful inflammatory process. In the foot, the talonavicular and subtalar joints are usually the site of attacks. Anti-inflammatory medications are recommended for acute synovitis. Surgery is reserved for advanced joint disease.

### *When to Call the Surgeon about Foot Arthritis*

- Unbraceable deformity
- Soft tissue ulcer from bony pressure
- Intractable pain

## KERATOTIC DISORDERS

Friction or pressure can result in corns or calluses. These are essentially localized keratoses caused by pressure from the shoe against resistance from the bones themselves. They occur on the projections of the bones. *Corns* are accumulations of the horny layers of the epidermis. Hard corns form on the surfaces of toes exposed to pressure. The lateral side of the fifth toe is the most common site for a hard corn. Soft corns form over a condyle of a phalanx between toes. *Calluses* have the same histologic appearance as corns and tend to form over or under any bony prominence. When the callus is located under a metatarsal head, it is often referred to as an *intractable plantar keratosis* (IPK).

In general, corns and calluses can be treated conservatively. Daily filing of the accumulation of tissue will keep the size of the corn or callus under control and often completely controls symptoms. Changing the patient's shoes to ones with a toebox with enough depth to accommodate the foot also often provides significant relief. The symptoms from IPKs are often significantly improved by the application of a metatarsal pad proximal to the callus. If the corn is over the dorsal surface of a claw toe or hammertoe, correcting the deformity will resolve the symptoms from the corn. When simple conservative measures fail, often minor surgery will relieve symptoms. For example, partial condylectomy to remove a bony exostosis may relieve a hard corn in a nonweightbearing portion of the foot. For more extensive plantar calluses, partial condylectomy may not be enough, and the offending metatarsal may have to be shortened, dorsiflexed, or both. Surgical excision of the callus without addressing the underlying bony abnormality will provide only temporary relief.

*Bunionette deformities* are enlargements on the lateral side of the fifth MTP joints. In the past, these deformities were also known as "Tailor's bunions" because historically tailors sat with their legs crossed while sewing clothes, placing increased pressure on the fifth metatarsal heads. If a bunionette deformity is present and the shoe is not wide enough, increased pressure results. With time, a bursitis develops and symptoms increase. Since the symptoms are secondary to pressure, pain is often relieved when walking barefoot or in loose-fitting socks or slippers. The treatment of a bunionette deformity initially is a broad toebox, with occasional donut-shaped pads within the shoe to relieve pressure. In more severe cases, operative intervention is warranted. Surgery involves removal of the bony prominence and often a metatarsal osteotomy.

## DISEASES OF THE NERVES OF THE FOOT

### Interdigital Plantar Neuromas

The causes of interdigital neuromas are controversial. The neuromas probably evolve in stages, but most authors of studies on the matter agree that an entrapment neuropathy occurs. The third web space is the most common site for a neuroma—probably because the common digital nerve supplying this web space receives branches from both medial and lateral plantar nerves and therefore is thicker than the common digital nerves supplying the other web spaces. This increase in size makes the third common digital nerve more susceptible to trauma and subsequent neuroma formation. The current theory is that the metatarsal heads are squeezed together, impinging the common digital nerve, either between the two metatarsal heads or against the transverse metatarsal ligament, leading to neuritic symptoms. Women are more susceptible to developing neuromas than men by a ratio of 4:1, a risk probably related to their shoe types. Neuromas are unilateral 85% of the time and usually exist singularly in a foot. Interdigital neuromas in the first and fourth web spaces are rare. Patients with neuromas complain of burning pain on the plantar surface of the foot. This pain is worsened with activity while wearing shoes, especially high heels, and may be totally absent when walking barefoot. Numbness is a complaint only 40% of the time. A key in examining such patients is to determine that the pain is localized. The neuromas can be palpated in one-third of the cases. Pain is also elicited if the examiner squeezes the metatarsals together. A negative "squeeze test" brings the diagnosis into doubt. The diagnosis is made solely on the basis of the history and physical exam, since radiographs and laboratory results are not helpful.

Patients with interdigital neuromas can often be treated successfully with conservative care. Shoes with adequate height and width in the toebox will often improve symptoms. Metatarsal pads placed proximal to the neuroma will alleviate pressure and often given symptomatic relief. Injection of the interspace with a combination of a local

*In general, corns and calluses can be treated conservatively.*

*A key in examining patients with neuromas is that the pain is localized.*

anesthetic and steroid medications may give long-lasting relief. If steroids are to be used, care must be taken to inject the fluid into the web space—not into the adjoining capsule of the MTP joint. An injection into the capsule could cause it to deteriorate, with subsequent divergence of the toe. Even with adequate conservative care, 75% of patients with an interdigital neuroma eventually require excision of the nerve.

### Tarsal Tunnel Syndrome

Tarsal tunnel syndrome is a condition analogous to carpal tunnel syndrome in the wrist. Excess pressure is placed against the posterior tibial nerve or one of its branches as it passes beneath the flexor retinaculum either at the ankle or more distally. A specific cause can be identified in about half the cases. Causes include direct trauma and nontraumatic causes such as ganglions, lipomas, or exostoses. Severe pes planus deformities can also cause tarsal tunnel syndrome. Patients usually complain of diffuse pain or numbness along the plantar aspect of the foot. Symptoms may include burning or tingling. Symptoms are aggravated by activity and improved with rest. Like patients with carpal tunnel syndrome, patients with tarsal tunnel syndrome often complain of night pain, relieved only by getting up and moving the affected extremity. The pain from tarsal tunnel syndrome can also radiate proximally. On examination, the patient must have a positive Tinel's sign over the tarsal tunnel area. Percussion over the tarsal tunnel should cause pain along the distribution of the medial and lateral plantar nerves. Failure to elicit this sign makes the diagnosis of tarsal tunnel syndrome questionable. Even though the patient has subjective complaints of numbness, the examiner will often fail to elicit decreased two-point sensation in the medial and lateral plantar nerve distributions. It is controversial whether positive electrodiagnostic studies are required to make the diagnosis of tarsal tunnel syndrome. Unlike carpal tunnel syndrome, where electrodiagnostic studies are usually positive, these studies in tarsal tunnel syndrome are positive only 50% of the time. Regardless, if the terminal latency of the medial plantar nerve to the abductor hallucis and of the lateral plantar nerve to the abductor digiti minimi is prolonged, it may indicate the presence of tarsal tunnel syndrome. Electrodiagnostic studies also can rule out lumbar disk disease as a cause of the patient's symptoms (see Chapter 18).

The initial treatment of tarsal tunnel syndrome is conservative. Anti-inflammatory medication coupled with foot orthotics will usually benefit the patient. Rarely, short-term cast immobilization will give relief. If patients fail to improve with conservative therapy, tarsal tunnel release should be considered. Typically, surgical release will improve symptoms 75% of the time. If a patient gets little or no relief from an adequate surgical release, a rerelease should not be considered. Re-exploration of the tarsal tunnel rarely, if ever, provides any benefit.

## ACCESSORY OSSICLES

### Sesamoids

Patients with symptomatic sesamoids usually complain of pain with weightbearing. Treatment consists of rest initially, followed by relief of excess pressure. Often an orthotic with a recess under the symptomatic sesamoid will afford good symptomatic relief. In intractable cases, excision of the sesamoid is indicated.

Sesamoids can also be fractured. Differentiation between a fractured sesamoid and a bipartite sesamoid can be difficult.

### Os Trigonum

When symptomatic, the os trigonum can cause pain in the retrocalcaneal space, anterior to the Achilles tendon. This pain is worse with ambulation and with plantarflexion of the ankle. Treatment includes a period of complete rest and appropriate anti-inflammatory medication. If this fails to relieve symptoms, excision is warranted.

### Accessory Navicula

When the accessory bone is asymptomatic, no treatment is warranted. With acute symptoms, the affected limb may be immobilized. For more chronic conditions, foot orthotics that gently support the arch will often give relief. If conservative care fails, excision of the accessory bone with advancement of the tibialis posterior tendon often corrects the problem permanently.

## THE DIABETIC FOOT

Patients are very commonly diagnosed with diabetes after a nonhealing ulcer is discovered on the plantar surface of the foot. The foot also is the most common site of infection leading to hospitalization in diabetics. Foot and ankle care in patients with diabetes now involves a multidisciplinary approach. The primary care provider or podiatrist provides routine care, with vascular surgeons, orthopedists, infectious disease specialists, and general surgeons readily available. Although amputations may be required, good preventive care can often avert the need for an amputation in a patient with diabetes.

Diabetic ulcers of the foot are common. The ulcers in an insensitive or dysvascular foot are classified based on the depth of the ulcer. Grade 0 ulcers may have a bony deformity, but the skin is intact. Grade 1 ulcers are localized and superficial. Grade 2 ulcers extend to the level of tendon, bone, joint, or ligament. Grade 3 ulcers represent either a deep abscess or osteomyelitis. Grade 4 ulcers involve gangrene of the toes or forefoot, and grade 5 ulcers involve gangrene of the entire foot. The treatment of diabetic ulcers is currently undergoing change. The old adage of doing one definitive procedure rather than weekly debridements is now considered passé. Conventional orthopedic procedures such as bunionectomies and correction of claw toes should be carried out to relieve bony pressure against the skin. Superficial ulcers should be treated with relief of pressure of weightbearing, serial debridements to healthy granulation tissue, and wet-to-dry dressing changes at least twice per day. These can be performed with sterile saline or with a number of solutions that promote healthy tissue growth while inhibiting bacterial overgrowth. In an ulcer that remains noninfected but is slow to heal, referral to a facility familiar with total contact casting will often result in a healed ulcer. Any patient with an ulcer that is Grade 3 or worse should be referred to a surgeon immediately.

*The old adage of doing one definitive procedure rather than weekly debridements to treat diabetic ulcers is now considered passé.*

Neuropathy is also a very common problem in the patient with diabetes and is usually manifested as a chronic sensory neuropathy. This is seen as dysesthesia or hyperesthesia, loss of position sense, loss of vibratory sense, loss of Achilles reflex, and an appreciable change in pain perception. The key to managing patients with a neuropathic foot is to maintain a plantigrade foot that is not prone to ulceration. Extra-deep, extra-wide shoes lined with plastizote inserts should be custom made for the patient with a neuropathic foot. All callosities should be kept pared down to prevent pressure. Patients should inspect their feet daily, and routine podiatric care of the nails should be done professionally every 8 weeks to avoid any ingrowing and subsequent infection. With this type of regimen, the more disastrous consequences of a peripheral neuropathy can usually be avoided.

Despite adequate medical and podiatric care, *Charcot's joints* are still the most common major manifestation of diabetes affecting the foot and ankle. Charcot's joints are neuropathic joints that frequently have fractures, dislocations, or both. Their onset may follow minimal trauma or surgery. At the onset, there is usually erythema, increased warmth, and swelling. Differentiation of an acute Charcot's joint from an infection can be very difficult. The care of an acute Charcot's joint involves protection from deformity via a nonweightbearing cast followed by a total-contact ankle-foot orthosis. A patient suspected of having an acute Charcot's joint should be referred to an appropriate foot and ankle specialist immediately.

Obviously the prevention of problems and subsequent treatment of the diabetic foot and ankle is beyond the scope of this book. If there is any question about the severity of an ulcer or the onset of an infection or Charcot's joint, immediate referral to a foot and ankle specialist is warranted.

## TRAUMATIC INJURIES

Traumatic injuries to the foot and ankle fall into either soft-tissue or bony classifications.

### Sprains

The most common soft-tissue injury to the foot and ankle is the ankle sprain. Three groups of ligaments surround the ankle (see Fig. 21–1). On the medial side is the deltoid ligament; on the lateral side, moving from anterior to posterior, are the anterior talofibular ligament, the calcaneofibular ligament, and the posterior talofibular ligament; and between the tibia and fibula is the syndesmotic ligament, which comprises the tibiofibular ligament and the interosseus membrane. Ankle sprains involve an injury to one or more of the ankle ligaments. A first-degree ankle sprain involves a partial or complete tear of the anterior talofibular ligament. A second-degree sprain is a partial or complete tear of both the anterior talofibular ligament and calcaneofibular ligament, and a third-degree sprain involves a tear in all three lateral ankle ligaments. First-degree tears are very common and are diagnosed when the patient has had an inversion, plantarflexion injury. On examination, the patient will have tenderness at palpation over the anterior talofibular ligament. Second-degree sprains are less common and involve tenderness at palpation over the anterior talofibular ligaments and peroneal tendons because the calcaneofibular ligament passes under the peroneal tendons. A third-degree sprain is rare but involves tenderness of the posterior talofibular ligament at palpation as well as to the anterior talofibular and calcaneofibular ligaments. Ankle sprains should be thought of as a continuum of injury. It is impossible to injure the calcaneofibular ligament or posterior talofibular ligament alone, so if patients have isolated tenderness over these areas, look for another injury rather than a routine ankle sprain.

When examining an ankle after an inversion injury, always palpate the region between the tibia and fibula anteriorly, just above the ankle mortise. This is the region of the syndesmotic ligament. Pain at palpation in this region portends a more serious injury. Testing for ankle instability can be difficult. The amount of inversion should be compared from the injured extremity to the uninjured extremity to determine the extent of damage present. Local anesthetic will often relieve enough pain to allow the examination to be performed, but rarely does testing for instability need to be done in the primary care setting, since the initial treatment of ankle sprains is the same, regardless of the degree.

Radiographs should be performed in suspected second- and third-degree sprains and should include anteroposterior, lateral, and mortise views. A mortise view is performed with the ankle rotated internally 30°. In a primary care setting, the purpose of the radiographs is to rule out a concomitant fracture. Fig. 21–6 shows several common fractures (talar dome, lateral process of the talus, anterior process of the calcaneus) that may mimic ankle sprains. Stress x-rays are useful in determining ankle instability, but they are painful in the acute setting and should probably be done by the specialist as part of the surgery decision process for chronic ankle sprains only.

The treatment for ankle sprains is aggressive. Rest, ice, compression, and elevation (RICE) constitute the initial treatment. This is quickly followed by limiting inversion/

*Ankle sprains should be thought of as a continuum of injury.*

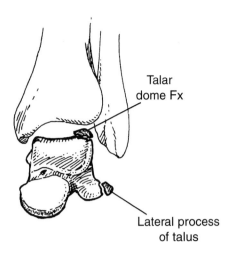

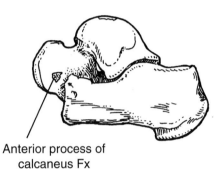

FIGURE 21-6
Some common fractures that may mimic ankle sprains.

Talar dome Fx

Lateral process of talus

Anterior process of calcaneus Fx

eversion with a protective functional brace and limited weightbearing with a normal heel-toe gait. The goal of early motion is to allow the ankle to obtain functional recovery while not losing proprioception. At approximately 5 to 10 days, patients can begin exercises against resistance. The brace can be removed when the patient can walk without pain, but the ankle may still require taping to avoid further injury. At this stage patients can resume athletics.

Injuries to the medial ankle ligaments are caused by a sudden eversion stress of the foot. This injury is rare by itself, but it can occur with an ankle fracture, so radiographs should be obtained. Usually sprains of the medial ankle ligaments are stable injuries and can be treated as outlined above. If there is any evidence of diastasis of the distal tibiofibular syndesmosis, surgical repair is warranted.

The other common ligamentous injury is the sprain of the first MTP joint, caused by stubbing the toe or by dorsiflexion. This condition has been called "turf toe." Examination reveals pain with motion and visible swelling of the joint. These injuries should be treated with taping and a rigid-sole shoe and will usually recover completely.

## Tendinitis

Tendons are also subject to trauma. The tibialis anterior and posterior tendons, Achilles tendon, and peroneal tendons are all commonly involved in either direct or indirect trauma. Direct laceration or rupture of any of these tendons necessitates repair. Achilles tendon ruptures in the elderly or very sedentary can be treated conservatively in an equinus case, but most should undergo operative repair. Repair has been shown to decrease the rate of recurrence and increase the function of the Achilles tendon. Fortunately, tendons in the foot and ankle more commonly develop a tenosynovitis as a response to trauma. The treatment for a tenosynovitis is rest from provocative motion and anti-inflammatory medication, followed by physical therapy with gentle strengthening and stretching. Only after failure of conservative therapy should surgery be contemplated. Often minor trauma results in a tendinitis. Common sites in the foot and ankle are the Achilles tendon, peroneal tendons, and tibialis anterior and posterior. Tendinitis in the foot should be treated with complete rest of the affected tendon and anti-inflammatory medications. After 2 to 3 weeks of rest, changing shoes, using heel lifts, or using orthotics should be considered prior to resuming full activity. Corticosteroid injections should be avoided except as a last attempt to avoid surgery. If the conservative management already mentioned fails, surgery includes debridement and tenosynovectomy, and, rarely, tendon transfers.

### Fractures

*In the midfoot and forefoot, many fractures or subtle fracture dislocations are missed.*

Bony and joint injuries are also very common in the foot and ankle. All displaced ankle fractures, talus fractures, and calcaneus fractures should be referred immediately to a surgeon with experience in dealing with these injuries. It is the surgeon's duty to determine which injuries are stable and which require operative intervention. In children, these fractures can involve the growth plate, resulting in overgrowth or undergrowth of the affected physis. For this reason, children with these fractures should undergo consultation with an orthopedic surgeon early, even if the injuries appear stable. In the midfoot and forefoot, many fractures or subtle fracture dislocations are missed. Metatarsal fractures are very common and can cause prolonged disability if initially overlooked. The third metatarsal is the most commonly fractured and the fourth the least commonly fractured. If there is minimal displacement, most metatarsal fractures can be treated conservatively with cast immobilization or a rigid, hard-sole shoe and progressive weightbearing as tolerated. If there is displacement, operative fixation is warranted.

Beware of fractures involving the base of the fifth metatarsal. Typically, two types of fractures occur at that location. The most common is an avulsion fracture occurring in the metaphysis of the bone. If nondisplaced, this injury can be treated as other metatarsal fractures. The more uncommon injury is a transverse fracture at the metaphysis-diaphysis junction. This fracture, also known as a Jones fracture, has a propensity for nonunion. When recognized, this fracture should be immobilized in a cast. If there is any displacement, referral to a surgeon is warranted.

## SYMPTOMS

### Flatfoot (Pes Planus)

Patients can have a unilateral or bilateral pes planus for a number of reasons. Children often have a flexible flatfoot. As long as the foot is supple and nonpainful, a normal shoe with a well-built arch is all that is warranted. A child can also have a flatfoot secondary to tibial torsion or femoral anteversion. If a more proximal malrotation exists, an orthotic to correct the arch will help the rotation problem.

In adolescents, a flatfoot that has been more flexible and asymptomatic may become rigid and painful. Often minor trauma precedes the onset of symptoms. Rigid flatfeet tend to have more symptoms and lead to more disability. When a flatfoot becomes more rigid, the examiner should suspect a tarsal coalition. A *tarsal coalition*, or persistent union between the talus and navicular, calcaneus and talus, calcaneus and navicular, or (rarely) calcaneus and cuboid, can be the source of a fair amount of pain. The union can be fibrous, cartilaginous, or bony. The onset of symptoms in an adolescent often corresponds to the time when the tarsal coalition ossifies, thus making it more rigid. A suspected tarsal coalition can be diagnosed by a combination of plain x-rays, bone scanning, and computed tomography (CT) scanning.

The initial treatment of a symptomatic tarsal coalition includes immobilization for 6 weeks in a short-leg walking cast. An orthotic made of semirigid material that accommodates the foot only and does not try to re-establish an arch may be helpful. If symptoms persist, referral to a surgeon is advised. Depending on the type of coalition and the state of the surrounding joints, surgical options include resection of the coalition or fusion of the affected joints.

Patients can also develop a painful flatfoot secondary to injury to the posterior tibial tendon. The patient will complain of medial hindfoot pain. This pain is due to a tenosynovitis along the course of the posterior tibial tendon. With time, the tendon can become insufficient, leading to the development of a flatfoot. The initial treatment again is immobilization in a short-leg walking cast. The patient then graduates to an orthotic that supports the arch and keeps the hindfoot in neutral. If the patient continues to have difficulties, surgical options include tendon debridement, tendon transfers, or bony osteotomies to correct the condition. In advanced cases, arthrodeses of the affected joints may have to be considered.

Finally, patients can develop a flatfoot secondary to degenerative arthritis in the midfoot, which collapses. Pain at palpation and crepitus will be noted along the midfoot. Appropriate anti-inflammatory medications and orthotics will often give relief temporarily. A rocker-bottom sole can be added to the shoe to decrease motion across the affected joints and often will result in an increased ability to perform activities of daily living. When symptoms warrant it, a surgical fusion of the affected joints will often provide significant pain relief.

### Heel Pain

Heel pain is a problem that continues to increase in frequency. Patients often complain of severe pain or burning with the first several steps of the day or after prolonged sitting. The pain then eases but does not disappear. Heel pain has several causes. The most common is plantar fasciitis. The plantar fascia can become inflamed when initial footstrike occurs not on the plantar fat pad but more distally at the origin of the plantar fascia. This can occur with a tight heel cord, which is found in the vast majority of patients complaining of heel pain. Heel pain can also be caused by calcaneal spurs or by entrapment of a small nerve supplying the adductor digiti quinti muscle, but these causes are less common.

The treatment for heel pain should be conservative, and 80% to 90% of patients should have complete recovery. Initially, treatment is with anti-inflammatory medication and an aggressive heel cord-stretching program. Until the tight heel cord is stretched back to length, symptoms will not improve. Hard heel cups, designed to contain the plantar fat pad under the weight-bearing axis, can also be beneficial. On occasion, patients may benefit from a soft foot orthosis, designed to relieve pressure under the insertion of the plantar fascia. Corticosteroid injections rarely, if ever, provide long-lasting relief of chronic heel pain. Only 10% to 20% of patients with heel pain will ever require surgery. Surgical referral for heel pain should be sought only after the patient has failed conservative care for at least 6 months. If the heel cord has not been sufficiently lengthened, results from surgery will be just as disappointing as those of the conservative care that preceded it.

*Until the tight heel cord is stretched back to length, heel pain will not improve.*

### When to Call the Surgeon about General Foot Problems

- Intractable foot pain
- Diabetic foot infection
- Nonhealing foot ulcer (may be vascular etiology)
- Fractures

# Foot and Ankle Procedures for the Primary Care Practitioner

## DIGITAL BLOCK

A digital block may be needed for treatment of ingrown toenail or other surgical procedures. Fig. 21–7 shows that there are both superficial and deep digital nerves that need to be anesthetized. Our preferred technique is to use a medial and lateral approach. Enter the skin at the 5 o'clock position, infiltrate the inferior nerve close to the bone, and slowly tract out to the skin. While the needle is still under the skin but very superficial, redirect it superiorly and medially; the superior superficial nerve is infiltrated and a field block is simultaneously performed. The same procedure is then done on the opposite side of the digit, entering at 7 o'clock. We recommend using a 5 mL syringe, an appropriate anesthetic *without* epinephrine, and a 25- or 27-gauge, ⅜ inch-long needle. We suggest placing 0.75 to 1.0 mL at each digital nerve.

## INGROWN TOENAIL REMOVAL

Ingrown toenails commonly occur because an embedded nail or a spicule of nail hooks into the nail groove, leading to local inflammation that may become secondarily infected. In mild cases, soaking, antibiotics, and elevation of the nail margin from the nail groove may prove successful. In more severe cases, surgical removal of the embedded nail is indicated. The key to success with nail removal is to have adequate anesthesia and the proper equipment. Using block anesthesia, a tourniquet is applied if the patient has adequate vascular supply to create a bloodless surgical field. With standard sterile techniques, English nail nippers are used to cut an incision down the entire nail into the insertion of the nail. Using a nail elevator, the excised nail is popped out and easily withdrawn with a hemostat. Exuberant granulation tissue, if present, is removed using a scalpel. If a matrixectomy is to be performed, we recommend removing the germinal nail matrix by scraping down to periosteum using a bone curette. Afterward, a nonadherent dressing is applied to the wound edge, the tourniquet is released, and a pressure compression dressing is applied to control bleeding.

## ANKLE TAPING

Ankle taping may be useful in preventing ankle sprains and is recommended for up to 6 months after a first degree lateral ankle sprain. Our preferred method is to use heavy

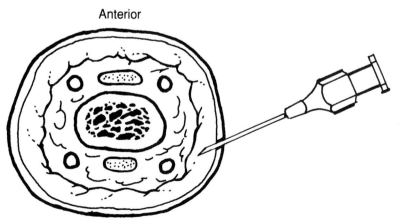

Anterior

Posterior

FIGURE 21–7
Both superficial and deep digital nerves need to be anesthetized.

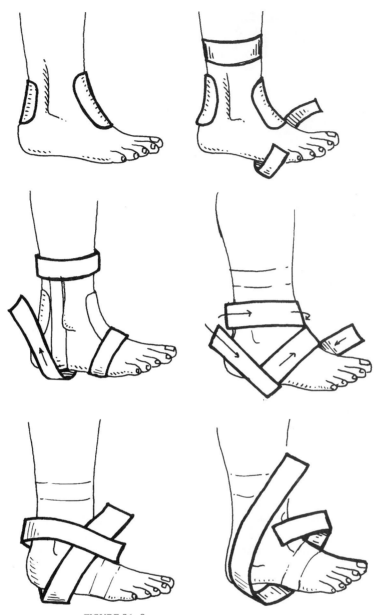

**FIGURE 21–8**
Ankle taping following a lateral inversion sprain.

athletic tape, 1½ inches wide. After skin shaving and with the ankle dorsiflexed, apply heel and lace pads. Next, apply two circumferential anchor strips at the midfoot and approximately 6 to 8 inches above the ankle mortise (Fig. 21–8). Then apply three to six stirrup strips, starting medially, passing under the heel and ending laterally. Then apply two or three heel locks in each direction, starting laterally across the tibia just above the medial malleolus. Pass behind the ankle along the lateral calcaneus and under the foot; then pass over the top of the forefoot. The process is reversed for a medial heel lock. Start at the top of the forefoot, cross in front of the lateral malleolus, go downward under the calcaneus and up behind the medial malleolus; then cross the Achilles tendon and continue to the top of the forefoot. Apply two or three figure-eight strips to force the foot into slight foot eversion. This is done by starting the tape at the medial malleolus, passing the tape under the foot and up the outside of the foot, and then going up and around the foot and then the lower leg. Finally, anchor the components with fill-in strips placed circumferentially, working up from the figure-eight strip.

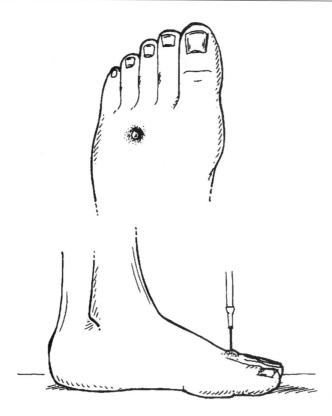

**FIGURE 21–9**
Interdigital neuroma block. Being able to palpate the neuroma increases the probability of success by this technique.

## INTERDIGITAL NEUROMA BLOCK

Injection of an interdigital neuroma may give significant relief to patients who fail to improve with conservative treatment or who have moderate pain on initial presentation. Being able to palpate the neuroma increases the probability of success by this technique (Fig. 21–9). First, localize the neuroma on the *plantar* surface between the metatarsal heads. Then place your fingers on the dorsal surface superior to the neuroma and mark this spot. After prep, use ethylchloride spray to anesthetize the skin. Enter the neuroma and inject directly at 90° 1 cc of steroid and 1 cc of local anesthetic premixed, using a 25-gauge needle.

## PLANTAR FASCIA INJECTION

Injection of plantar fascia near the insertion of the calcaneus (i.e., heel spur) can be quite helpful to treat plantar fasciitis if the diagnosis is correct and the underlying biomechanical problems have been adequately treated. We favor the medial approach rather than the inferior approach because the skin is less callused and therefore injections appear to be less painful. After prepping the area and spraying with ethylchloride, inject from the medial side toward the point of maximal tenderness (usually ¾ inch distal to the origin of the plantar fascia, between the fascia and the calcaneus). Inject 1 cc of steroid and 1 cc of local anesthetic premixed, using a 1½-inch, 25-gauge needle.

## SINUS TARSI INJECTION

The subtalar joint (talocalcaneal joint) is prone to arthritis and may respond to steroid injection. Palpate the sinus tarsi tunnel (Fig. 21–10) by palpating the depression just

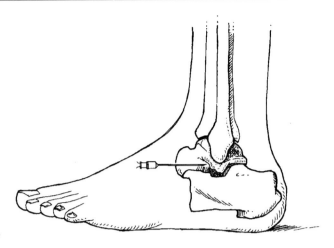

FIGURE 21–10
The subtalar joint (talocalcaneal joint).

below the tip of the lateral malleolus and 1 cm anterior with the ankle passively inverted 15°. Inject 1 cc of steroid and 1 cc of local anesthetic premixed, using a 1½-inch, 22-gauge needle.

## TIBIOTALAR ASPIRATION AND INJECTION

The ankle joint may need to be aspirated for diagnostic purposes or injected with steroids for symptomatic relief of osteoarthritis. Have the patient dorsiflex the great toe to locate the large extensor hallucis longus tendon. Palpate the joint line (tibiotalar) just medial to this landmark. Prepare the site and, using sterile technique, inject local anesthetic, angling the needle 30° from midline, keeping the syringe parallel to the ground, as shown in Fig. 21–11. Aspirate the synovial fluid using a 20-cc syringe and a large-bore (20- or 18-gauge) needle. If steroids are to be injected, use a hemostat to hold the needle after aspiration, change syringes, and inject 3 to 5 cc of steroid. If only injecting and not aspirating, using a 22-gauge needle is less painful and equally effective.

FIGURE 21–11
Tibiotalar aspiration or injection.

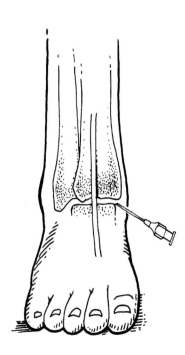

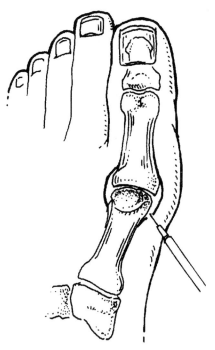

**FIGURE 21–12**
Aspiration or injection of the first metatarsophalangeal (MTP) joint. Enter medially on the metatarsal side of the joint line.

## ASPIRATION AND INJECTION OF THE FIRST MTP JOINT

Gout and osteoarthritis are both associated with pain in the first MTP joint. Synovial analysis can help differentiate these two conditions and tailor therapy appropriately. Also, steroid injection may improve symptoms. Enter medially on the metatarsal side of the joint line (Fig. 21–12). Use a ⅝-inch, 21-gauge needle to aspirate and a 25-gauge needle for injection only. The usual depth is ⅜ inch to ½ inch, depending on swelling. Use 1 to 2 mL of anesthetic and 0.25 mL of steroid.

## RECOMMENDED READING

Hoppenfeld, S: Physical Examination of the Spine and Extremities. Appleton-Century-Crofts Publishers, Norwalk, Connecticut, 1976.

Mann, RA, and Coughlin, MJ: Surgery of the Foot, ed 4. CV Mosby, St. Louis, Missouri, 1995.

# Chapter 22

# Skin Lesions

CHENICHERI BALAKRISHNAN, MD,
and JASON CHAO, MD

Because skin is the largest organ of the body, the variety of skin lesions exceeds that of any other organ. Deciding which skin tumors are benign or malignant can be challenging.

Pathophysiology of skin lesions is related to both environmental and genetic factors. Exposure to a variety of chemicals contained in coal tar, pitch, soot, and petroleum products has been recognized as a cause of skin cancer. Prolonged sun exposure, creosote oil, arsenicals, and radiation are also implicated in the production of skin tumors. Although patients often give a history of injury to explain a skin tumor, the validity is often difficult to substantiate. The tendency to develop some skin tumors may be genetically determined, but their appearance may be delayed until puberty. Certain skin tumors, like multiple neurofibromatoses and nevoid basal cell epitheliomas, follow a direct hereditary pattern.

Medical treatment can be helpful for many skin lesions. If there is doubt in the diagnosis—particularly if a malignancy is considered in the differential diagnosis of a lesion—the primary care provider should perform a biopsy. Treatment of large lesions that are not amenable to primary closure and defects after Moh's surgery should be carried out by a specialist, as should dermabrasion, laser treatment, and radiation.

*If there is doubt in the diagnosis, a biopsy should be performed by the primary care provider.*

## Common Dermatologic Procedures

### INCISION AND DRAINAGE

Incision and drainage are limited to infected cysts and abscesses because attempted removal of an infected cyst results in recurrence and depressed scars. An incision is made over the most fluctuant area. The cavity is drained and lightly packed to control bleeding.

## CURETTAGE

Removal of a lesion under local anesthesia using a small curette leaves a flat surface that will re-epithelialize in a few days. This procedure is useful for removal of small flat or moderately raised lesions. The specimen can be analyzed histologically for malignant changes. Electrocautery should be used as little as possible to prevent excessive scarring.

## EXCISION

A skin lesion can be removed by excising it along with a minimal amount of normal skin around it. The specimen can be examined histologically for diagnosis and excision margins. The excised specimen should be marked for orienting the anatomic margins for the pathologist. The method commonly used is to place a suture at the 12 o'clock position and draw a figure on the pathology request form. All excisions of skin lesions should follow skin tension lines, especially on the face. Office surgery can be used for excision of lesions that can be repaired without distortion of the anatomy. Excision of large lesions that require a local flap or skin graft is best carried out by a surgeon.

## BIOPSY

Small lesions can be subjected to excision biopsy and, if small enough, can be entirely removed with a punch biopsy. If lesions are large, an incisional biopsy or a punch biopsy should be carried out. The biopsy should be from a suspicious area, typically near the border, in order to prevent sampling error. An incisional biopsy does not increase the chances of spread of a malignant tumor. Conversely, it prevents unnecessarily wide excisions of benign lesions.

## CRYOSURGERY

Many large superficial lesions can be removed by briefly freezing them. However, biopsy should be considered before cryotherapy of any lesion in which malignancy, especially melanoma, is considered. Liquid nitrogen or nitrous oxide commonly has been used for cryosurgery. Freezing can be combined with curettage. The cure rate is related to the size of the tumor. An absolute contraindication for cryosurgery is intolerance to cold, as in cryoglobulinemia and the morphea type of basal cell carcinoma.

## *Benign Neoplasms and Hyperplastic Lesions*

### VERRUCA VULGARIS

The common wart (*verruca vulgaris*) (Fig. 22–1*A*) is caused by a papillomavirus. It is found on the surface of the skin, in the vagina and rectum, and infrequently on the oral mucosa. Since warts are benign lesions that tend to regress spontaneously, the primary care provider should strive for minimal destruction of normal tissue, thereby reducing the scarring. Treatment modalities for warts include local application of acids, cryotherapy, cauterization, laser ablation, immunotherapy, and excision. Extensive perineal warts (Figure 22–1*B*) or recalcitrant plantar warts require surgical consultation.

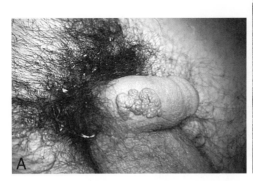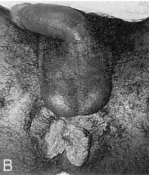

**FIGURE 22–1**
(*A*) Verruca vulgaris. (*B*) Perineal wart (condyloma). See color photographs in Color Section 2.

## Seborrheic Keratosis

*Seborrheic keratoses* (Fig. 22–2) present in middle-aged and older patients as a light- to dark-brown raised papular lesion on the face, on the neck, on the thorax, and over the dorsum of the hands. The surface of the lesion varies from smooth to wart-like and may be pedunculated. Although the cause is unknown, there is a familial predisposition with an autosomal mode of inheritance. The *Leser-Trélat sign* is the sudden eruption of seborrheic keratoses with an internal malignancy. As seborrheic keratosis and most kinds of cancer occur in older persons, some investigators express caution in linking the temporal association of the two. The differentiation of flat seborrheic keratosis from senile lentigo, a form of melanoma, may be difficult without a biopsy.

## Epidermal Nevus

An *epidermal nevus* is a circumscribed anomaly caused by the overproduction of surface or adnexal epithelium present at birth or shortly thereafter. They may be associated with other congenital defects. The individual lesions are flesh colored and favor the extremities. Epidermal nevi grow for a variable period of time and then become quiescent. Rarely has basal cell epithelioma developed from pre-existing epidermal nevi.

**FIGURE 22–2**
Seborrheic keratosis. See Color Section 2.

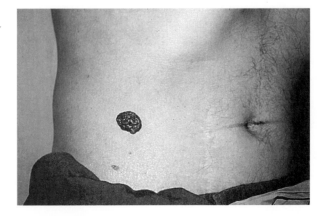

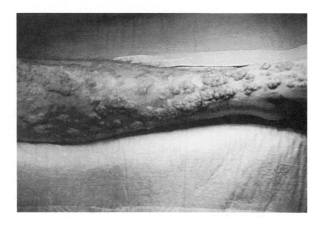

**FIGURE 22–3**
Linear nevus. See Color Section 2.

## INFLAMMATORY LINEAR VERRUCOUS EPIDERMAL NEVUS

*Inflammatory linear verrucous epidermal nevus* (Fig. 22–3) is a pruritic, erythematous verrucous lesion present at birth or appearing before puberty. It is commonly seen on the lower extremities and may be disfiguring. Treatment is excision with primary closure or skin grafting.

## KERATOACANTHOMA

*Keratoacanthomas* (Fig. 22–4) are self-healing, rapidly developing, benign epithelial tumors. They are rare in Asians and individuals under 20 years of age and may be mistaken for squamous cell carcinoma. Spontaneous regression may result in a disfiguring scar. Treatment in suspicious cases is by excisional biopsy.

## COMMON MELANOCYTIC NEVUS (MOLE)

*Melanocytic nevocellular nevi* (Fig. 22–5) are small (<1.0 cm), circumscribed, acquired pigmented macules or papules made up of groups of melanocytic nevus cells located in the epidermis, dermis, or both. They are named accordingly as:

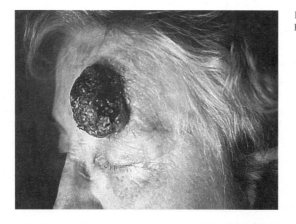

**FIGURE 22–4**
Keratoacanthoma. See Color Section 2.

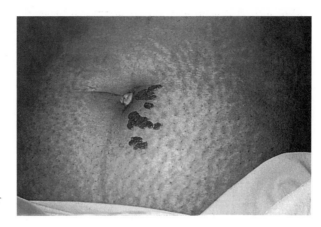

**FIGURE 22-5**
Common melanocytic nevi. See Color Section 2.

I. Junctional melanocytic nevus: cells at the dermoepidermal junction above the basement membrane

II. Dermal melanocytic nevus: cells exclusively in the dermis

III. Compound melanocytic nevus: a combination of the histologic features of the junctional and dermal nevi.

## GIANT HAIRY NEVUS

*Giant hairy nevi* (Fig. 22-6) are rare, large, disfiguring congenital nevi affecting the torso. They are also called "garment" or "bathing trunk" nevi. The incidence of melanoma in this type of nevus ranges from 8% to 10%. Staged excision with skin grafting is recommended.

## HALO NEVOMELANOCYTIC NEVUS

*Halo nevomelanocytic nevi* (Fig. 22-7) are pigmented nevi encircled by a halo of leukoderma. The leukoderma is caused by a decrease in melanin in the melanocytes at the dermoepidermal junction. These lesions usually undergo spontaneous resolution. A high proportion of patients with these lesions, like patients with melanoma, have circulating antibodies against melanoma cells.

**FIGURE 22-6**
Giant hairy cell nevus. See Color Section 2.

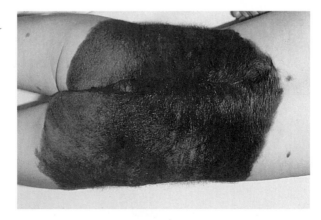

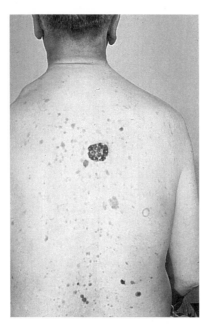

FIGURE 22–7
Halo nevus. See Color Section 2.

## COMMON BLUE NEVUS

A *blue nevus* is an acquired benign, firm, dark-blue to black, sharply defined papule or nodule caused by a localized proliferation of dermal melanocytes.

## SPITZ NEVUS

*Spindle and epithelioid nevus (juvenile melanoma, spitz nevus)* is a clinically benign, histologically malignant-appearing nevus that occurs frequently in childhood. Eosinophilic globules, which are presumably degenerated nevus cells or keratinocytes, may help differentiate these lesions from melanoma.

FIGURE 22–8
Nevus sebaceous of Jadassohn. See Color Section 2.

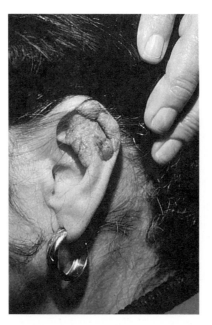

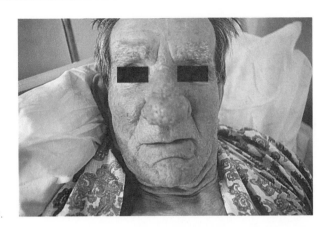

**FIGURE 22–9**
Rhinophyma. See Color Section 2.

## NEVUS SEBACEOUS

*Nevus sebaceous* of Jadassohn (Fig. 22–8) evolves through several stages and may be associated with a range of skin tumors. They appear at or soon after birth, usually on the head and neck. With puberty, these lesions become thickened and verrucous. The reported incidence of basal cell epithelioma arising from these nevi ranges from 6.5% to 50%. Suspicious lesions should be subjected to excision biopsy.

## RHINOPHYMA

Although various etiologies have been suggested for *rhinophyma*, including alcohol ingestion and acne, no consistent causative factor has been identified. Most investigators agree that rhinophyma represents a severe stage of acne rosacea. There may be an increase in the number and size of sebaceous glands, accompanied by an increase in the amount of dermal collagen present (Fig. 22–9). Dermabrasion is a useful technique if acne medications, especially erythromycin, are ineffective. In advanced cases, the nose may be shaved down to normal size and allowed to re-epithelialize.

## CYLINDROMA

*Cylindromas* (Fig. 22–10) are benign adnexal tumors, multiple when inherited as an autosomal dominant or solitary when nonfamilial. Clinically these tumors appear as

**FIGURE 22–10**
Cylindroma. See Color Section 2.

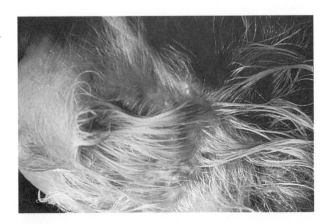

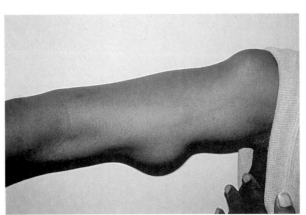
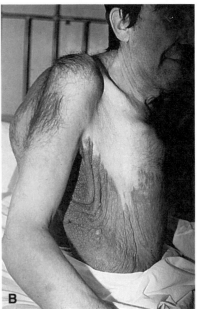

**FIGURE 22–11**
Neurofibroma. (*A*) von Recklinghausen's disease. (*B*) Plexiform neurofibroma. See Color Section 2.

smooth, firm, pink dermal tumors measuring a few millimeters to a few centimeters in size. They may even cover the entire scalp. The origin of these tumors is controversial. They may ulcerate or even undergo malignant transformation. Excision, including excision of the entire scalp, has been used to cure these unusual tumors.

## NEUROFIBROMA

*Neurofibromas* are benign encapsulated growths of the multicellular elements of peripheral nerves. They may occur as multiple lesions, as in von Recklinghausen's disease (Fig. 22–11*A*). Plexiform lesions (Fig. 22–11*B*) are locally invasive and may cause significant deformity. Sudden increase in size and severe localized pain is seen in malignant transformation. Treatment of symptomatic lesions is by surgical resection.

## LIPOMA

*Lipomas* are fatty tumors that are soft, generally lobulated, and well encapsulated (Fig. 22–12). Because there may be fluctuation on palpation, they may be difficult to differ-

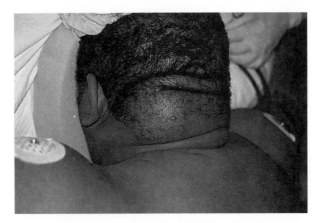

**FIGURE 22–12**
Lipoma. See Color Section 2.

entiate from hemangiomas. Most lipomas require no treatment unless there are other symptoms or they show signs of growth.

# Hemangiomas and Vascular Malformations

Vascular tumors are classified, based on endothelial characteristics, into hemangiomas and vascular malformations. *Hemangiomas* are vascular tumors that enlarge by rapid cellular proliferation followed by involution. *Vascular malformations* are congenital abnormalities with a normal rate of endothelial cell turnover.

## PORT-WINE STAIN

*Port-wine stains* (Fig. 22–13) are capillary malformations characterized by ectatic vessels in the dermis. These stains are pink to purple and macular, and they blanch completely with pressure. The most common site is the face, and many facial lesions have a quasidermatomal distribution. About 5% of patients with port-wine stain have the Sturge-Weber syndrome, vascular malformations of the upper facial dermis, choroid plexus, and ipsilateral meninges. There may be associated overgrowth of connective tissue and skeleton, causing midfacial hypertrophy and focal or generalized seizures. Port-wine stains grow proportionately with the child and do not regress. Treatment using lasers produces favorable results.

## HEMANGIOMA

*Hemangiomas* (Fig. 22–14) are common tumors of infancy, usually not present at birth. Most appear within the first 2 or 3 months of life. They expand beyond the child's growth, with the rapid growth phase lasting 3 to 6 months. Most lesions occur on the head and neck. Capillary or strawberry hemangiomas usually occur in the dermis. Cavernous hemangiomas are ill defined, occurring in the subcutaneous tissue. Potential complications are ulceration and bleeding. With ulceration, secondary infection may occur. Certain hemangiomas in infants may be associated with thrombocytopenic purpura, known as Kasabach-Merritt syndrome. Clinical indications for treatment of hem-

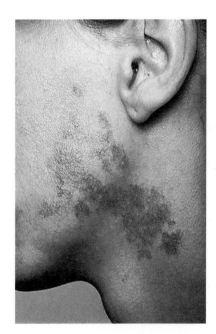

**FIGURE 22–13**
Port-wine stain. See Color Section 2.

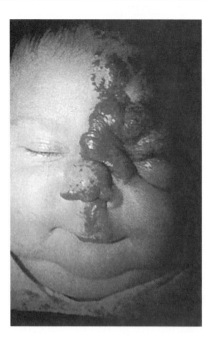

**FIGURE 22–14**
Hemangioma. See Color Section 2.

angiomas are impairment of vision, bleeding, coagulopathy, ulceration, and infection. Rapidly growing hemangiomas of infancy can be treated successfully with intralesional and oral corticosteroid. Surgery is usually used for correction of residual deformity and incompletely resolved lesions. Laser surgery has been useful in inducing early regression of hemangiomas.

## SENILE ANGIOMA

*Senile angiomas* (Fig. 22–15) are also known as cherry angiomas or De Morgan spots. Multiple domed, red to purple lesions measuring 1 to 3 mm usually appear over the trunk and proximal extremities. Following initial enlargement, these lesions persist indefinitely without change. They require no treatment. Although not necessarily related to old age, they do not appear until adulthood.

## PYOGENIC GRANULOMA

A *pyogenic granuloma* (Fig. 22–16) is an acquired, solitary lesion occurring in any area and at any age, although the greatest tendency is in childhood. Despite its name, it is

**FIGURE 22–15**
Senile angioma. See Color Section 2.

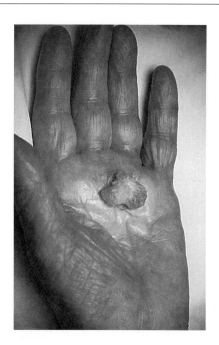

**FIGURE 22-16**
Pyogenic granuloma. See Color Section 2.

not an infective process. It usually begins as a small, erythematous papule that rapidly enlarges. It is usually friable, and minor trauma may produce considerable bleeding. After removal or destruction of a solitary lesion, multiple satellite lesions can form around the original treatment site. Pyogenic granulomas may be excised or treated with laser or electrocautery. They may recur after incomplete removal.

## DERMATOFIBROMA

*Dermatofibroma* is one of the most common benign dermal tumors of the skin seen on the extremities, especially on the legs of women. They are small and vary in color from skin-colored to dusky brown. Sometimes they are black and may be confused with melanoma. The histogenesis of dermatofibroma is controversial. Recurrence can be seen if the lesions extend into the subcutis.

## FIBROMATOSIS

*Fibromatosis* is a group of disorders involving the fibroblasts. The most common such disorder seen in adults is the Dupuytren's contracture affecting the palm (Fig. 22-17). These tend to recur after excision. Recurrent cases may require excision with replace-

**FIGURE 22-17**
Dupuytren's contracture. See Color Section 2.

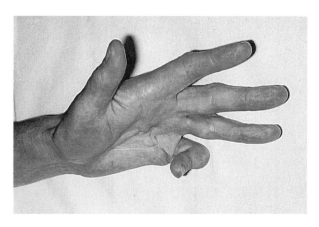

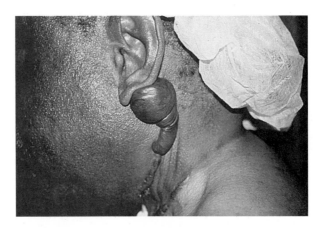

**FIGURE 22–18**
Keloids. See Color Section 2.

ment of skin. Surgery should be carried out by a specialist trained in hand surgery to prevent damage to the neurovascular bundles.

## HYPERTROPHIC SCARS AND KELOIDS

*Pressure, silicone gel, steroids, surgery, and radiation have been used as treatment modalities for keloid scars.*

*Hypertrophic scars* are wide, red, uniformly elevated scars. *Keloid scars* are wide, raised scars that continue to grow beyond the limits of the original scar (Fig. 22–18). The exact etiology of the keloid scar is unknown. Pressure, silicone gel, steroids, surgery, and radiation have been used as treatment modalities for keloid scars.

# *Mucocutaneous Cysts and Pseudocysts*

## EPIDERMOID CYST

*Epidermoid cysts* (Fig. 22–19) are common cysts lined by squamous epithelium. They vary in size and affect both sexes equally. They may be single or multiple and usually cause no symptoms unless secondarily infected. These cysts are benign, but rare malignancy has been described.

## EPIDERMAL INCLUSION CYST

An *epidermal inclusion cyst* (Fig. 22–20) is usually secondary to traumatic implantation of epidermis within the dermis. These cysts contain thick, dense keratin and commonly

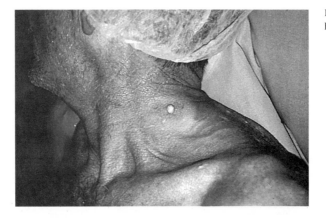

**FIGURE 22–19**
Epidermoid cyst. See Color Section 2.

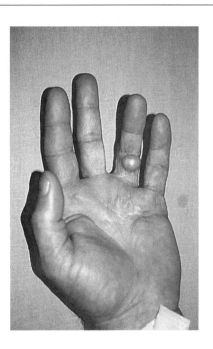

FIGURE 22–20
Epidermal inclusion cyst. See Color Section 2.

affect the palms and soles. Secondary infection may occur in these cysts. Treatment is excision if the cysts become infected or are otherwise symptomatic.

## GANGLION CYST

The *ganglion cyst* (Fig. 22–21) is the most common tumor found in the hand. Ganglion cysts are commonly seen over the dorsum of the wrist, the radial aspect of the wrist close to the radial artery, and at the base of the volar aspect of the fingers. The most common complaint is pain. They originate in the connective tissue near joints. The most popular nonoperative modalities include cyst rupture by external compression with a heavy book and needle aspiration, but recurrence is common. Large symptomatic cysts require excision.

## DIGITAL MUCOUS CYST

A *digital mucous cyst* (Fig. 22–22) is a pseudocyst occurring over the distal interphalangeal joint of the finger. Extrusion of mucin from the underlying joint is believed to

FIGURE 22–21
Wrist ganglion. See Color Section 2.

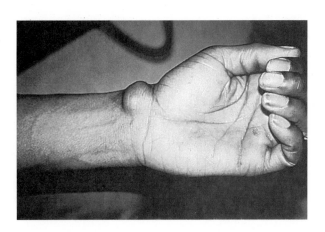

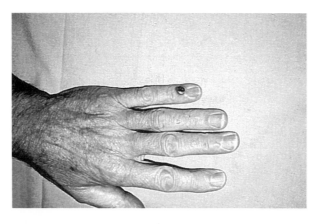

**FIGURE 22–22**
Digital mucous cyst. See Color Section 2.

be the cause. They are solitary with no true cyst lining and may cause nail dystrophy. Recurrence is common after excision.

## HIDRADENITIS

*Hidradenitis* (Fig. 22–23) is an inflammatory disease of the apocrine glands. It is seen most commonly in young adults. The most frequent site is the axilla, but the groin and perineum can also be involved. Early acute phases can be treated with local wound care and antibiotics. An abscess will require incision and drainage with long-term antibiotic therapy because of chronic infection of surrounding glands. Progression to the chronic stage of the disease will require wide excision of the involved area. This disease may recur and may involve multiple sites (e.g., both axilla and groin).

## ACNE VULGARIS

*Acne vulgaris* is a common disorder of the adolescent and young adult. The lesions are small comedones and cysts, which may become secondarily infected. The disease can be severe, with deep cysts and chronic infection causing severe facial scarring. Millions of dollars are spent on over-the-counter treatments. Topical antimicrobial agents, topical or systemic retinoids, and careful skin hygiene, combined with long-term systemic antibiotics, have been helpful in controlling the disease. Although cosmetic makeup helps to camouflage acne scarring, dermabrasion is used for the most recalcitrant cases.

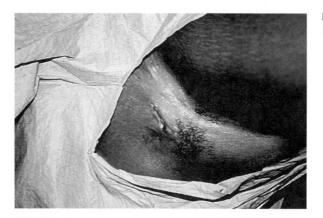

**FIGURE 22–23**
Hidradenitis. See Color Section 2.

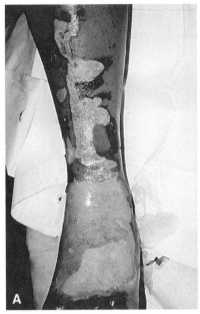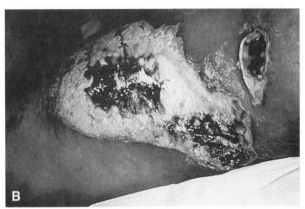

**FIGURE 22-24**
Thermal injuries. See Color Section 2.

## Thermal Injuries

As the largest organ of the body, skin is subjected to the effect of sun, flame, cold, and chemicals. Burns (Fig. 22-24) are common and cause considerable pain and suffering. In *first-degree burns* only the epidermal layer is injured; these heal without any scarring. In *second-degree burns* the epidermis and part of the dermis is injured. These include superficial partial-thickness burns, in which the epidermis and a thin layer of dermis is destroyed, and deep partial-thickness burns, in which the epidermis and most of the dermis are injured. The deep dermis, although injured, will provide tissue for spontaneous healing if protected. In full-thickness or *third-degree burns*, epidermis, dermis, subcutaneous tissue, and possibly muscle are damaged. Spontaneous healing is not possible owing to the loss of all skin appendages, so skin grafting is necessary.

Because fluid is lost from the body through the burn wound, burn patients require fluid resuscitation. Children with burns over more than 10% of their body surface; adults with burns over 20% of their body surface; patients with burns of the face, hands, feet, or perineum; patients with electrical or chemical burns; and patients with smoke inhalation injury should be transferred to a burn center. Burn patients with any significant injury should be referred to a specialist. Wound care is important to prevent wound infection and sepsis. Commonly used topical antimicrobials are silver sulfadiazine, mafenide, nitrofurazone (Furacin), and bacitracin ointment. Minor second-degree partial-thickness burns should be debrided nonsurgically and treated with topical microbials. Deep burns require surgical debridement and skin grafting.

*Children with over 10% body surface area burn; adults with over 20% body surface area burn; patients with burns of the face, hands, feet, or perineum; patients with electrical or chemical burns; and patients with smoke inhalation injury should be transferred to a burn center.*

### When to Call the Surgeon about Burn Injuries

- Major burns involving more than 20% of body surface in adults and more than 10% of body surface in children
- Third-degree burns
- Burns involving face, hands, feet, or perineum

- Burns associated with inhalation injury
- Infected burns
- Electrical and chemical injuries
- Burns associated with abuse or neglect

## *Premalignant Lesions*

### SOLAR KERATOSIS

*Actinic keratosis* or *solar keratosis* is the most common premalignant skin tumor. These lesions are seen in older people with sun-damaged skin. They are irregular, scaly lesions with surrounding erythema. Histologically they may vary from cellular atypia to carcinoma in situ. Left untreated, actinic keratosis may progress to squamous cell carcinoma. The incidence of malignant transformation is debated. Some of these lesions may undergo spontaneous regression. Treatment modalities include curettage, cryosurgery, chemotherapy with topical fluorouracil (5-FU), laser ablation, and excision.

> • ▬▬
> *Left untreated, actinic keratosis may progress to squamous cell carcinoma.*

### LEUKOPLAKIA

*Leukoplakia* are white patches or plaques of varying appearance that do not rub off easily. They are more common in men and in older persons. Although the exact cause is unknown, external irritants can influence location. Biopsy and histologic examination divide them into dysplastic and nondysplastic categories, depending on cellular atypia. Treatment is by removal of any causative factor, along with excision, electrodesiccation, or carbon dioxide laser.

### BOWEN'S DISEASE

*Bowen's disease* (Fig. 22–25) is characterized by cutaneous plaques of intraepidermal squamous cell carcinoma secondary to chronic sun exposure. These occur in older adults with fair complexion. They appear as a solitary lesion in two-thirds of patients and slowly enlarge in most cases. Five percent evolve into invasive squamous cell carcinoma. Histologic examination can differentiate this disease between hyperkeratosis and parakeratosis. The dermis usually shows a heavy inflammatory infiltrate. Treatment is by surgical excision, curettage, or electrodesiccation.

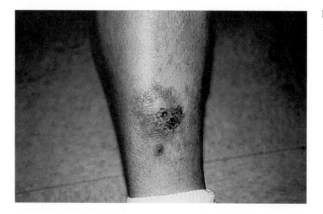

FIGURE 22–25
Bowen's disease. See Color Section 2.

# *Malignant Tumors*

## BASAL CELL CARCINOMA

*Basal cell carcinoma* (BCC) (Fig. 22–26) is the most common malignant skin tumor affecting white people. BCC arises from the basal cells of the surface epidermis or the external sheath of the hair follicle. It is uncommon among black and Asian people. Sun exposure plays an important role in the cause, and the highest incidence is on the face. Arsenicals, x-ray exposure, burns, and vaccinations have been implicated in the cause. Clinical forms of basal cell carcinoma are superficial, cystic, noduloulcerative, pigmented, and sclerosing (morphea-like). *Noduloulcerative BCC* typically appears as a single, pearly papule with telangiectatic vessels across the surface. These lesions are seen most frequently on the face. They enlarge slowly and if neglected will ulcerate (rodent ulcer). These lesions can erode through nose, eyes, and skull. *Superficial BCC* is often multiple and commonly affects the trunk. *Pigmented BCC* can mimic melanoma. The *sclerotic* type presents as a depressed sclerotic plaque without a distinct border.

A number of therapeutic modalities such as surgery, radiation, electrosurgery and curettage, and Moh's surgery have been used to cure BCC. Moh's surgery (microscopically controlled surgery) is helpful for lesions where tissue preservation is required—as on the eyelid, ear, or nose—and for recurrent lesions or lesions with poorly defined borders. Topical 5-fluorouracil may be effective with curettage. Small BCCs may be excised by the primary care provider. If lesions are large or the excision is incomplete, the patient should be referred to a specialist.

## SQUAMOUS CELL CARCINOMA

Squamous cell carcinoma (SCC) (Fig. 22–27) arises from the epidermal keratinocytes. The causative factors for this disease include solar exposure, x-ray therapy, nitrogen mustard, chimney soot (Percivall Pott), xeroderma pigmentosa, albinism, and chronic skin lesions (Marjolin's ulcer, discussed next). An increased incidence of SCC has been seen in organ transplant patients, which raises the question of the relationship of immunosuppression and skin cancers. SCC commonly occurs in sun-exposed areas, with surrounding skin showing actinic change. SCC of the lower lip usually is related to sun exposure or pipe smoking. The measure of malignancy may be judged by invasiveness and ability to metastasize. Metastatic spread is usually to the regional lymph nodes. Occasionally SCC may be difficult to differentiate clinically from keratoacanthoma and BCC.

Three methods of treatment are available for SCC: radiation, excision, and Moh's

*Occasionally squamous cell carcinoma may be difficult to differentiate clinically from keratoacanthoma and basal cell carcinoma.*

**FIGURE 22–26**
Basal cell carcinoma. See Color Section 2.

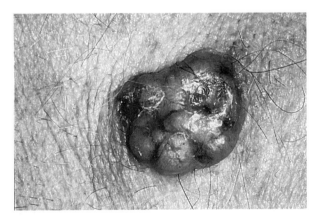

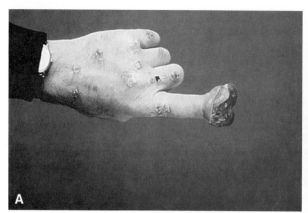
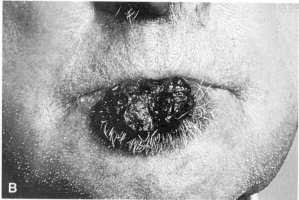

**FIGURE 22–27**
Squamous cell carcinoma. See Color Section 2.

surgery. Cure depends on early recognition and aggressive treatment. Suspicious lesions should be subjected to biopsy. SCC may be reported in biopsy specimens done by the primary care provider. Oncology consultation should be obtained for further management.

## MARJOLIN'S ULCER

Neoplastic changes in scar tissue of chronically ulcerating wounds are commonly known as *Marjolin's ulcer*. These lesions consist of malignant, verrucous ulceration occurring in chronic scar tissue or at the epithelial edge of a chronic benign ulcer. They have been reported following burns, chronic venous stasis ulcers, osteomyelitis, urinary fistulae, and chronic hidradenitis suppurativa and at skin-graft donor sites. These primary lesions have a varying incidence of metastatic spread and twice the incidence when on a lower extremity. If suspicious, multiple incision biopsies of the lesion should be carried out. Wide excision is the treatment of choice.

## MALIGNANT MELANOMA

*Cutaneous melanomas* (Fig. 22–28) arise from the melanocytic system. Although the incidence is equal between sexes, mortality is higher in men. Risk factors for melanoma (Table 22–1) include white race, a family history, phenotype (blue eyes, blonde hair, light complexion), increased number of nevocytic nevi, and sun sensitivity. Genetic factors are especially important; persons with a family history of melanoma have more than a 10-fold risk of developing the disease themselves. Patients with familial dysplastic syndrome (an autosomal dominant trait) also have a much higher risk of developing melanoma than the general population. Familial melanoma is usually diagnosed when patients are 10 to 20 years younger than melanoma in those with no such family history. Pregnant patients have a significantly shorter disease-free interval. Although the incidence of regional lymph node metastasis is higher in pregnant patients, survival rate is similar to that of nonpregnant patients. Standard surgical treatment is advised in pregnant patients with melanoma.

The early recognition of malignant melanoma is the key to possible cure. The American Academy of Dermatology stresses the mnemonic "ABCD" for evaluating any pigmented lesion (Table 22–2). Melanoma should be considered when there is change in color, size, or surface characteristics, or there are symptoms like itching and development of satellite lesions. Most melanomas have an initial radial growth phase, during

*Melanoma should be considered when there is change in color, size, or surface characteristics, or symptoms like itching and development of satellite lesions.*

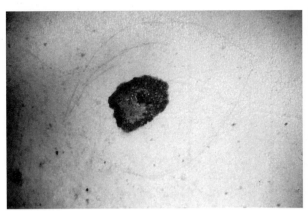
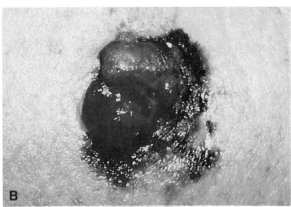
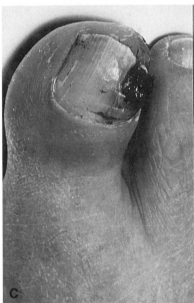

FIGURE 22-28
Malignant melanoma. See Color Section 2.

which they are confined to the epidermis and papillary dermis. Eventually, they invade the reticular dermis and the subcutaneous tissue—the vertical growth phase. With the transition from the radial to the vertical growth phase, the prognosis becomes less favorable.

There are four major types of malignant melanomas: lentigo malignant melanoma, superficial spreading melanoma, nodular melanoma, and acral-lentiginous melanoma.

TABLE 22-1

### Risk Factors for Cutaneous Melanoma

Changing mole
Pigmented lesions
    Dysplastic nevus and familial melanoma
    Dysplastic nevus
    Lentigo maligna
Congenital nevus
White race and phenotypic characteristics
Previous cutaneous melanoma
Immunosuppression
Cutaneous melanoma in parent or sibling
Sun sensitivity

**TABLE 22–2**

## Evaluation of Pigmented Lesions ("ABCD")

**A**symmetry: two halves of the lesion are not identical
**B**order irregularity: scalloped, notched, or poorly circumscribed
**C**olor variegation: pure black or combinations of red, white, brown, and black
**D**iameter: >0.6 cm

Microscopic classification has been used to evaluate tumor depth. The American Joint Committee on Cancer has divided melanoma into four stages: Stages I and II are confined to the skin, stage III includes involvement of regional lymph nodes, and stage IV is advanced local disease or systemic disease. The prognosis of melanoma depends on the anatomic location, the thickness of the lesion, and the presence or absence of metastasis.

Suspected lesions should be subjected to biopsy. Small lesions can be excised with primary closure. Incision biopsy should be carried out from the most suspicious area of the lesion. This does not increase the incidence of spread. Large lesions and lesions where primary closure will distort the features should be referred to a specialist. All patients with a confirmed malignant melanoma should be referred to an oncologist for follow-up. Wide local excision by a surgical specialist is the treatment of choice for malignant melanoma. Prophylactic lymph node dissection in melanoma patients is controversial. Radiation, immunotherapy, and chemotherapy have been tried as adjuvant therapy. All patients with malignant melanoma should be followed indefinitely with yearly physical examination, chest x-rays, and liver function tests.

## KAPOSI'S SARCOMA

*Kaposi's sarcoma* (Fig. 22–29) is a multicentric tumor characterized by endothelium-lined channels and vascular spaces in a stroma of spindle-shaped cells. Kaposi's sarcoma was first described by Moritz Kaposi in 1872. Significant evidence links multiple-lesion Kaposi's sarcoma and AIDS. The combination of Kaposi's sarcoma and AIDS is usually fatal within several months. Kaposi's sarcoma is essentially a malignant degeneration of the reticuloendothelial system, primarily affecting the skin. Early lesions are irregular, reddish-brown macules. These may become papular or nodular and coalesce to form patches. Early wide excision of a solitary lesion may produce gratifying results. Controlled radiation in small doses is also used in the treatment of Kaposi's sarcoma. Poor prognosis is usually related to delayed recognition.

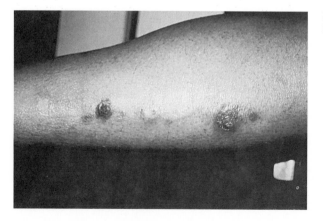

**FIGURE 22–29**
Kaposi's sarcoma. See Color Section 2.

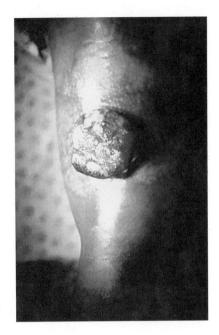

**FIGURE 22–30**
Tumor metastatic to skin. Adenocarcinoma from lung to arm.
See Color Section 2.

## TUMORS METASTATIC TO THE SKIN

The incidence of visceral carcinoma metastasizing to skin (Fig. 22–30) ranges from under 1% to approximately 5%. The most common primary sites appear to be the breast in women and the lung in men. The colon is the second most common primary site. Other primary tumors include malignant melanoma, kidney tumors, stomach tumors, and ovarian tumors. The scalp has been reported as the preferable cutaneous metastatic site for renal cell carcinoma and breast cancer. Adenocarcinoma from the lung has been reported to metastasize to a recent burn scar. The umbilical nodule seen in intra-abdominal malignancy is known as the Sister Mary Joseph nodule.

### *When to Call the Surgeon about Skin Lesions*

- Lesions at an anatomic location where tissue preservation is important (e.g., vermilion of lip, eyelids)
- Lesions greater than 5 cm in diameter where primary closure is difficult
- Lesions associated with lymphadenopathy
- Recurrent lesions of skin where wide excision may be needed
- Suspicious lesions and lesions where histology suggests malignancy

### RECOMMENDED READING

Balch, CM: The role of lymph node dissection in melanoma: Rationale, results, controversies. J Clin Oncol 6:163, 1988.

Bercovitch, L: Topical chemotherapy of actinic keratosis of the upper extremity with tretinoin and 5-fluorouracil: A double-blinded controlled study. Br J Dermatol 116:549, 1987.

Breslow, A: Thickness, cross-sectional areas and depth of invasion in the prognosis of cutaneous melanoma. Ann Surg 172:902, 1970.

Brotherston, TM, et al: Long term follow-up dermofaciectomy for Dupuytren's contracture. British J of Plastic Surg 47:440, 1994.

Cohen, M: Mastery of Plastic and Reconstructive Surgery. Little Brown and Company, Boston, 1994, pp 295–407.

Fleming, ID, and Amonette, R: Principles of management of basal and squamous cell carcinoma of the skin. Cancer 75:699, 1995.

Goldberg, LH: Basal cell carcinoma. Lancet 347:663–667, 1996.

Goldsmith, LA, et al: Adult and Pediatric Dermatology: A Color Guide to Diagnosis and Treatment. FA Davis, Philadelphia, 1997.

Marks, R: Squamous cell carcinoma. Lancet 347:735–738, 1996.

McCarthy, JG: Plastic Surgery. WB Saunders, Philadelphia, 1990, pp 3191–3274; 3560–3662.

McGrath, MH, and Turner, ML: Dermatology for plastic surgeons. Clin in Plastic Surg, vol. 21, Jan 1994.

Moschella, SL, and Hurley, HJ: Dermatology, ed 3. WB Saunders, Philadelphia, 1992, pp 1721–1808.

Reeves, JRT, and Maibach, H: Clinical Dermatology Illustrated—A Regional Approach, ed 3. FA Davis, Philadelphia, 1998.

Rockwell, WB, et al: Keloids and hypertrophic scars: A comprehensive review. Plast Reconstr Surg 84:827, 1989.

Smith, JW, and Aston, SJ: Plastic Surgery, ed 4. Little Brown and Company, Boston, 1991, pp 731–851.

Sober, AJ: Precursors to skin cancer. Cancer 75:645–650, 1995.

Watson, JD: Hidradenitis suppurative: A clinical review. Br J Plast Surg 38:567, 1985.

Zacarian, SA: Cryosurgery of cutaneous carcinomas: An 18-year study of 3022 patients with 4228 carcinomas. J Am Acad Dermatol 9:947, 1983.

# Index